D0847827

Energy Metabolism, Indirect Calorimetry, and Nutrition

Simon Bursztein, M.D.

Associate Professor of Surgery and Critical Care Medicine, School of Medicine and Department of Bio-Medical Engineering, Technion-Israel Institute of Technology; Director, Department of General Intensive Care, Rambam Medical Center, Haifa, Israel

David H. Elwyn, Ph.D.

Senior Research Scientist, Department of Anesthesiology, Albert Einstein College of Medicine of Yeshiva University and Montefiore Medical Center, Bronx, New York

Jeffrey Askanazi, M.D.

Associate Professor of Anesthesiology, Albert Einstein College of Medicine of Yeshiva University; Associate Attending in Anesthesiology, Montefiore Medical Center, Bronx, New York

John M. Kinney, M.D.

Professor Emeritus in Surgery, Columbia University; Visiting Professor, Rockefeller University; Attending in Medicine and Surgery, St. Luke's-Roosevelt Hospital Center, New York, New York

Vladimir Kvetan, M.D.

Assistant Professor of Anesthesiology and Medicine, Albert Einstein College of Medicine of Yeshiva University; Director, Critical Care Medicine, Department of Anesthesiology, Montefiore Medical Center, Bronx, New York

Michael M. Rothkopf, M.D.

Clinical Assistant Professor of Anesthesiology/Critical Care, VMD—New Jersey, Medical School, Newark, New Jersey; Chief, Section on Critical Care/Nutrition, Medical Service Veterans Administration Medical Center, East Orange, New Jersey

Charles Weissman, M.D.

Assistant Professor of Anesthesiology and Medicine, Columbia University; Assistant Attending in Anesthesiology and Medicine, Presbyterian Hospital, New York, New York

Energy Metabolism, Indirect Calorimetry, and Nutrition

Simon Bursztein, M.D.
David H. Elwyn, Ph.D.
Jeffrey Askanazi, M.D.
John M. Kinney, M.D.

with the collaboration of

Vladimir Kvetan, M.D.

Michael M. Rothkopf, M.D.

Charles Weissman, M.D.

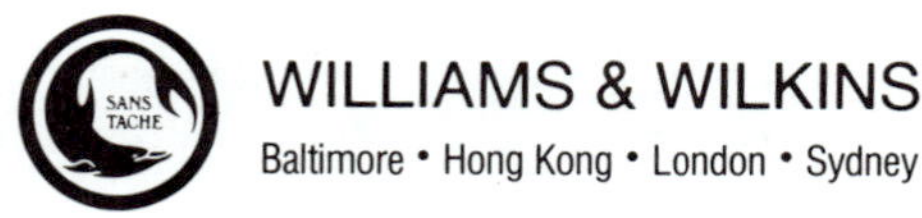

WILLIAMS & WILKINS
Baltimore • Hong Kong • London • Sydney

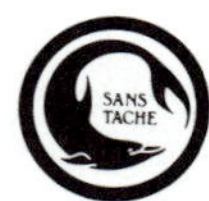

Editor: Timothy H. Grayson
Associate Editor: Carol Eckhart
Copy Editor: Shelly Hyatt-Blankman
Design: Saturn Graphics
Illustration Planning: Ray Lowman
Production: Anne G. Seitz

Williams & Wilkins
428 East Preston Street
Baltimore, Maryland 21202, USA

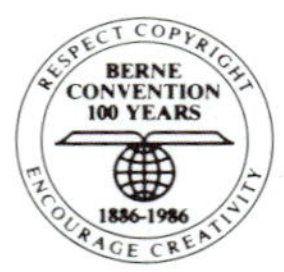

Printed in the United States of America

Library of Congress Cataloging-in-Publication Data

Energy metabolism, indirect calorimetry, and nutrition.

Includes index.
1. Energy metabolism—Measurement. 2. Indirect calorimetry. 3. Nutrition.
4. Artificial feeding. I. Bursztein, Simon.
QP176.E54 1989 615.8'55 88-20792
ISBN 0-683-01141-3

89 90 91 92 93
1 2 3 4 5 6 7 8 9 10

This book is dedicated to Rivka Sevy, without whose effort and advice it would never have been finished, and to Sylviane Bursztein and Lisbe Elwyn for their encouragement.

Foreword

The rapid growth in the use of enteral and parenteral forms of nutrient supply for critically ill patients and for those who cannot ingest, digest, or absorb an adequate supply of energy and nutrients for other reasons, has made it necessary to have available a quantitative means of assessing the nature and progress of an illness and the form of intensive care required.

The value of using measurements based on indirect calorimetry is that it could possibly reduce the prescribed amount of total parenteral nutrition by as much as 22% for the patients in general hospitals.

The resurgence of interest in measuring energy expenditure was focused initially on certain obvious problems, such as proper adjustment of the reducing diet for the refractory obese patient or on designing the correct energy intake for the acutely ill patient in the intensive care unit. Less obvious, but of equal importance, is monitoring the delicate balance of the patient with chronic pulmonary disease who is losing weight and needs better nutrition, yet cannot tolerate the additional demands for ventilation that might arise from overly enthusiastic efforts at nutritional support.

Dr. John Kinney and his collaborators have worked in this field for many years, and probably few teams have had a comparable wealth of experience in designing and using the most effective methods to monitor the course and progress of an acute illness. I well remember discussing with Dr. Kinney his aspirations some 35 years ago when he was then under the guidance of Dr. Francis Moore.

Specific clinical conditions in which the patient's resting energy expenditure has been reported include: the obese patient before and during energy restriction; the depleted patient; the patient with trauma or sepsis; the patient with head injury; the burned patient; the patient with inflammatory bowel disease; the patient with chronic pulmonary disease; the patient with cardiac failure; the patient with multiple organ failure; and the patient with cancer with or without weight loss.

Weight gain or loss is largely treated by dietary means, but this may be only partially successful since the underlying metabolic state of the patient may tend to resist a return to normal body weight. Indirect calorimetry may play a central role in establishing the proper energy balance.

Technological advances now offer the promise of simplifying measurements of both energy expenditure and body composition, so that the future supply of energy and demand per unit of body cell mass can become a routine part of patient management.

This book, lucidly written and well illustrated, is virtually a first class textbook, completely up to date on the intermediary metabolism of protein, fat, and carbohydrate in those who have been the victims of a traumatic accident or who have had to undergo major surgery. Further, there is provided a wealth of detail on the techniques available for measuring energy expenditure, the calculations involved, their interpretation, and the possible complications that may arise and how they can be overcome.

It is good that the energy exchange is given in the traditional kilocalories with joule values in parentheses (1000 kcal = 4.186 MJ (megajoules), for in Europe the term calorie is disappearing from the school textbooks).

There is an account of some of the new and exciting studies on the pharmacological effects of lipids, and these represent only the beginning of a new field of investigation mediated by prostaglandins, thromboxanes, and leucotreines, some of which are inflammatory, immunostimulatory, and vasodilatory. The amounts and proportions of these hormone-like substances can be strongly influenced by the composition and amount of administered lipids. This raises the possibility for the future of using disease-specific lipid regimens for therapeutic purposes in many types of illness. The chapter on hypermetabolic, hypercatabolic, stressed states is especially useful.

The authors point out that parenteral nutrition is used more frequently than enteral nutrition in the USA, whereas in Western Europe the enteral route seems to be preferred, and that has mainly come about for historical rather than rational reasons. Enteral feeding, when it is possible, is after oral feeding, the most physiological, the safest, and the most economical way to supply artificial nutrition. The advantages of the jejunal route over the gastric route and the problems of inadequate mixing of both bile and pancreatic enzymes seem to be avoided when elemental diets are used.

The authors agree with the present writer's view that the losses following accidental injury are greater than those after elective operation, even with operations as traumatic as total hip replacement. They also found that sepsis was not in this respect more stressful than accidental injury.

It is obvious that the power of the therapist is so complete in enteral and parenteral nutrition that it is extremely important to be well informed and to exercise it according to the best available criteria. One of the most important criteria for establishing the appropriate amounts of carbohydrate, fat, and protein that should be given is the quantitative effect of each of these nutrients on maintenance of the body's cell mass, usually as measured by N balance. But it is also necessary that the supply of vitamins, minerals, and other essentials not be limiting factors for the optimal recovery of health that the patients' injuries, operations, or diseased state will permit.

Sir David P. Cuthbertson, M.D., D.Sc., L.L.D.

Glasgow University
Royal Infirmary
Glasgow, Scotland

Preface

In the past decade, there has been a resurgence of interest in energy metabolism associated with two major areas. On the one hand, there has been a growing public awareness of the importance of diet and exercise in maintaining physical fitness. On the other hand, there is increasing concern with estimating the caloric requirements of critically ill patients receiving parenteral or enteral nutrition. At the same time there has appeared a new generation of instruments for measuring indirect calorimetry, which remains, as for the last 100 years, the prime method for measuring energy expenditure. These instruments have appeared in response to the new interest in energy metabolism, and because of their utility they have served to fuel this interest as well.

As far as we know, there has not been a major treatise on energy metabolism, indirect calorimetry, and nutrition since Swift and French's *Energy Metabolism and Nutrition,* which was published in 1954. Major developments in our knowledge of energy metabolism and introduction of important improvements in methods of calculating energy expenditure and fuel utilization have been contributed by Weir (Weir JBDeV: New methods for calculating metabolic rate with special reference to protein metabolism. *J Physiol* 109:1–9, 1949) and Consolazio, Johnson, and Pecora (Consolazio CF, Johnson RE, Pecora LJ: *Physiologic Measurements of Metabolic Functions in Man.* New York, McGraw-Hill, 1963, pp 313–339). Recently, a major text on the detailed theory and practice of both direct and indirect calorimetry has been published (McLean JA, Tobin G: *Animal and Human Calorimetry.* Cambridge, Cambridge University Press, 1987). This is an important source book.

The three-plus decades since 1954 have also seen the transformation of artificial nutrition from a hopeful dream to a life-saving reality that has become an essential part of medical practice. The pioneering work of Dudrick in the United States, Wretlind in Sweden, and their colleagues in the 1960s, demonstrated that a complete and adequate diet could be given intravenously. It is now evident to all that parenteral or enteral nutrition has dramatic effects in saving the lives of patients with abdominal fistulae, short bowel syndrome, or severe malnutrition. Nevertheless, although there is considerable evidence to show that artificial nutrition can reduce morbidity and mortality significantly, for some obscure reasons this aspect of patient management has not yet acquired its proper status in modern medicine.

When studies have demonstrated that malnourished patients given, preoperative nutrition results, postoperatively, in a 2.5-fold reduction in complication rate, a 7-fold reduction in infection rate, and a 5-fold reduction in mortality (Chapter 7), it becomes malpractice when a patient is not given the benefit of such treatment.

Nutrition never appears to be a priority. When dealing with acute hemodynamic or respiratory disturbances, the time is usually counted in minutes, whereas with acute renal failure the time may be counted in hours or up to 1 or 2 days. When dealing with the multiple consequences of malnutrition in severely ill patients, whether reduction in host defense mechanisms, delayed or absent wound healing, or reduced serum albumin with water maldistribution, the time is much longer and counted in many days or sometimes in weeks. This is probably why nutritional aspects of a patient's management are often neglected or totally ignored until the situation becomes catastrophic, although the condition may become life-threatening long before the alarming signs appear.

For patients who are unable to feed themselves normally, water and electrolyte needs are roughly evaluated and are supplied according to certain rules; calorie and nitrogen intake deserve the same consideration.

The most useful tool for estimating the nutritional needs of critically ill patients is indirect calorimetry. The early work of Kinney and colleagues in the United States and Glaser and Nedey in France in adapting indirect calorimetry for patient use is now paying off; highly accurate equipment is available for use by clinicians everywhere.

In this volume we attempt to provide insight into the development of our present concepts of energy metabolism; a detailed critique of the theory and practice of indirect calorimetry and the related measurements of nitrogen balance and body composition; a discussion of the role of nutrition in the evolution of plants and animals; a summary of the interrelations between food intake and metabolism in normal and pathological states; and some simple guidelines for estimating energy expenditure and nutritional requirements of patients given artificial nutrition.

We hope that this book will be of theoretical and practical use for all new practitioners of indirect calorimetry, who have not yet had time to master the voluminous literature in this field. Our particular emphasis has been on the problems of the critically ill patient although we have presented a comprehensive approach to energy metabolism, indirect calorimetry, and nutrition needs.

Simon Bursztein
David H. Elwyn

Contents

CHAPTER

1

Indirect Calorimetry: History and Overview

INTRODUCTION

Indirect calorimetry is the method by which the type and rate of substrate oxidation and heat production are measured in vivo starting from gas exchange measurements. This method provides a unique sort of information, is noninvasive and can be combined with other measurement techniques to investigate numerous aspects of nutrient metabolism, heat production, energy requirements of physical activity, and the altered energy metabolism of disease and injury. The development and interpretation of gas exchange has represented a fundamental milestone for chemistry, biology and medicine. Yet, the field has been largely ignored in modern medical education and clinical care. Thus, it is appropriate to review the basis of indirect calorimetry in order to emphasize the theoretical approach and the assumptions that must be made to translate the measurement of gas exchange into units of heat production and fuel utilization for clinical application.

The resurgence of interest in indirect calorimetry over the past decade has resulted from the confluence of various factors. The rapid growth of lay attention to food and exercise as important ways to improve life-style has been associated with increasing awareness of nutrition as an important part of treating hospitalized patients. The commercial availability of improved equipment for bedside measurement of gas exchange has paralleled the growth in commercial products for the treatment of acute and chronic malnutrition. At the same time, measurements of energy expenditure have assumed new importance in investigating and managing obesity. Historical developments from 1650 to 1950 were directed primarily toward the measurement of the basal metabolic rate. The new interest in calorimetry has moved from focusing attention on the basal state to the influence on energy expenditure associated with food intake and physical activity. Diet-induced thermogenesis is being examined following the intake of carbohydrate and lipid, rather than assuming that it is predominantly related to amino acid intake. The energy requirements of physical activity are being measured in relation to physical fitness and in relation to stress-testing in cardiopulmonary disease. As the use of energy measurements is being broadened, it is important to understand the limitations and errors of indirect calorimetry, both in terms of technical measurements and theoretical assumptions, in order for the measurements to be properly adapted to the investigation and management of clinical conditions. Such information is of particular importance at the present time when bedside measuring equipment includes small, efficient computers, which offer the convenience of making immediate calculations and presenting the measurement of gas exchange in terms of calories per unit of body size. Such instruments offer the temptation to utilize the output data without careful and frequent calibration of the measuring equipment and without proper effort to understand the calculations which are being employed to convert units of O_2 uptake and CO_2 production into units of heat production. However, with proper calibration, bedside measurements can be performed much more readily than before.

HISTORICAL DEVELOPMENT

Discussions of gas exchange often start with references to Lavoisier and his contemporaries, who established O_2 and CO_2 as the important gases in the process of combustion and in the metabolism of animals and man. It is unfortunate that the background of the preceding 100 years is seldom acknowledged in the history of gas exchange.

William Harvey not only revolutionized medicine with his recognition of the circulation of the blood, but also attracted around him a talented group of younger men interested in experimental medicine (1). The activities of this group became prominent in Oxford where Harvey was serving as the personal physician to Charles I of England. Preeminent in this group of investigators was the chemist William Boyle. Before his time, the nature and behavior of gases were not clearly understood. Some felt that gases were composed of incompressible materials which were separate from solid materials. Others felt that gases were composed of particles of a nature which could be expanded or compressed. Boyle developed a device for producing a vacuum and proceeded to examine aspects of combustion and metabolism in evacuated glass containers. In the process, he established the relationship between gas volume and pressure and also revealed that a bird could not survive when placed in this evacuated container. Since a candle would not burn in the same evacuated container, he and his associates proposed that removing the gas in the container somehow deprived both the candle and the bird of some necessary gaseous element needed for the support of the flame and the support of life. Incidental investigations also revealed that leaving a green plant in the evacuated container for a period of time would then allow a flame to burn, or an animal to live, for a limited period of time. These studies of Boyle and his associates did much to lay the foundation for modern chemistry, as well as providing dramatic preliminary information about the advances which were to follow 100 years later.

Joseph Black, while still a medical student in Glasgow, became interested in the fact that bladder stones, when treated with acid, would release a gas which became known as "fixed air." After obtaining his medical degree in 1754, he continued his research into fixed air and observed that an atmosphere of fixed air would not support either a flame or animal life (2). Some 20 years later, an English minister, Joseph Priestley (3), and a Swedish apothecary, Carl Scheele (4), conducted experiments which pointed to the existence of oxygen as being the necessary factor for both combustion and animal life. However, they both failed to understand the significance of their studies because of the then-popular phlogiston theory, which stated that for a substance to burn there had to be the escape of a fictitious material known as "phlogiston." During this same decade, Lavoisier in Paris was studying the combustion and oxidation of metals (5). He gave the name "oxygene" to the material absorbed by the metal when heated in air. While Lavoisier was struggling to explain fire, he introduced the term "calorique" to describe heat. In collaboration with the physicist, Laplace, he conducted studies of the heat released in combustion, which laid the foundation for thermal chemistry. Later, Lavoisier carried out elegant experiments to relate the uptake of oxygen by an animal to the output of CO_2 and heat. The heat production was measured by an ice calorimeter and helped to establish the science of calorimetry.

The first half of the 1800's represented a period of time when techniques for the chemical measurements of foods and other biological materials were being developed. However, the revolutionary concepts of Lavoisier continued to be a source of scientific controversy for several decades. The second half of the 1800's represented the ascendency of organic chemistry, followed by biochemistry. The gas exchange of nutrients upon oxidation was related to heat production in a bomb calorimeter. Such studies were extended to animals and then to man by the use of direct and indirect calorimetry. Carl von Voit established a center for investigators in Germany and studies there led the way in establishing the relationship between gas exchange and calorimetry of the whole body. The most outstanding of these investigators was Max Rubner (6). Such studies had widespread influence on the growth of calorimetry in Europe, as well as in the United States where Atwater (7), Benedict (8), Lusk (9), and Du Bois (10) were particularly influential in advancing the field.

The decade of the 1920's represented a transition from the strong nutritional interest in energy expenditure to identification of vitamins, enzymes and the related steps in metabolic pathways. The extensive studies of Du Bois and colleagues (10) on the influence of various medical conditions on the basal metabolic rate (BMR) provided much interesting background information. This was particularly true in relation to the influence of fever on energy expenditure. However, the one clinical area where measurement of the BMR became part of the standard medical care was in thyroid disease. The majority of hospitals established an area for performing BMR tests, which were used both to diagnose and manage thyroid disease. This use of the BMR continued for approximately 25 years, but was then replaced by measurement of thyroid metabolites in the urine or in the blood. In the 1950's, hospitals began to close down their BMR facilities and an era began when patients were treated on the basis of an assumed energy expenditure which was never measured. It is interesting to note that when energy expenditure, like any other clinical variable, is not measured, it leads to clinicians gaining erroneous ideas about normal values which are never corrected in the course of daily practice.

Safe and effective total parenteral nutrition (TPN) was introduced in the 1960's by Wretlind and co-workers in Sweden (11) and by Dudrick and co-workers in the United States (12). During the 1970's, it became appropriate to provide nutritional support in amounts which were determined in relation to a patient's assumed or measured energy expenditure. New nutritional products became available for both parenteral and enteral feeding of hospital patients and, in selected cases, this specialized nutrition could be continued at home.

The stimulus of nutritional support for the measurement of energy expenditure had to do with the desire to estimate the energy requirements on a daily basis. Another stimulus arose from the need to measure the energy expenditure during short-term periods of exercise to determine the cardiac or pulmonary response to progressive increases in demand for gas exchange (13). It is self-evident that a significant limitation in exercise tolerance may exist which compromises a particular life-style yet may not be a major influence on the total energy expenditure per day. Therefore, commercial instruments which were introduced to measure gas exchange as part of exercise stress-testing proceeded to find a market in the field of nutritional management (14).

THERMAL METABOLISM

Indirect calorimetry, by its very nature, keeps attention focused on gas exchange. The thermal considerations associated with energy metabolism tend to be ignored in indirect calorimetry, which is primarily concerned with fuel needs and the ratio of gas exchange to the oxidation of a given food. This is somewhat ironic since the term "calorie" derives from the term "calorique," or heat, in the pioneering studies of Lavoisier (5). The use of the word calorie as a unit of heat was proposed to be replaced by "joule" on the recommendation of the British National Committee of Nutritional Science of the Royal Society (15): "The joule should be adopted as the unit for energy in nutritional work and the calorie should fall in disuse."

This change was considered by some to be an important improvement in the move toward metric units. However, Kleiber (16) published a spirited defense of the use of the "calorie," pointing out that the calorie is part of the metric system as a unit of heat since it is based on a temperature difference expressed in degrees centrigrade and on mass expressed as kilograms. Since heat is one of the various forms of energy, it follows that the calorie should be used as a unit of heat and not for energy in general.

The excellent correlation of direct and indirect calorimetry was first demonstrated by Rubner (17) in animals. Since the direct measurement of heat loss avoids the various assumptions of indirect calorimetry, sometimes it has been considered to be the preferred measurement for energy expenditure if the physical difficulties of measurement could be overcome. This idea overlooks the fact that indirect calorimetry is devoted to substrate oxidation (and associated heat production), while direct calorimetry measures heat loss with no indication of the tissue fuel utilized to produce the heat. Thus, direct calorimetry is an important measurement for studies of thermoregulation, but is of relatively less value for nutritional purposes (18). Furthermore, the study of thermoregulation has progressed much faster in studies of small animals than in studies of man. This is related in part to the fact that the human body represents such a large heat sink in relation to its intrinsic rate of heat production. Hence, small changes in body temperature, or body heat content, are less evident in man for a given addition or subtraction of body heat.

Body temperature is a convenient reflection of body heat content. Fever can be looked upon as a temporary period when heat production exceeds heat loss. Studies on reptiles, amphibians, and fishes support the notion that the observed elevation in their body temperature during infection is the result of an elevated thermoregulatory set point (19). Since these animals are ectotherms and must raise or lower their body temperature by behavioral means, the selection of warmer ambient temperature resulting in the elevation of their deep body temperature is consistent with a raised thermoregulatory set point. Lizards placed in a simulated desert environment were allowed to move about between cool and warm areas of sand to maintain a preferred body temperature of about 38° C. During infection, the lizards developed a fever and then selected a warmer portion of the chamber resulting in a 2° to 3° C increase in deep body temperature and an improved survival. Future clinical management of fever can be expected to monitor and treat heat production and heat loss separately.

INDIRECT CALORIMETRY

The measurement of gas concentration before World War II was largely gravimetric for chamber, or room, calorimeters, versus volumetric when measuring the BMR of an individual. The classic portable BMR apparatus of Benedict (20) depended on a closed system, in which a container of oxygen would decrease in volume in proportion to the uptake of oxygen by the subject, while the CO_2 was absorbed but not measured. The oxygen consumption was then translated into calories per hour by assuming an amount of expired carbon dioxide, which would yield a nonprotein respiratory quotient (RQ) of 0.82 and hence a caloric equivalent for oxygen of 4.825 kcal (20.19 kJ) liter^{-1}.

The wartime events of the early 1940's provided stimulus to develop more rapid and accurate methods of gas analysis, particularly for the new demands of combat aviation at higher altitudes. Following World War II, physical methods of gas analysis began to dominate the field of gas exchange. Mass spectrometry was introduced for measuring both O_2 and CO_2, as well as paramagnetic analyzers for O_2 and infrared analyzers for CO_2.

Any analytical system must be calibrated against gas mixtures of known composition. It is not wise to trust commercial sources for gas standards, since even the most prestigious companies sometimes provide gas mixtures that lack the precise composition needed for calibrating an analyzer over the appropriate range. It is interesting to realize that the standard atmospheric air contains more than water, O_2, N_2, and CO_2 (21). The international civil aviation organization lists 17 different gases as possible constituents of clean, dry air at sea level. The content of these unusual gases obviously will vary from time to time and from place to place, but they are usually present only in trace amounts.

The use of gas exchange for indirect calorimetry is based on assumptions that go back to the investigations of Lavoisier in the late 18th century (5). The standard gas equations will be reviewed elsewhere in this volume. They are based on the assumption that all gas exchange occurs across the lungs, although the skin can allegedly be the site of small amounts of gas exchange in the presence of large gradients. The gas equations treat O_2 and CO_2 as ideal gases. Johnson (21) pointed out that this is correct for O_2 and N_2, but is only partially true for CO_2, thus introducing a small error. A more important potential error is related to water vapor, where the expired air is assumed to be saturated and complete drying is required for use of the gas equations, although neither of these conditions may be totally correct. The gut of ruminants (and occasionally of man) may be the site of gas production which passes into the bloodstream and then is exhaled by the lung. Expired air can, of course, also be contaminated by ethyl alcohol and acetone.

Our experience with acutely ill surgical patients has shown that many of these patients have a mild degree of hyperventilation at rest. This is associated not only with some increase in minute ventilation, but also with an increase in alveolar ventilation. Thus, in such patients, the arterial PCO_2 is often 2 to 4 mm of mercury less than the normal value. We have the impression that whenever a patient has some degree of hyperventilation at rest, any tight-fitting apparatus that is attached to the face, or introduced into the upper airway, will tend to accentuate the hyperventilation. This will cause an R value for the expired air, which is higher than the RQ of the tissue metabolism because the patient is excreting a portion of his body stores of CO_2. This effect is much more significant for CO_2 than O_2; in part, because the body gas stores of CO_2 are generally about 30 to 40 times as large as the body stores of O_2 (Table 2.14).

Transparent head enclosures can avoid the spurious hyperventilation which may occur with a mask, or mouthpiece, when used with an acutely ill patient (22). Such head enclosures may function by a negative pressure at the outlet, drawing in room air into the enclosure beneath some sort of plastic apron. It is possible to isolate the patient from room air by ventilating the head enclosure with a continuous stream of outside air, introduced on one side of the enclosure by positive pressure and withdrawn from the other side by negative pressure. An airtight seal with a properly designed foam rubber collar will allow the patient to remain comfortable while breathing air independent of the composition of room air (Figure 5.13). This is important if the patient is surrounded by staff or family in a poorly ventilated area in which the ambient air no longer has the composition of ordinary room air. The advantage of such a system is that it can be modified to perform continuous spirometry along with gas exchange (23). This is made possible by balancing the airflow into and out of the head enclosure, so that the pressure in the canopy remains neutral. If this balance is achieved, then a sensitive pressure transducer can be used to reflect pressure changes that occur in the canopy in association with each breath, which can be translated into airflow.

Respiratory gases must be collected in a leak-free manner and analyzed in a way which corresponds to the calibration procedure. The collection step presents possibilities for error from loss, dilution, or addition of gases. Different types of errors occur in the presence of a leak depending on whether the leak is inboard or outboard. One of the few completely satisfactory devices for gas collection is a full-body, leakproof suit, such as those made for astronauts, which permits expired air and gases from the skin and the gut to be collected (24). A leakproof respiration chamber also permits an accurate inventory of all gases entering and leaving the body (25,26).

Calculations of daily energy expenditure by extrapolating from a BMR measurement and adding an estimated factor for diet-induced thermogenesis and another factor estimated for physical activity are relatively unsatisfactory. Some improvement in the calculation can be made by making multiple measurements of at least 30 minutes throughout the day. However, the energy requirements for physical activity between measurements can only be grossly estimated and may introduce major errors in the calculated total daily energy expenditure. It is for such reasons that four prominent nutritional investigators stated in an editorial: "We do not know how much food man requires" (27). Measurements of energy expenditure utilizing a respiration chamber over periods of 24 hours, or longer, provide a much more accurate indication of daily energy expenditure than isolated measurements of gas exchange at rest (28). The 24-hour energy expenditure of any given adult individual is surprisingly constant, with a coefficient of variation reported to be only 21.4%. However, interpersonal variations are considerable, even when corrected for fat-free mass. A large portion of the variability has been linked to the degree of spontaneous physical activity, which might account for values from 100 to 800 (400 to 3300kJ) kcal day^{-1}. How representative such respiration chamber studies are of the normal energy requirements of the individual depend, of course, upon how closely the type and amount of physical activity in the chamber resembles that which the person normally performs in regular, daily life.

The use of oxygen-18 has been proposed to measure body water because it avoids the exchange of the label with nonaqueous hydrogen in the body associated with hydrogen isotopes, which can result in overestimation of body water by 1% to 5%. Schoeller and co-workers (29) extended this approach by administering both ^{18}O- and ^{2}H- labeled water and following the decay rates of each isotope in body water over 1 to 2 weeks. The difference in the decay rates then allowed the calculation of the CO_2 production over that time period. Comparison of this isotopic method with total CO_2 production measured by indirect calorimetry has shown good agreement in normal man (30). More recent studies have been directed toward investigating the time required for equilibration of each isotope in various clinical conditions, together with the statistical variability inherent in each isotope determination. Although plasma or serum tracer concentrations are commonly used to calculate body water, saliva concentrations may be useful in some conditions. Implementation of this technique is currently difficult outside of a specialized research laboratory because of the need for laborious procedures and specialized equipment, including a mass spectrometer, together with the high cost of the oxygen-18 isotope.

Many factors affect a person's daily energy expenditure, but physical activity has by far the most profound effect. Since the requirements of direct calorimetry prevent all but the most limited exercise, some form of gas exchange has been used over the decades to measure the energy expenditure associated with specific forms of physical activity. In the interval between 1940 and 1980, efforts were made to escape the confinement of a treadmill and a Tissot apparatus for measurement of energy expenditure during physical activity. A large, portable Douglas bag was often used with a mouthpiece and noseclip attached to a respiratory gas valve for collecting the total expired air during the period of physical work. The Douglas bag would then be taken to the laboratory for measurement of volume and gas composition. Meteorological balloons for expired air collections were large and lightweight, but were found to have gas diffusion losses if the contents were not analyzed promptly.

In order to avoid large collections of expired air during physical activity, the Kofranyi-Michaelis meter was devised (31). This is a dry gas meter worn as a lightweight backpack through which the exercising subject's expired air is passed. An aliquot of each expired breath is collected and stored in a small rubber bag for subsequent analysis. The meter is less than half the weight of a 100-liter gas bag and is much less clumsy to use. A further step in measuring the energy expenditure of exercise is represented by a device named the "Oxylog" (32). This is a small, convenient oxygen analyzer which can be worn on the belt and gives a direct readout of O_2 consumption. The output of such a device can be continuously stored on a tape recorder, which also is worn on the belt.

For some investigations, the very high precision of gas measurements is not required. The more vigorous the activity, the easier it is to measure the energy cost. Athletes performing at high levels of exertion are good subjects to measure. They give reproducible results by various indirect methods, including heart rate. Sedentary individuals pose greater difficulties since the conditions of the measurement may introduce significant error due to the total energy expenditure being significantly smaller (33).

Despite the advances made in measuring gas exchange during physical activity, the tight-fitting attachments to the face may be uncomfortable or interfere with whatever activity is being undertaken. The most indirect approach to measuring energy expenditure during physical activity is through the use of activity diaries, surveys, and activity-related means (pedometers, cumulative heartbeat, and so forth) (34). Not only must the measuring devices be calibrated properly, but the psychological, physiological, and sociological variables which may interfere with measurement accuracy must also be considered. Such variables include body size, growth, sex, climate, environment, disability, and occupation, along with the use of leisure time. A temporal activity diary, together with average caloric values for each activity, has been widely used. The many obvious sources of error in the diary method have led to estimates of energy expenditure from proportional physiological sources, such as heart rate.

A linear relationship exists between heart rate and oxygen consumption for normal individuals throughout a large portion of the aerobic work range. Portable equipment has been used to record heart rate for prolonged periods of time in order to estimate energy expenditure during highly variable daily activities. Considerable data on energy expenditure have been obtained by this method for running, fast walking, cycling, and swimming. This relationship is linear for most people, but the slope of the O_2 heart rate correlation differs considerably among individuals (35). Since factors other than O_2 consumption, such as temperature, emotions, and body position can also influence pulse rate, the relationship of O_2 consumption to pulse rate with exercise must be established with care and made to resemble the exercise to be studied as closely as possible. A similar approach involves measuring the rate of pulmonary ventilation for representative activity and relating this to O_2 consumption (36). Utilizing the linear relationship between minute ventilation and O_2 consumption to calculate energy expenditure indirectly has several undesirable aspects. Some device must be attached to the face in order to measure the minute ventilation; a requirement which favors the use of the pulse rate, where no connection with the airway is required. Furthermore, measuring ventilation to represent energy expenditure is reported not to be valid outside the range of 15 to 50 liters per minute, which is above the range associated with many low-level but common activities. A comparison between estimating O_2 consumption from heart rate and from ventilatory rate has suggested that the percentage error is somewhat less with the latter (37). However, various clinical conditions, particularly with fever or abnormal catecholamine levels, appear to influence both the heart rate and ventilatory rate independent of O_2 consumption. This dissociation can be marked in the presence of cardiac or pulmonary disease.

METABOLIC BODY SIZE

The evaluation of the BMR of any individual requires comparison with normal values from a group of individuals. It has long been apparent that body size is a major determinant of the BMR. Therefore, energy expenditure could be compared with normal values more readily if it were expressed as calories per unit of body weight. Unfortunately, the use of body weight as a reference for indirect calorimetry poses various questions. What is the normal or desirable weight for an adult? Do other changes in energy metabolism occur before significant changes in body weight have occurred? Further, patients may have their energy expenditure expressed per unit of body weight, with no indication of probable changes in body composition and no indication of how the use of normal, or reference, body weight would have influenced the result.

The question of what is normal weight has received more attention from investigators interested in obesity than those interested in other areas of medicine, as reviewed by Simopoulos and van Itallie (38). They note that the scientific literature abounds with inadequately defined terms, such as "ideal body weight" and "desirable body weight," resulting in the publication of data that are difficult to interpret and impossible to compare with the findings in other studies.

Numerous studies of malnutrition and experimental starvation have shown that dietary restriction causes a reduction in energy expenditure, when expressed as calories per unit of body weight. One of the most complete studies of prolonged human starvation was conducted by Benedict in 1912 (39). A normal, 40-year-old male received only distilled water for 31 days. By day 21 of the fast, this individual had reduced his energy expenditure by 30% at a time when he had lost 16.7% of his body weight. Keys and co-workers (40) also observed a more rapid decrease in energy expenditure than in weight loss during partial starvation. Over a period of 6 months their subjects lost an average of 24% of their body weight, while their energy expenditure had decreased by 39%. The investigators calculated that whereas the BMR had decreased by 39% per individual, the reduction amounted to 31% when calculated per square meter of body surface and 19.5% when calculated per kilogram of body weight. Kinney and Weissman (41) reviewed evidence which suggests that the slow weight loss of partial starvation is associated with a relatively constant extracellular fluid volume (ECF); hence, there is a relative expansion of the ECF compared with intracellular water or other indicators of the body cell mass. This situation appears to differ from acute catabolic states where there is a variable degree of ECF expansion relative to a shrinking cell volume.

Rubner and Voit (42) believed that heat produced from metabolism within the body had to be lost through the surface of the body to the environment and that the level of heat production appeared to bear a constant relationship to the body surface area. This led Rubner to a simple rule: fasting homeotherms have a daily heat production of 1000 Calories (4180 kJ) per square meter of surface area.

Tables and nomograms have been prepared to represent the surface area of each sex, based upon the data from Aub and Du Bois (43), the Mayo Clinic (44), and Fleisch (45). More recently, in London, Robertson and Reid (46) prepared an extensive series of new standards on normal individuals which are about 10% below those of the Mayo Clinic. In general, 90% to 95% of normal adults are expected to fall between ±10% of the mean value, or more recently between +5%, and −15% of the traditional mean values.

Harris and Benedict (47) attempted to avoid hypotheses, such as the ill-defined "body surface area," or "surface law," and therefore derived equations from the study of 249 normal subjects which involved not only height and weight, but sex and age as well.

Long and associates (48) observed that the results calculated from the Harris-Benedict equations were in close agreement with those obtained by gas exchange measurements in normal adult males and females. However, Daly and co-workers (49) conducted a study of the BMR of 201 healthy adult men and women, using both direct and indirect calorimetry, and reported that the Harris-Benedict equation overestimated the measured expenditure by 10% to 15%. These authors also reported on 15 other studies in which the BMR of healthy, adult individuals was compared with a value predicted from the Harris-Benedict equation. A striking range of variations was obtained from +19% to −14%. The reasons for the variability could not be determined. However, the variability emphasized the importance of making standardized measurements with carefully calibrated equipment. Data from the normal subjects studied by Harris and Benedict have been analyzed recently by Cunningham (50). Body weight and age were used with the prediction equations of Moore and co-workers (51) for total body water. The estimated lean body mass was found to be the best single predictor of the BMR, while the influence of sex and age added little to the estimation. These findings suggested that estimations of the BMR based on body surface area owed their usefulness to a hidden correlation with lean body mass in each sex. This would be in agreement with Benedict's own suggestion, made in 1915, that the "active body mass" determined the BMR.

The metabolic body size is that portion of the body composition to which the metabolic rate is proportional. Kleiber (52) presented an entertaining critique of the theories that have been advanced in support of the "surface law" and gives extensive evidence that a power function of weight, such as weight to the 3/4 power, would be more appropriate than the use of body surface area. Kleiber concluded that: "For all practical purposes, one may assume that the mean standard metabolic rate of mammals is 70 times the 3/4th power of their body weight in kilograms per day, or about 3 times the 3/4th power of their body weight in kilograms per hour." The Kleiber equations predict the metabolic rate of humans with about the same accuracy as the empirical regression equation of Harris and Benedict. The advantage of the Kleiber equations is that all of the terms have a physiological meaning. The mean BMR of all mammals is about 70 $\pm$1.2 kcal (293 $\pm$ 5kJ) $kg^{-3/4}$. The use of a power function for calculating the normal metabolism of an individual is cumbersome. Therefore, while his calculation may be the most correct for comparison between species covering a wide range of body weight, the use of body weight appears to be reasonably satisfactory when comparing individuals of the same species.

The significance of body size, surface area, and body composition for metabolic rate is still under lively discussion. The observation that poikilothermic animals show levels of metabolism that are proportional to surface area continues to puzzle those who lean toward a causal relationship between surface area and heat production. Zeuthen (53) presented evidence that the relative decrease of surface area with increasing size has nothing to do with establishing the level of heat production. It seems probable that the apparent relationship of surface area to heat production is a secondary one, which is not causal; rather, it must derive from some unrecognized correlation between surface area and the virtual size of the metabolically active tissues in the body.

Grande and Keys (54) presented evidence that the fat-free body should be a better reference for metabolic body size than either body weight or surface area. Moore and co-workers (51) utilized total exchangeable potassium to calculate the body cell mass, as over 98% of body potassium is located within cells. Roza and Shizgal (55) reevaluated the data on normal subjects used by Harris and Benedict to derive their equations for basal metabolism of normal subjects. The body cell mass for each subject was calculated using the regression equations developed by Moore (51). These workers found that malnutrition is associated with an increase in resting oxygen consumption which becomes apparent when the oxygen consumption is expressed as a function of the body cell mass. This is in contrast to the decrease in resting O_2 consumption which occurs with partial starvation if the O_2 consumption is expressed per unit of body weight. Roza and Shizgal concluded that the Harris-Benedict equations accurately predict resting energy expenditure in normally nourished individuals with a precision of $\pm 14\%$, but are unreliable in the malnourished patient.

The use of neutron activation has enabled investigators to measure total body nitrogen in normal subjects and in patients with various diseases. McNeill (56) and Cohn (57) proposed that the simultaneous measurement of whole body potassium and nitrogen may allow better estimates of whole body protein. These measurements should provide new insights into the processes associated with weight loss and the response to nutritional therapy. Whether this work will lead to a new approach to metabolic body size remains an interesting possibility.

The controversy over the proper reference for the metabolic body size continues up to the present day. Owen and co-workers (58), in a recent study, reported that body weight is just as satisfactory as surface area or fat-free mass when comparing the energy expenditure of normal adult men and women. This finding, if confirmed by others, will probably relate more to the limitations in defining body composition than to any inherent superiority of body weight as a reference for energy expenditure.

The use of body potassium as a reflection of the body cell mass (51) is an appealing idea, although not widely available for clinical conditions. Recent reports have emphasized that potassium may be lost faster than predicted during catabolic nitrogen loss and that, similarly, potassium may be gained faster than nitrogen during nutritional repletion (59, 60). It remains to be shown how much of such discrepancies relate to the loss and gain of potassium in relation to glycogen stores. Another consideration is the difference in potassium/nitrogen ratios for cellular tissues, such as muscle, and the high collagen containing tissues, like the skin. Although muscle protein breakdown is well-established in most catabolic states, the contribution of high collagen tissues to the nitrogen loss is still poorly understood.

DIET-INDUCED THERMOGENESIS

The stimulating effect of food on energy expenditure was observed over a century ago by Rubner (61), who named it the "specific dynamic action" (SDA). It was originally thought to be related to the process of digesting and absorbing nutrients. However, subsequent studies revealed comparable effects when nutrients were administered by vein. The most prominent stimulus of food to energy expenditure was associated with the intake of protein or amino acids, where the SDA could vary between 10% and 35% of the ingested food energy, in contrast to much lower values for the intake of carbohydrate or fat. Initial beliefs that the SDA was somehow a response to the mass action effect of ingested amino acids were revised when it was recognized that the SDA was observed in relation to amino acid catabolism, rather than to amino acid incorporation into protein. Krebs (62) suggested that the energy losses following the administration of protein were somehow linked to urea production. However, studies by Garrow and Hawes (63) did not demonstrate any association between the amount of urea produced and the increase in metabolic rate after a meal. It was then suggested that the increased energy metabolism after a protein meal was perhaps more related to protein synthesis than to protein catabolism.

The thermic response to food and to cold were initially thought to be independent. However, in animals in which brown adipose tissue is the main organ responsible for nonshivering thermogenesis it has been found that the thermogenic activity can be stimulated by feeding. Thus, the somewhat vague term "specific dynamic action" has given way to the term "diet induced thermogenesis" (DIT). Rothwell and Stock (64) proposed that brown adipose tissue may perform a regulatory function in response to overfeeding. These authors and others have studied rats that have become obese when eating a highly palatable diet instead of their normal rat chow. Under these circumstances, the brown adipose tissue of the rats showed a marked increase in weight, together with a substantial increase in thermogenesis. This response is remarkably similar to that shown by cold-induced thermogenesis, and both types of response are felt to involve stimulus of the sympathetic nervous system.

Diet-induced thermogenesis can be divided into obligatory and adaptive components (65). *Obligatory thermogenesis*, formerly known as specific dynamic action, is the energy cost of food intake and the subsequent conversion of food substrates. This is thought to be partly due to the synthesis of glycogen and fat from carbohydrate, in contrast to the adaptive diet-induced thermogenesis (formerly known as Luxuskonsumption), which represents the dissipation of energy over and above that associated with the basal metabolic activity and the obligatory DIT. There has been considerable controversy recently regarding the existence of adaptive DIT in both humans and large mammals in general. The evidence for adaptive DIT relies upon the demonstration of an apparent discrepancy between estimates of energy intake as food, energy expenditure, and energy storage or change in body fat. Unfortunately, most of these studies have not involved actual measurements of energy balance. Rothwell and Stock (64) suggested that perhaps the capacity for DIT enables an animal to consume adequate quantities of a poor quality diet in order to obtain sufficient essential nutrients without compromising energy balance by depositing excess energy intake as fat.

PHYSICAL ACTIVITY AND EXERCISE TESTING

An extensive literature has built up over the past century relating to the energy expenditure of various forms of physical activity. Despite this, there is now renewed attention to the energy efficiency of physical activity which has arisen from diverse origins. A growing number of individuals wish to incorporate planned exercise into their usual daily activities as an important part of improving their health and life-style. Such individuals, as well as professional athletes, are seeking quantitative information on energy intake and energy utilization in various forms of exercise. Exercise stress-testing has become commonplace as a means of evaluating cardiopulmonary reserve, and the level of exercise stress is commonly expressed as some fraction of the "VO_2 max." The exercise physiologist is now engaged in relating the energy requirements in various forms of exercise to the energy needs of specific muscle fiber types, as well as to considerations of overall body composition (66). At the same time, workers struggling with the problems of global nutrition are seeking more quantitative information on the energy requirements and work efficiency of individuals in developing countries. Isolated reports have indicated a surprising variability in food requirements and work efficiency within a population of apparently healthy, active adults (67).

The energetics of physical activity are receiving new attention from those who deal with inactivity, especially those involved in the weightless environment of the space program (68). How much exercise and what exercise efficiency is required to maintain physical conditioning? Modern medicine is becoming concerned with the weakness and easy fatigue which is commonly present in patients leaving the hospital after having undergone major injury or severe illness (69). How much of this weakness and fatigue can be prevented with better nutrition while in the hospital? Can measurements of energy expenditure guide a program of special nutrition and exercise for such individuals as they seek to return to a full and effective life?

CALORIMETRY IN CLINICAL CONDITIONS

Measurements of gas exchange have now changed from attention to the BMR to the resting energy expenditure which is measured without regard for the time of day or the relation to food intake. Feurer and co-workers (70) compared the measured resting energy expenditure by bedside indirect calorimetry with the estimated resting energy expenditure (REE) calculated by the Harris-Benedict equations and the Kleiber formula in 200 clinically stable hospitalized patients and in 72 healthy control subjects. Mean predicted values were not significantly different from the measured REE for the male patients and control subjects; however, the measured REE was significantly overestimated by the Kleiber formula in the female patients and controls. These data revealed an important finding that has been confirmed in less extensive studies: it relates to the number of individuals who can be expected to fall within the normal range of ±10% of the mean value (sometimes considered as ±15% of the mean value). It is expected that 80% to 90% of normal adult individuals will fall within a prescribed normal range. Feuer and associates (70) found that their measured values for 80% of the healthy males and 81% of the healthy females fell within ±10% of values predicted by the Harris-Benedict formula. Both the male and female patients had similar mean values to that predicted as normal from the formula, but only 60% fell within the normal range, with the remainder divided between those who were hypometabolic (as low as 30% below predicted) and hypermetabolic (up to 70% above predicted). The authors concluded that since no method exists for identifying the clinically stable patient for whom the REE cannot be predicted by commonly employed equations or formulae, the bedside measurement of REE is appropriate whenever a knowledge of caloric balance is an important part of management. A study of acutely ill patients requiring mechanical ventilation was reported by Weissman and co-workers (71) where measured energy expenditure fell both above and below the predicted normal range and where the hypermetabolic patients could not be separated reliably from the hypometabolic patients by clinical evaluation.

Most physicians are familiar with the normal range of laboratory values for a remarkable number of materials in blood and urine. However, this array of information seldom includes normal values for human energy expenditure. Many physicians overestimate the REE of patients by 500 to 1500 kcal (2000 to 6000 kJ) per day. Therefore, the common practice of providing approximately 3000 kilocalories (12,000 kJ) of nutrient infusion to every patient does not appear excessive unless the REE is measured and found to be in the range of only 1300 to 1500 kcal (5400 to 6300 kJ) day^{-1}.

The respiratory quotient (RQ) is a helpful part of indirect calorimetry determination, since it establishes the caloric equivalent of oxygen. This is commonly done after subtracting the proportion of O_2 and CO_2

associated with the oxidation of protein as judged by nitrogen excretion. The RQ normally represents a range of 0.71 for the oxidation of fatty acids up to 1.0 for the oxidation of carbohydrate. The oxidation of an average protein has an RQ of approximately 0.81. Correcting the RQ for protein oxidation makes essentially no difference when the proportion of calories from fat and carbohydrate are approximately equal. This is because protein represents only about 15% of the total calories in the fuel mixture of the average daily diet and has an RQ in mid-range between fat and carbohydrate. Correction for protein oxidation does introduce a modest change when the RQ is very low with predominantly fat oxidation or very high with predominantly carbohydrate oxidation. Weir (72) emphasized the small correction represented by most protein oxidation and proposed a simple factor which avoids the need for knowledge of nitrogen excretion. RQ values above 1.0 represent lipogenesis from carbohydrate, and here the correction for protein oxidation to arrive at a nonprotein RQ is of greater importance if the extent of lipogenesis is considered significant in nutritional management.

The human body does not ordinarily encounter high carbohydrate loads which will produce an RQ of 1.0 or higher. A nonprotein RQ of 1.0 is commonly considered to represent the oxidation of carbohydrate as a sole fuel for all tissues. However, it may also indicate a balanced mixture of carbohydrate oxidation, fat oxidation, and lipogenesis. It is our opinion that as carbohydrate intake is increased, lipogenesis from carbohydrate begins in adipose tissue and liver at a time when fat oxidation is continuing in muscle or other tissues and that the combined effect of these two processes can yield an RQ of 1.0.

The influence of carbohydrate-loading has come under study as the result of administering high carbohydrate total parenteral nutrition (TPN) to patients. Askanazi and co-workers (73) compared the changes in O_2 consumption and CO_2 production in a group of depleted surgical patients with that found with the same type of nutrition in a group of acutely injured and septic patients. After 5 days of high carbohydrate TPN, the CO_2 output of the depleted patients had increased with no change in the O_2 consumption yielding an RQ above 1.0. The acutely ill patients had larger increases not only in CO_2 production, but in O_2 consumption as well. The RQ of the acutely ill patients remained at 0.94 because the TPN given to these patients produced a thermogenic response, as reflected by the increased O_2 consumption. Similar findings were reported by Stoner and co-workers (74) when studying the fuel mixture of septic patients.

Attention to the RQ has been considered important by some in evaluating nutritional support. Henneberg and co-workers (75) used gas exchange and the RQ to evaluate the substrate utilization of postoperative patients when given TPN of two different compositions. Some investigators have suggested that giving high carbohydrate TPN until the RQ rises above 1.0 indicates that an adequate number of calories have been provided since the body is now converting extra carbohydrate calories into fat. Other workers have taken the point of view that high carbohydrate loads may have certain undesirable side effects, such as stimulating CO_2 production (which may be a problem for the patient with pulmonary compromise) and producing hepatic steatosis in some other patients. Therefore, the administration of TPN which includes some lipid together with only moderate amounts of carbohydrate will yield an RQ between 0.8 and 0.9, which is preferable to an RQ of 1.0 or above. Foster and co-workers (76) conducted a detailed study indicating that the amount of TPN being prescribed in a general hospital population could be reduced by 22% if the amount were to be based upon measurements of indirect calorimetry.

The resurgence of interest in measuring energy expenditure was focused initially on certain obvious problems, such as the proper adjustment of the reducing diet for the refractory obese patient or designing the correct caloric intake for the acute patient in the intensive care unit. Less obvious, but of equal importance, is monitoring the delicate balance of the patient with chronic pulmonary disease who is losing weight and needs better nutrition but who cannot tolerate the additional demands for ventilation which might arise from overenthusiastic efforts at nutritional support. Specific clinical conditions where the resting energy expenditure has been reported include: the obese patient, before and during caloric restriction (77), the depleted patient (78), the patient with trauma or sepsis (79), the patient with head injury (80), the burned patient (81), the patient with inflammatory bowel disease (82), the patient with chronic pulmonary disease (83), the patient with ventilatory failure (71), the patient with multiple organ failure (84), and the patient with cancer of various types, with and without weight loss (85, 86). At the present time, the weight gain of obesity is treated largely by dietary restriction. Weight loss in various catabolic states is treated by increasing the dietary intake. Yet, both types of nutritional therapy are only partially successful since the underlying metabolic state of the patient may tend to resist a return to normal body weight. The rapid strides in pharmacology and molecular engineering may soon make it possible to alter, or abolish, certain aspects of the metabolic state which underlie abnormal losses or gains of body weight. If this should become a reality, then indirect calorimetry will play a central role in establishing the proper energy balance to restore a normal body weight (and body composition) and to monitor whether a normal energy balance is being maintained.

The history of calorimetry in general and of indirect calorimetry in particular has been the alternation between developing new concepts and inventing better technology. At various times in history, it appeared that concepts were ahead of technology and, at other times, the introduction of new technology was necessary to advance conceptual understanding. Technological advances now offer the promise of simplifying measurements of both energy expenditure and body compositon, so that in the future energy supply and demand per unit of body cell mass can become a routine part of patient management.

REFERENCES

1. Frank RG Jr: *Harvey and the Oxford Physiologists*. Berkeley, The University of California Press, 1980.
2. Read J: Joseph Black, M.D.: The teacher and the man. In Kent A (ed): *An Eighteenth Century Lectureship in Chemistry*, Glasgow, Jackson, Son and Company, 1950, pp 78–98.
3. Priestley J: *Experiments and Observations on Different Kinds of Air*, New York, Kraus Reprint Company, 1970, Vol 1.
4. Astrup P, Severinghaus JW: *The History of Blood Gases, Acids and Bases*. Copenhagen, Munksgaard International Publishers, 1986, pp 43–49.
5. Holmes FL: *Lavoisier and the Chemistry of Life*, Madison, The University of Wisconsin Press, 1985.
6. Lusk G: *The Elements of the Science of Nutrition* , ed 4. Philadelphia, W.B. Saunders Company, 1928.
7. Atwater WO, Benedict FG: *A Respiration Calorimeter with Appliances for the Direct Determination of Oxygen*. Washington DC, Carnegie Institute, Publication No 42, 1905, pp 1–193.
8. Webb P: *Human Calorimeters*. New York, Praeger Publishers, 1985.
9. "Graham Lusk". *JAMA* Editorial 210:2385, 1969.
10. DuBois EF: *Basal Metabolism in Health and Disease*. Philadelphia, Lea and Febiger, 1924.
11. Wretlind A: Current status of intralipid and other fat emulsions. In HC Meng, DW Wilmore (eds): *Fat Emulsions in Parenteral Nutrition*. Chicago, American Medical Association, 1975, pp 109–122.
12. Dudrick SJ, Wilmore DW, Vars HM, Rhoades JE: Can intravenous feeding as the sole means of nutrition support growth in the child and restore weight loss in an adult? An affirmative answer.*Ann Surg* 169:974-984, 1969.
13. McArdle WD, Katch KI, Katch VL: *Exercise Physiology*, ed 2. Philadelphia, Lea and Febiger, 1986, pp 131–146.
14. Norton AC: Portable equipment for gas exchange. In Kinney JM (ed): *Assessment of Energy Metabolism in Health and Disease*. Columbus, Ross Laboratories, 1980, pp 36–41.
15. Ames SR: The Joule-unit of energy. *J Am Diet Assoc* 57:415–416, 1970.
16. Kleiber M: Joules vs calories in nutrition. *J Nutr* 102:309-312, 1972.

17. Kleiber M: *The Fire of Life*. Huntington NY, Robert E Krieger Publishing Company, 1975, pp 123–124.
18. Kinney JM: Summary. In Kinney JM (ed): *Assessment of Energy Metabolism in Health and Disease*. Columbus, Ross Laboratories, 1980, pp 151–153.
19. Kluger MJ: *Fever: Its Biology, Evolution and Function*. Princeton, The Princeton University Press, 1979, pp 8–14.
20. Benedict FG: A portable respiration apparatus for clinical use. *Boston Med Surg J* 178:667-678, 1918.
21. Johnson RE: Techniques for measuring gas exchange. In Kinney JM (ed): *Assessment of Energy Metabolism in Health and Disease*. Columbus, Ross Laboratories, 1980, pp 32–36.
22. Kinney JM, Morgan AP, Domingues FJ, Gildner KJ: A method for continuous measurement of gas exchange and expired radioactivity in acutely ill patients. *Metabolism* 13: 205-211, 1964
23. Spencer JL, Zikria BA, Kinney JM, et al.: A system for the continuous measurement of gas exchange and respiratory functions. *J Appl Physiol* 33:523-528, 1972.
24. Webb P, Annis JF, Troutman SJ Jr: Human calorimetry with a watercooled garment. *J Appl Physiol* 32:412-418, 1972.
25. Jéquier E: Studies with direct calorimetry in humans: Thermal body insulation and thermoregulation responses during exercise. In Kinney JM (ed): *Assessment of Energy Metabolism in Health and Disease.* Columbus, Ross Laboratories, 1980, pp 15–20.
26. Schoffelen PFM, Saris WHM, Westerterp KR, ten Hoor F: Evaluation of an automated indirect calorimeter for measurement of energy balance in man. In van Es AJH (ed): *Human energy metabolism: Physical activity and energy expenditure measurements in epidemiological research based upon direct and indirect calorimetry*. Report of an EC Workshop, Wageningen, The Netherlands, 24–26, October 1984.
27. Durnin JVGA, Edholm OG, Miller DS, Waterlow JC: How much food does man require? *Nature* (London) 242:418, 1973.
28. van Es AJH (ed): *Human Energy Metabolism: Physical Activity and Energy Expenditure Measurements in Epidemiological Research Based upon Direct and Indirect Calorimetry*. Euro-Nut Report 5, EC Workshop, Wageningen, The Netherlands, 24–26 October 1984.
29. Schoeller DA, van Santen E, Peterson DW, et al.: Total body water measurements in humans with ^{18}O and ^{2}H labelled water. *Am J Clin Nutr* 33:2686-2693, 1980.
30. Schoeller DA, Webb P: Five-day comparison of the doubly labelled water method with respiratory gas exchange. *Am J Clin Nutr* 40:153-158, 1984.
31. Consolazio CF, Johnson RE, Pecora LJ: *Physiological Measurements of Metabolic Functions in Man*. New York, McGraw-Hill Book Company, 1963, pp 40–50.
32. Humphrey SJE, Wolff HS: The Oxylog. *J Physiol* 267:12 P, 1977.
33. McArdle WD, Katch FI, Katch VL: *Exercise Physiology* . Philadelphia, Lea and Febiger, 1986, pp 147–165.
34. Buskirk ER, Hodgson J, Blair D: Assessment of daily energy balance: Some observations on the methodology for indirect determinations of energy intake and expenditure. In Kinney JM (ed): *Assessment of Energy Metabolism in Health and Disease.* Columbus, Ross Laboratories, 1980, pp 113–117.
35. Andrews RB: Indices of heart rate as substitutes for respiratory calorimetry. *Am Ind Hyg Assoc J* 27:526-532, 1966.

36. Durnin JVGA, Edwards RG: Pulmonary ventilation as an index of energy expenditure. *Quart J Exper Physiol* 40:370-377, 1955.
37. Sharkey BJ, McDonald JF, Corbridge LG: Pulse rate and pulmonary ventilation as predictors of human energy cost. *Ergonomics* 9:223-227, 1966.
38. Simopoulos AP, Van Itallie TB: Body weight, health and longevity. *Ann Intern Med* 100:285-295, 1984.
39. Benedict FG: *A Study of Prolonged Fasting* . Washington DC, Carnegie Institute, Publication No. 203, 1915.
40. Keys A, Brozek J, Henschel A et al: *The Biology of Human Starvation* . Minneapolis, The University of Minnesota Press, 1950, Vol 1.
41. Kinney JM, Weissman C: Forms of malnutrition in stressed and unstressed patients. In Askanazi J (ed): *Clinics in Chest Medicine* .7:19-28,1986.
42. Voit E: Uber Die Grosse des Energiebedarfs der Tiere in Hungerzustande.*Z Biol* 23:113-154, 1901.
43. Aub JC, Du Bois EF: Clinical calorimetry. The basal metabolism of old men. *Arch Int Med* 19:823-831, 1917.
44. Boothby WM, Berkson J, Dunn HL: Studies of the energy metabolism of normal individuals: A standard for basal metabolism with a nomograph for clinical application. *Am J Physiol* 116:468-484, 1936.
45. Fleisch A: Le metabolisme basal standard et sa determination au moyen du "Metabocalculator". *Helvet Med Acta* 18:23-44, 1951.
46. Robertson JD, Reid DD: Standards for the basal metabolism of normal people in Britain. *Lancet* 1:940-943, 1952.
47. Harris JA, Benedict FG: *A Biometric Study of Basal Metabolism in Man* . Washington DC, Carnegie Institute of Washington, Publ. 279, 1919.
48. Long CL, Schaffel N, Geiger JW, et al.: Metabolic response to injury and illness: estimation of energy and protein needs from indirect calorimetry and nitrogen balance. *JPEN* 3:452-456, 1979.
49. Daly JM, Heymsfield SB, Head CA, et al.: Human energy requirements: overestimation by widely used prediction equations. *Am Soc Clin Nutr* 42:1170-1174, 1985.
50. Cunningham JJ: A reanalysis of the factors influencing basal metabolic rate in normal adults. *Am J Clin Nutr* 33:2372-2374, 1980.
51. Moore FD, Olesen KH, McMurrey FD, et al.: *The Body Cell Mass and its Supporting Environment: Body Composition in Health and Disease.* Philadelphia, W.B. Saunders Company, 1963.
52. Kleiber, M: *The Fire of Life.* Huntington NY, Robert E. Krieger Publishing Company, 1975, pp 179–222.
53. Zeuthen E: Oxygen uptake as related to body size in organisms. *Quart Rev Biol* 28:1-12, 1953.
54. Grande F, Keys A: Body weight, body composition and calorie status. In Goodhart RS, Shils ME (eds): *Modern Nutrition in Health and Disease*, ed 6. Philadelphia, Lea and Febiger, 1980, pp 3–34.
55. Roza AM, Shizgal HM: The Harris-Benedict equation reevaluated: Resting energy requirements and the body cell mass. *Am J Clin Nutr* 40:168-182, 1984.
56. McNeill KG, Mernagh JR, Harrison JE, et al.: In vivo measurements of body protein based on the determination of nitrogen by prompt gamma analysis. *Am J Clin Nutr* 32:1955-1961, 1979.
57. Cohn SH, Vartsky D, Yasumura S, et al.: Indexes of body cell mass: Nitrogen versus potassium. *Am J. Physiol* 244:E305-E310, 1983.

58. Owen OE, Holup JL, D'Alessio DA, et al.: A reappraisal of the caloric requirements of men. *Am J Clin Nutr* 46:875-885, 1987.
59. Wood CD, Goumas W, Pollard M, Brinker JAE: Tissue nitrogen and potassium variation in trauma, starvation and realimentation. *JPEN* 8:665-667, 1984.
60. Almond DJ, King RFGJ, Burkinshaw L, et al.: Potassium depletion in surgical patients: Intracellular cation deficiency is independent of loss of body protein. *Clin Nutr* 6:55-50, 1987.
61. Rubner M: *Die Gesetze des Energieverbrauchs bei der Ernahrung.* Leipzig, Deutiche, 1902.
62. Krebs HA: The metabolic fate of amino acids. In Munro HN, Allison JB(eds): *Mammalian Protein Metabolism,* Vol I. New York, Academic Press, 1964, p 125.
63. Garrow JS, Hawes SF: The role of amino acid oxidation in causing specific dynamic action in man. *Br J Nutr* 27:211-219, 1972.
64. Rothwell NJ, Stock MJ: Diet-induced thermogenesis. In Girardier L , Stock MJ: *Mammalian Thermogenesis.* London, Chapman and Hall, 1983, p 208.
65. Girardier L, Stock MJ: Mammalian thermogenesis: An introduction. In Girardier L, Stock MJ: *Mammalian Thermogenesis.* London, Chapman and Hall, 1983, p 1.
66. McArdle WD, Katch FI, Katch VL: *Exercise Physiology,* ed 2. Philadelphia, Lea & Febiger, 1986, pp 289–304.
67. Edmundson W: Individual variations in basal metabolic rate and mechanical work efficiency in East Java. *Ecol Food Nutr* 8:189-195, 1979.
68. Sandler H, Vernikos J (eds): *Inactivity: Physiological Effects.* Orlando FL, Academic Press, 1986.
69. Christensen T, Kehlet H: Postoperative fatigue and changes in nutritional status. *Br J Surg* 71:473-476, 1984.
70. Feurer ID, Crosby LO, Mullen JL: Measured and predicted resting energy expenditure in clinically stable patients. *Clin Nutr* 3:27-34, 1984.
71. Weissman C, Kemper M, Askanazi J, et al.: Resting metabolic rate of the critically ill patient: Measured versus predicted. *Anesthesiology* 64:673-679,1986.
72. Weir JB de V: New methods for calculating metabolic rate with special reference to protein metabolism. *J Physiol* 109:1-9, 1949.
73. Askanazi J, Carpentier YA, Elwyn DH, et al.: Influence of total parenteral nutrition on fuel utilization in injury and sepsis. *Ann Surg* 191:40-46, 1980.
74. Stoner HB, Little RA, Frayn KNB, et al.: The effect of sepsis on the oxidation of carbohydrate and fat. *Br J Surg* 70:32-35, 1983.
75. Henneberg S, Eklun A, Stjernstrom H, et al.: Post-operative substrate utilization and gas exchange using two different TPN-systems: Glucose versus fat. *Clin Nutr* 4:235-242, 1985.
76. Foster GD, Knox LS, Dempsey DT, Mullen JL: Caloric requirements in total parenteral nutrition. *J Am Coll Nutr* 6:231-253, 1987.
77. Ravussin E, Burnand B, Schutz Y, Jéquier E: Energy expenditure before and during energy restriction in obese patients. *Am J Clin Nutr* 41:753-759, 1985.
78. Chikenji T, Elwyn DH, Gil KM, et al.: Effects of increasing glucose intake on nitrogen balance and energy expenditure in malnourished adult patients receiving parenteral nutrition. *Clin Sci* 72:489-501, 1987.
79. Little RA: Heat production after injury. *Br Med Bull* 41:226-231, 1985.
80. Clifton GL, Robertson CS, Grossman RG et al.: The metabolic response to severe head injury. *J Neurosurg* 60:687-696, 1984.
81. Saffle JR, Medina E, Raymond J, et al.: Use of indirect calorimetry in the nutritional management of burned patients. *J Trauma* 25:32-39, 1985.

82. Barot LR, Rombeau JL, Feurer ID, Mullen JL: Caloric requirements in patients with inflammatory bowel disease. *Ann Surg* 195:214-218, 1982.
83. Goldstein SA, Thomashow B, Askanazi J: Functional changes during nutritional repletion in patients with lung disease. In Askanazi J(ed): *Clinics in Chest Medicine, Nutrition in Respiratory Disease.* WB Saunders Company, Philadelphia, 1986, Vol 7, No. 1, pp 141–152.
84. Bartlett RH, Dechert RE, Mault JR, et al.: Measurement of metabolism in multiple organ failure. *Surgery* 92:771-779, 1982.
85. Bozzetti F: Determination of the caloric requirement of patients with cancer. *Surg Gyn Obst* 149:667-670, 1979.
86. Knox LS, Crosby LO, Feurer ID, et al.: Energy expenditure in malnourished cancer patients. *Ann Surg* 197:152-162, 1983.

CHAPTER

2

The Theoretical Framework of Indirect Calorimetry and Energy Balance

- Energy Balance
  - Energy Out
  - Energy In
  - Energy In Minus Energy Out
  - Carbohydrate and Fat Balances
  - Energy Balance and Obesity

In the human body the unique source of energy is food, which may be expressed as caloric intake. Energy expenditure, which may also be expressed as caloric loss, consists of heat loss or mechanical work.

When humans or animals ingest carbohydrates, proteins, or fats, they either oxidize them to produce energy, or transform these nutrients to forms that may be stored as potential energy. Energy is stored mainly as fat. A normal 70 kg man has about 16 kg of fat in adipose tissue (between zero and the sky is the limit), which can yield 150,000 kcal (630,000 kJ) on oxidation. This is sufficient, at least theoretically, to allow a sedentary individual to survive for 2 months, if he is in good health, if he does not use more than 2500 kcal (10,000 kJ) a day (2500 kcal $day^{-1} \times 60$ days = 150,000 kcal) and if he is able to oxidize all his fat stores. The fasting demonstrators in Ireland, who were normal young men, died after about 60 days of starvation. Mahatma Ghandi, who was not in the best nutritional condition, nearly died from a fast of 40 days.

Fat loss during starvation is accompanied by obligatory breakdown of another major body constituent, protein. A normal man contains about 11 kg of protein of which approximately 7 kg are intracellular and 4 kg are extracellular. The extracellular proteins, mainly in bone, ligaments, tendons, cartilage and connective tissue, are very stable and are not available for metabolic needs. Intracellular proteins serve various functions as enzymes or contractile and structural elements of the cell; there are no storage proteins as such. Nevertheless, these functional proteins are continuously synthesized and degraded, and about 5 kg, most of which comes from muscle, can be mobilized during prolonged fasting. All organs and tissues, except the brain, lose proteins, and this loss soon becomes harmful, since it reduces host defense mechanisms and the healing process and compromises resistance to infection. Most people dying from starvation are, at the final stages, infected by all kinds of pathogenic microorganisms. These 5 kg of proteins represent a small amount of energy, 22,000 kcal (92,000 kJ), compared to fat stores. However, protein unlike fat can be almost entirely converted to glucose, which is required by the brain. This process of glucogenesis takes place mainly in the liver and kidneys. These biochemical aspects of body composition and energy utilization in different physiological and pathophysiological states are discussed in Chapter 4.

Besides fat and proteins, we also have between 1000 and 3000 kcal of carbohydrate stored in the liver and muscles as glycogen. This is immediately available for needs such as exercise, but is of little long-term value. Other compounds in the body, such as phospholipids and nucleic acids, are able to provide small amounts of energy but are not usually taken into account when evaluating energy balance.

Alcohol is not an important body constituent, but for a high percentage of men comprises an important, if not the main part, of their normal energy intake, providing 7 kcal (29 kJ) g^{-1}. Today alcohol is not advised by nutritionists. But in the sixties and the beginning of the seventies, alcohol was administered intravenously by many physicians and serious publications appeared in the literature about the benefits of alcohol in total parenteral nutrition (TPN), without mentioning that very ill patients under this treatment were at the very least euphoric (1).

Since "energy may neither be created nor destroyed" the human body is busy transforming energy, combusting foodstuffs from its own reserves or from dietary intake, and producing heat and mechanical work. According to conditions, the environment, age, sex, nutritional status, physical activity, the moment of the day or the night, psychological condition, and, in fact, to all that is happening, the human body will modify energy metabolism or, in other words, lose more or less heat and so be obliged to produce more or less energy to cover its needs. This confirms Max Kleiber's comment that "energy expenditure is the most representative parameter of the life process" (2).

BASAL ENERGY EXPENDITURE—RESTING ENERGY EXPENDITURE

Basal energy expenditure (BEE) or basal metabolic rate (BMR) is defined as the heat expended by an individual at least 10 hours after the last meal, resting in a lying position, awake, at a normal body and ambient temperature, and without physical or psychological stress. Usually measured after an overnight sleep, the BMR, expressed in kcal per day per square meter, is remarkably constant for normal subjects of similar age, height, and sex. The 10 hours after the last meal is to reach the postabsorptive state defined as the situation where the digestive process is completely terminated. At this time there is no influence on energy expenditure of "diet-induced thermogenesis" (DIT), known until recently as "specific dynamic action of nutrients" (SDA). There remains an argument as to when the postabsorptive state is reached, somewhere between 8 and 18 hours (3), and for other reasons as well it is difficult to insure that basal conditions obtain. Most reports of measurements claimed to be made under basal conditions were probably made, instead, under resting conditions. Resting energy expenditure (REE) is defined as the energy expenditure obtained at rest in a lying position. The major difference from BEE is that REE includes diet-induced thermogenesis. Therefore, to a first approximation:

$$REE = BEE + DIT \tag{1}$$

However, resting conditions are defined less rigorously than basal conditions; therefore, REE will include components due to physical or psychological stress and variation in ambient or body temperature. Operationally, REE is a more useful measurement than BEE. From a practical view, it is sometimes hard to distinguish between the two, and they are therefore discussed together in this section.

Body Surface Area and Energy Expenditure

Since heat is mostly lost via the skin it seems appropriate to relate energy expenditure to body surface area expressed in standard units of kilocalories per square meter (kcal m^{-2}). Measurement of body surface area is not, however, an easy procedure. To determine body surface area as a function of height and weight, Du Bois and Du Bois clothed 8 men and 2 women in very tight underwear, and applied melted paraffin and paper strips to prevent modifications of the surface (4). The treated cloth was then removed and cut into flat pieces to allow precise measurements of body surface area. From those measurements Du Bois and Du Bois derived the following empirical formula:

$$SA = H^{0.725} \times W^{0.425} \times 71.84 \qquad (2)$$

where SA = body surface area in cm, H = height in cm, and W = weight in kg. Figures 2.1 and 2.2 are nomograms derived from this formula facilitating the calculation of body surface area, which can also be calculated as shown in Table 2.1. This formula was slightly modified for Japanese subjects by Takahira (5).

$$SA = H^{0.718} \times W^{0.427} \times 74.49 \qquad (3)$$

A formula useful for animal investigations is that of Meeh for calculating body surface area (in m^2) of the dog as a function of weight only (6)

$$SA = 0.112\ W^{2/3} \qquad (4)$$

The technique used by Du Bois and Du Bois for body surface calculation has been criticized. Harris and Benedict, instead, proposed formulas for predicting energy expenditure directly from sex, age, height, and weight based on measurements in 136 men, 103 women, and 94 infants (7).

$$\textit{Men:}\quad EE\ (kcal) = 66.5 + 13.75\ W + 5.003\ H - 6.775\ A \qquad (5)$$
$$EE\ (kJ) = 278 + 57.5\ W + 20.93\ H - 28.35\ A$$

$$\textit{Women:}\quad EE\ (kcal) = 655.1 + 9.563\ W + 1.850\ H - 4.676\ A \qquad (6)$$
$$EE\ (kJ) = 2741 + 40.0\ W + 7.74\ H - 19.56\ A$$

where A=age, and the other terms are as defined above.

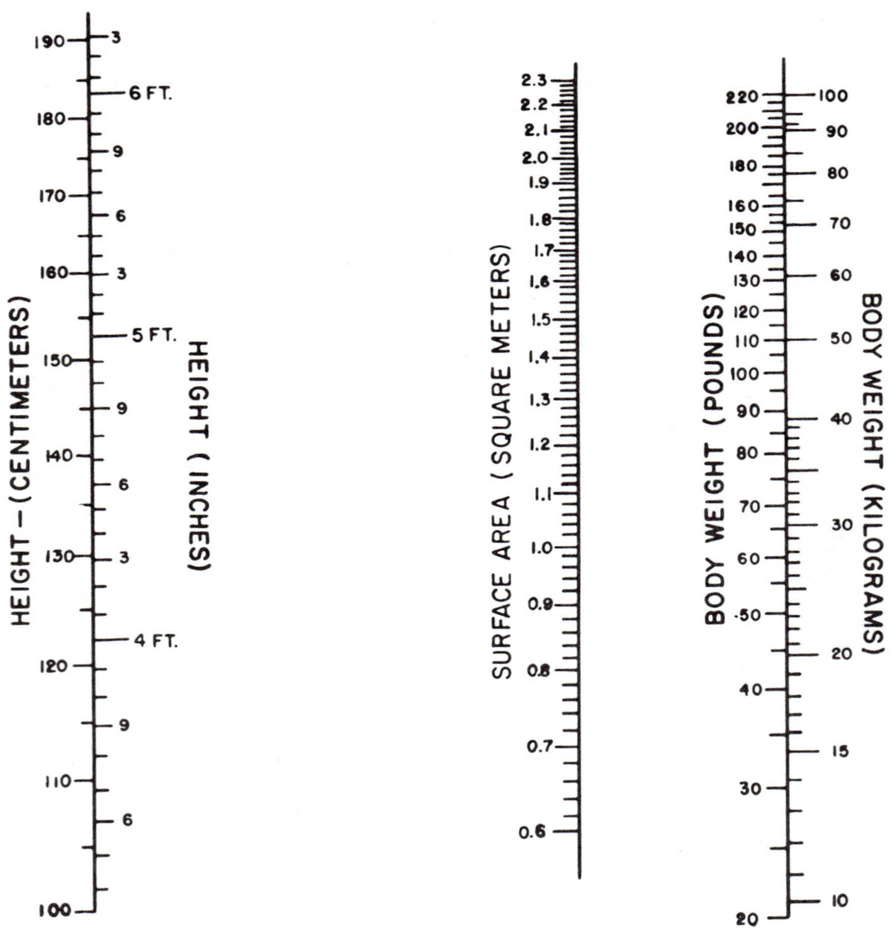

Figure 2.1. Data of Du Bois and Du Bois. Reproduced from Wilmore DW: *The Metabolic Management of the Critically Ill.* New York, Plenum Medical Book Company, 1977, p 21. With permission of Plenum Medical Book Company. Body surface area from height and weight.

Although these formulas were published in 1919, they are still widely used by clinicians. Since they are based on studies in untrained volunteers, the values are slightly elevated compared to values of Boothby, et al. (8), Fleisch (9), or even to Harris and Benedict's own values obtained from individuals who where trained for these uncomfortable tests, which include the inconvenience of a mouthpiece and noseclip (10).

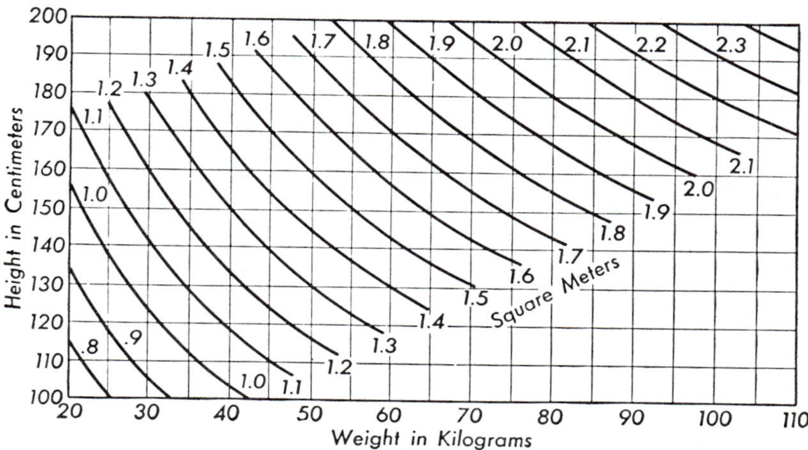

Figure 2.2. Reproduced from Du Bois D and Du Bois EF: Clinical calorimetry. A formula to estimate the approximate surface area if height and weight be known. *Arch Intern Med* 17:863-871, 1916. With permission of *Archives of Internal Medicine.* Chart for determining surface area of man in square meters from weight and height.

Table 2.1.
Surface area in square meters for different heights and weights.[a]

Height in	Weight in Kilograms																
Centimeters	25	30	35	40	45	50	55	60	65	70	75	80	85	90	95	100	105
200							1.84	1.91	1.97	2.03	2.09	2.15	2.21	2.26	2.31	2.36	2.41
195						1.73	1.80	1.87	1.93	1.99	2.05	2.11	2.17	2.22	2.27	2.32	2.37
190				1.56	1.63	1.70	1.77	1.84	1.90	1.96	2.02	2.08	2.13	2.18	2.23	2.28	2.33
185				1.53	1.60	1.67	1.74	1.80	1.86	1.92	1.98	2.04	2.09	2.14	2.19	2.24	2.29
180				1.49	1.57	1.64	1.71	1.77	1.83	1.89	1.95	2.00	2.05	2.10	2.15	2.20	2.25
175	1.19	1.28	1.36	1.46	1.53	1.60	1.67	1.73	1.79	1.85	1.91	1.96	2.01	2.06	2.11	2.16	2.21
170	1.17	1.26	1.34	1.43	1.50	1.57	1.63	1.69	1.75	1.81	1.86	1.91	1.96	2.01	2.06	2.11	
165	1.14	1.23	1.31	1.40	1.47	1.54	1.60	1.66	1.72	1.78	1.83	1.88	1.93	1.98	2.03	2.07	
160	1.12	1.21	1.29	1.37	1.44	1.50	1.56	1.62	1.68	1.73	1.78	1.83	1.88	1.93	1.98		
155	1.09	1.18	1.26	1.33	1.40	1.46	1.52	1.58	1.64	1.69	1.74	1.79	1.84	1.89			
150	1.06	1.15	1.23	1.30	1.36	1.42	1.48	1.54	1.60	1.65	1.70	1.75	1.80				
145	1.03	1.12	1.20	1.27	1.33	1.39	1.45	1.51	1.56	1.61	1.66	1.71					
140	1.00	1.09	1.17	1.24	1.30	1.36	1.42	1.47	1.52	1.57							
135	0.97	1.06	1.14	1.20	1.26	1.32	1.38	1.43	1.48								
130	0.95	1.04	1.11	1.17	1.23	1.29	1.35	1.40									
125	0.93	1.01	1.08	1.14	1.20	1.26	1.31	1.36									
120	0.91	0.98	1.04	1.10	1.16	1.22	1.27										

[a]Reproduced from Du Bois D and Du Bois EF: Clinical calorimetry. A formula to estimate the approximate surface area if height and weight be known. *Arch Intern Med* 17:863-871,1916. With permission of *Archives of Internal Medicine.*

Standard values of basal metabolic rate as measured by several laboratories are shown in Table 2.2.

Table 2.2.
Standard basal metabolic rate in kcal m^{-2} $hour^{-1}$.[a] To obtain kJ from kcal multiply by 4.184

	Males				Females			
Age, yr	Fleisch	Robertson and Reid	Boothby et al.	Aub and Du Bois	Fleisch	Robertson and Reid	Boothby et al.	Aub and Du Bois
6	48.3	54.2	53.0		47.0	51.8	50.5	
7	47.3	52.1	52.4		45.4	50.2	48.5	
8	46.3	50.1	51.5		43.6	48.4	46.7	
9	45.2	48.2	49.9		42.8	46.4	46.1	
10	44.0	46.6	48.0		42.5	44.3	45.7	
11	43.0	45.1	47.2		42.0	42.4	45.1	
12	42.5	43.8	46.8		41.3	40.6	43.9	
13	42.3	42.7	46.5		40.3	39.1	42.5	
14	42.1	41.8	46.4		39.2	37.8	41.1	
15	41.8	41.0	46.1		37.9	36.8	39.7	
16	41.4	40.3	45.5	46.0	36.9	36.0	38.6	43.0
17	40.8	39.7	44.4		36.3	35.3	37.6	
18	40.0	39.2	42.9	43.0	35.9	34.9	37.0	40.0
19	39.2	38.8	42.2		35.5	34.5	36.6	
20	38.6	38.4	41.6	41.0	35.3	34.3	36.3	38.0
25	37.5	37.1	40.3		35.2	34.2	36.0	
30	36.8	36.4	39.6	39.5	35.1	34.1	35.8	37.0
35	36.5	35.9	38.9		35.0	33.5	35.7	
40	36.3	35.5	38.3	39.5	34.9	32.6	35.5	36.5
45	36.2	34.1	37.6		34.5	32.2	35.3	
50	35.8	33.8	37.0	38.5	33.9	31.9	34.4	36.0
55	35.4	33.4	36.3		33.3	31.6	33.4	
60	34.9	33.1	35.7	37.5	32.7	31.3	32.8	35.0
65	34.4	32.7	—		32.2	31.0	—	
70	33.8	—	—	36.5	31.7	30.7	—	34.0
75	33.2	—	—		31.3	—	—	
80	33.0	—	—	35.5	30.9	—	—	33.0

[a]Reproduced from Du Bois EF: Energy metabolism. *Ann Rev Physiol* 16:125-134, 1954. With permission of *Annual Review of Physiology*.

The introduction by Kinney's group in the sixties of a noninvasive canopy system, eliminating the need for mouthpieces, noseclips, or face masks, made measurements of energy expenditure more comfortable and thus also more reliable, particularly for ill patients (11).

At the beginning of the century, many other formulas for predicting energy expenditure were presented. These gave quite similar results as can be seen from the following three calculations cited by Lusk (12):

9 *normal men (Du Bois)*:	*Mean value*: 39.7 *kcal* (166 *kJ*) $hr^{-1}m^{-2}$
9 *normal men (Means)*:	*Mean value*: 39.6 *kcal* (166 *kJ*) $hr^{-1}m^{-2}$
82 *normal men (Harris-Benedict)*:	*Mean value*: 38.9 *kcal* (163 *kJ*) $hr^{-1}m^{-2}$

For almost all normal subjects measured values of BEE or REE are ±10% of predicted values. Additional factors are required for hospitalized patients. Injury, sepsis, and burns increase REE, as much as 100% for severe burns; malnutrition may decrease REE as much as 40%. Normal predicted values may be corrected with appropriate factors for such patients. Such corrections provide reasonable mean values for groups of patients. However variability is much greater than for normal subjects(13–15). Predicted REE for individual patients may vary as much as 50% from measured values and is of little use for clinical evaluation in establishing a nutritional program for patients given parenteral or enteral nutrition (Chapter 7).

To evaluate basal energy expenditure of children, Dreyer, in 1920, reanalyzed the data of Harris and Benedict and Aub and Du Bois, and suggested other formulas that would fit males and females from the age of 5 (16).

$$\textit{Male}: EE = \frac{W^{1/2}}{0.1015 \times A^{\,0.1333}} \tag{7}$$

$$\textit{Female}: EE = \frac{W^{1/2}}{0.1127 \times A^{\,0.1333}} \tag{8}$$

Where: EE = kcal per 24 hours, W = weight in grams, and A = age in years. Values of BEE for children between the ages of 1 and 18 are shown in Table 2.3 (17).

In modern usage BMR, BEE, and REE are expressed as kcal or kJ per individual; per m^2 or per kg; and per min, per hour, or per day. According to classical terminology, BMR is the difference between the measured and standard metabolic rates, expressed as a percentage of the standard rate:

$$BMR = \frac{(\textit{Measured BMR - Standard BMR}) \times 100}{\textit{Standard BMR}} \tag{9}$$

This ratio is represented in Figure 2.3. Results are expressed as the percentage difference from predicted; ±10% is considered as the normal range. Traditionally, as used primarily to evaluate thyroid function, measured values of BMR were calculated from O_2 consumption and body surface area as shown in Figure 2.3. Predicted values for BMR

Table 2.3.
Basal energy metabolism of children.[a]

Age in Years	Calories per Kilogram Body-Weight per Hour Boys	Girls
1	2.33	2.33
2	2.29	2.29
3	2.13	2.00
4	1.96	1.83
5	1.88	1.75
6	1.79	1.67
7	1.71	1.63
8	1.67	1.58
9	1.58	1.54
10	1.54	1.50
11	1.46	1.42
12	1.42	1.33
13	1.67	1.29
14	1.71	1.54
15	1.50	1.33
16	1.38	1.25
17	1.25	1.17
18	1.25	1.08

[a]Reproduced from Sherman, HC: *Chemistry of Food and Nutrition*, *ed 8.* MacMillan Company, New York, 1952. With permission of the Macmillan Company.
[b]In the older terminology, Calories with a capital C represents kcalorie or kilogram calories, whereas calorie represents gram calories. To convert Calories to kJ multiply by 4.184.

can be obtained from the formulas of Harris and Benedict or of others, or from tables as represented by Tables 2.2 and 2.4 (10,18).

Table 2.4.
Normal standards of basal metabolism.[a] **To obtain kJ from kcal multiply by 4.184.**

Age in Years	Cal per sq. m. of body surface per hour Males	Females
14–16	46.0	43.0
16–18	43.0	40.0
18–20	41.0	38.0
20–30	39.5	37.0
30–40	39.5	36.5
40–50	38.5	36.0
50–60	37.5	35.0
60–70	36.5	34.0
70–80	35.5	33.0

[a]Reproduced from Aub JC, Du Bois EF: Clinical calorimetry. The basal metabolism of old men. *Arch Int Med* 19:823-831, 1917. With permission of *Archives of Internal Medicine.*

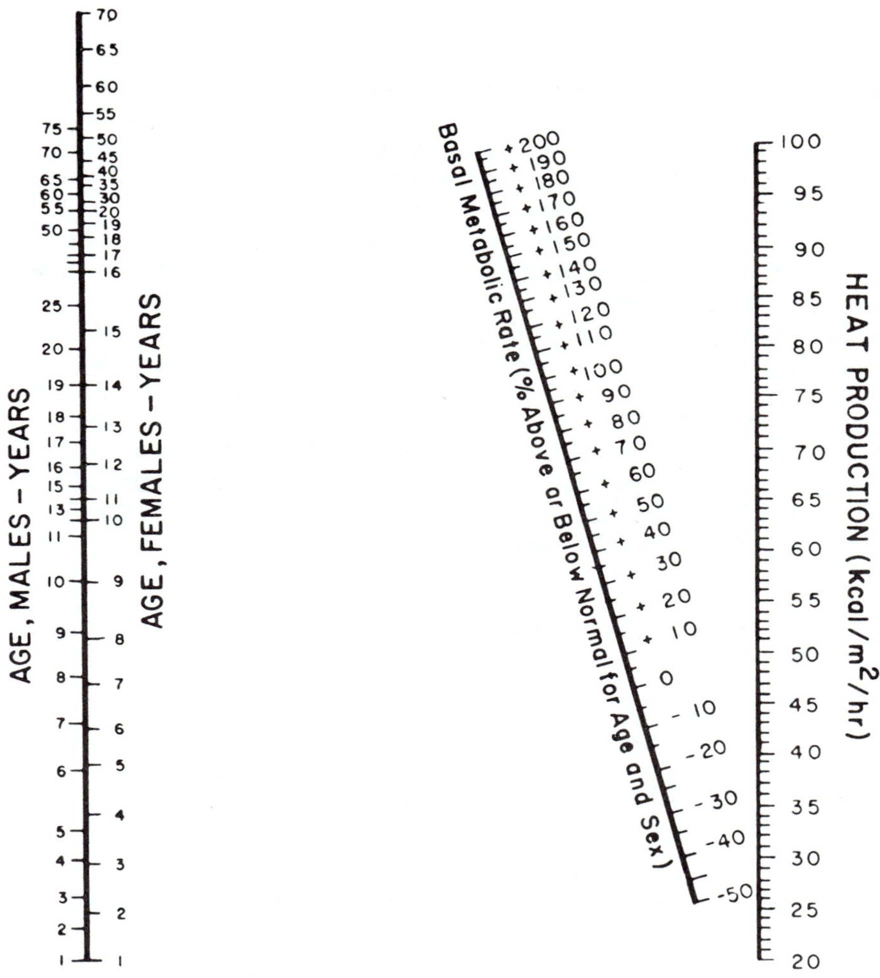

Figure 2.3. Data of Boothby. Reproduced from Wilmore DW: *The Metabolic Management of the Critically Ill.* New York, Plenum Medical Book Company, 1977, p 19. With permission of Plenum Medical Book Company. Basal metabolic rate from heat production, age and sex.

Influence of Various Factors on Energy Expenditure

A normal 70-kg man has a daily resting energy expenditure of about 1800 kcal (7500 kJ). Since by definition 1 kilocalorie or 1 great calorie (1 kcal or 1 Cal) is the amount of heat necessary to raise 1000 ml of water by 1° C, the amount of heat expended or lost by our man corresponds to the amount necessary to raise 18 liters of water from 0° to 100° C, from ice cold to boiling. With severe injury a patient may increase REE by 30%, or 540 kcal (2260 kJ). This is equivalent to the amount of heat spent by running for 75 min, or for energetically cleaning house for about 4 hours. The injured patient has this huge increase in REE, even when he lies quietly in his bed.

The big consumers of energy at rest are the liver, the brain, the heart and the kidneys; representing only 6% of the body weight, they utilize between 60% and 70% of REE. Skeletal muscle, comprising up to 40% of body weight, utilizes only 18% of REE, of course while at rest (Table 2.5) (19). A variety of cellular processes contribute to BMR, like ion pumps, synthesis and degradation of cell constituents, biochemical cycles, and leakage of protons across the mitochondrial membrane. According to Grande the sodium pump and protein turnover may account for two-thirds of the BMR (19). In the nervous system, ion pumping related to electrical conduction is most important, whereas in the liver, protein synthesis may be the major energy consumer (20-22).

Table 2.5.
Approximate energy expenditure of organs in human adults.[a]

Organ	% of REE
Liver	29
Brain	19
Heart	10
Kidney	7
Total	65
Muscles	18

[a]Adapted from Grande(19).

Although, as we observed above, almost everything influences energy expenditure, a few general factors need to be especially emphasized. These include age; sex; body temperature; ambient temperature; and the very important but poorly understood factor, food intake, which produces this mysterious heat called *diet-induced thermogenesis*. These will be taken up before we discuss the specific effects of physical activity and disease.

Age and Energy Expenditure

If we look at a standard metabolic rate table like the one given by Fleisch (Table 2.6), we can see that the values vary from 53 kcal (222 kJ)$m^{-2}hr^{-1}$ at the age of 1, to 31 kcal (131 kJ) m^{-2} hr^{-1} at the age of 75, so that there is a non-negligible influence of age on energy expenditure (9). The literature is well-furnished with data concerning the variations of energy expenditure with age, in all kind of animals and with a lot of simple or complicated formulas expressing heat production per m^{-2}, per kg, or even per kg $^{2/3}$; some studies have compared the variation of energy expenditure from birth to puberty between rats and girls. The only interpretation that could be found to explain that young pregnant women had a relatively higher increase of metabolic rate than young pregnant rats was the fact that the psychological stress in juvenile pregnant women was greater than in precocious pregnant rats (23). However, it is not explained how the stress in precocious pregnant rats was evaluated. Benedict was able to measure energy expenditure in some individual patients over many year periods (24). He observed:

- A women studied between the ages of 24 and 36 had remarkably constant values of energy expenditure.
- Two men studied between the ages of 30 and 57 showed progressive decreases in energy expenditure, the most marked decrease appearing in one at the age of 42 and in the other at the age of 47.
- One man was studied between the ages of 43 and 59. His metabolic rate remained essentially constant; this was explained by Benedict on the grounds that the man had gained weight and had improved his physical condition.

Sex and Energy Expenditure

The magnitude of energy expenditure is a function of the amount of active cells in the body or body cell mass (BCM). Women have more adipose tissue and less muscle than men, and therefore have a lower metabolic rate than men, whether expressed per m^2 or per kg (Tables 2.3, 2.4, and 2.6). These differences begin to appear at age 3, and increase rapidly at puberty, when there is a marked increase in skeletal muscle in boys and in adipose tissue in girls. Indeed when expressed per kg, energy expenditure actually increases in boys at age 13 and 14 (Table 2.3). At the age of 20 these sex differences in relative amounts of muscle and adipose tissues start to decrease and the difference in EE between men and women becomes progressively smaller (Table 2.6).

Body Temperature and Energy Expenditure

Human body temperature is constant, as it is for all homeothermic species who are normally able to regulate their core temperature independently of environmental temperature. Thus, the parrot of the tropi-

Table 2.6.
Standard metabolic rates.[a]

Age in years	kcal/m²/hr		kJ/m²/hr	
	Men	Women	Men	Women
1	53.0	53.0	222	222
2	52.4	52.4	219	219
3	51.3	51.2	215	214
4	50.3	49.8	211	208
5	49.3	48.4	206	203
6	48.3	47.0	202	197
7	47.3	45.4	198	190
8	46.3	43.8	194	183
9	45.2	42.8	189	179
10	44.0	42.5	184	178
11	43.0	42.0	180	176
12	42.5	41.3	178	173
13	42.3	40.3	177	169
14	42.1	39.2	176	164
15	41.8	37.9	175	159
16	41.4	36.9	173	154
17	40.8	36.3	171	152
18	40.0	35.9	167	150
19	39.2	35.5	164	149
20	38.6	35.3	162	148
25	37.5	35.2	157	147
30	36.8	35.1	154	147
35	36.5	35.0	153	146
40	36.3	34.9	152	146
45	36.2	34.5	152	144
50	35.8	33.9	150	142
55	35.4	33.3	148	139
60	34.9	32.7	146	137
65	34.4	32.2	144	135
70	33.8	31.7	141	133
75 and over	33.2	31.3	139	131

[a]Reproduced from Fleisch A: Le metabolisme basal standard et sa determination au moyen du "Metabocalculator." *Helv Med Acta* 18:23-44, 1951. With permission of *Helvetica Medica Acta*.

cal Brazilian jungle and the penguin of the Antarctic have the same body temperature as the elephant of Africa and the polar bear. The body temperature of poikilotherm species, such as reptiles and fishes, rises and falls with changes in temperature of the environment. In these species, changes in metabolic rate accompany changes in temperature, conserving energy at low temperatures. There is a third category of animals, such as the marmot, who behave as homeotherms when it is warm and hibernate during the winter. Animals sleep during hibernation and their body temperature falls as with poikilotherms.

Rubner compared the metabolic rate in a 3.15-kg marmot when he was awake and during his winter sleep (Table 2.7).

Table 2.7.
Metabolic rate and temperature of the marmot either awake or asleep during hibernation.[a]

	Body Temperature °C	Metabolic Rate			
		kcal kg^{-1}	$kJkg^{-1}$	kcal m^{-2}	kJm^{-2}
Marmot awake	36.7	67.74	283.4	1160	4850
Marmot asleep	10.0	2.87	12.0	47.5	199

[a]Adapted from Lusk (12) quoting Rubner.

In homeotherms there are circadian changes in body temperature, usually in the range of no more than 0.5° C.

Body temperature is regulated in the brain by complex mechanisms, starting at the level of peripheral receptors and terminating at the level of vasoactive reactions modulating blood flow, (therefore, heat loss in the skin). As early as 1944, it was known that cultured slices of rat brain when separated from the rest of the body behave like slices of the brain of poikilotherms (25). One of the severe complications of high severe spinal injury or of severe brain damage is the loss of thermoregulatory control. Decreasing temperature and a tendency to behave like a poikilotherm is one of the symptoms used to identify brain death. Early in the century, Du Bois summarized his studies of the influence of body temperature on metabolic rate, stating that metabolic rate increased 13% per degree Celsius or 7.2% per degree Fahrenheit(10). Since metabolic rate is correlated with VO_2, a fever of 40° C may easily increase VO_2 and metabolic rate by 30%. Similarly, a decrease in body temperature reduces oxygen demands and decreases energy expenditure. Artificially induced hypothermia is frequently used to reduce cerebral metabolism during open heart surgery, neurosurgery, or carotid surgery. Some years ago, in an attempt to reduce cerebral metabolic needs, hypothermia was often used for treatment of cerebral damage or other very critical conditions, but without proven benefit. When hypothermia is induced incorrectly, it will produce shivering, which in turn causes an increase rather than a decrease in energy expenditure. This shivering and its ill effects are avoided during anesthesia by curarization of the patient during the cooling procedure, even when the temperature is reduced as much as 16° C. After the surgical procedure, during rewarming, as the influence of neuromuscular blocking agents wears off, shivering is often observed with a large increase in oxygen consumption and a parallel increase in energy expenditure (26, 27). This shivering can be prevented by morphine (28). The effect of increasing body temperature on metabolic rate is related to acceleration of the rates of biochemical reactions.

Ambient Temperature and Energy Expenditure

Of the 1500 people who died during the Titanic catastrophe, more probably died from hypothermia than from drowning. The temperature of the water was estimated to be around 12° C, which is not compatible with life for more then 1 hour. Mice die when their skin temperature reaches 12 ° C. The cause of death in either mice or men seems to be circulatory failure related to the deep hypothermia resulting from loss of the ability to keep body temperature within acceptable limits. Since death occurs at a temperature not low enough to cause tissue damage, it seems to be caused by circulatory failure producing: (*a*) irreversible central nervous injury due to anoxia; and (*b*) a toxic effect of excessive amounts of catecholamines on the myocardium, producing heart block or ventricular fibrillation. The excess catecholamine results from a lowered rate of degradation at low temperatures.

When the ambient temperature rises progressively, energy expenditure will decrease, reaching a minimum in normal subjects at around 27° C. With a further increase in ambient temperature, the energy lost due to cooling by sweating or panting increases, and there is an increase in energy expenditure. At sufficiently high ambient temperature, the body's ability to maintain core temperature near 37° C becomes overwhelmed and core temperature starts to rise. At approximately 42° C death will ensue. The ambient temperature at which energy expenditure is at a minimum was termed the "critical" temperature by Rubner at the beginning of this century. The more usual term today is the zone of thermal neutrality. This is defined as the ambient temperature above which resting energy expenditure of nude subjects begins to rise in order to maintain body temperature and heat balance within normal limits. This is 27° to 29° C in normal men (29, 30). Injured patients have a higher zone of thermal neutrality. For instance, in severely burned patients the minimum metabolic rate was obtained when ambient temperature reached 32° C (31). When burn patients were allowed to regulate ambient temperature themselves, using a manual thermostat, they felt most comfortable at 32° C.

When the ambient temperature decreases below the zone of thermal neutrality, there is an increase in energy expenditure, termed cold-induced thermogenesis. This occurs in two forms, shivering and nonshivering thermogenesis. Nonshivering thermogenesis involves increased rates of metabolic reactions involving hydrolysis of ATP. In rodents most of this occurs in a special organ, brown adipose tissue (BAT) (29, 32). While BAT is found in humans, it is not known whether it is mainly responsible for nonshivering thermogenesis or whether reactions in other tissues, yet poorly defined, may play a major role. When skin temperature decreases to 12° to 19° C, shivering will allow a further increase of heat production. In dogs, energy expenditure was shown to increase by 7% before shivering and by 30% after 20 minutes of shivering (33). As ambient temperature decreases further, the body can no longer maintain core temperature at 37° C, and energy expenditure decreases as body temperature decreases. Careful therapeutic reduction of body temperature can reduce metabolic rate to as low as half the initial value. This was demonstrated as early as 1956 in anesthetized, curarized, ventilated dogs who, when cooled to a rectal temperature of 29° C, decreased their energy expenditure to 52% (34).

Body temperature is mainly regulated centrally through several mechanisms. Blood flow to the skin can be increased by vasodilatation, inducing greater heat loss, or decreased by vasoconstriction, inducing less heat loss. Erection of hair or feathers in animals, increasing the insulation layer, is an important factor, as reported by two nice experiments quoted by Lusk (12). One by E. Voit in 1903 showed the metabolic rate of a pigeon to double after removal of his feathers. In a second experiment, Morgulis in1924 measured energy expenditure of a dog, at an ambient temperature of 10° C, before and after shaving. Heat production of the dog rose from 59 to 112 kcal (247 to 469 kJ) kg^{-1} day^{-1}. Thus nakedness had an almost identical effect on the dog as on the pigeon. Since human beings are no longer covered with hair or feathers they use their central nervous system to dress themselves with various kinds of clothing, which represents an important contribution to the world's culture and economy. Other factors influencing body temperature regulation are:

- secretion of sweat glands
- water evaporation from the skin, dependent on wetness of the skin and humidity of the air
- water loss by evaporation from the respiratory tract

Food Intake and Energy Expenditure (Diet-Induced Thermogenesis, Specific Dynamic Action)

Rubner measured by indirect calorimetry the energy expenditure of a 24-hr fasting dog and found it to be 742 kcal (12). During the following 24 hr, he fed the dog with 2 kg of meat containing 1926 kcal of what he called chemical energy, which we would now term "metabolizable" energy. The energy expenditure during those 24 hr of the dog when fed was 1046 kcal. The difference of 304 kcal (1046 minus 742) was considered by Rubner as the "chemical work of glands in metabolising absorbed nutrients." Zuntz called the same phenomenon "work of digestion." Whatever it was called, it is clear that when the dog absorbed 1926 kcal (8058 kJ) of meat his metabolic rate increased by 304 kcal. This increase of 304 kcal (1272 kJ) is 16% of the amount ingested, thus the specific dynamic action (SDA) associated with a meat meal is 16%. Meat energy consists of roughly ⅓ protein and ⅔ fat. Since the SDA of fat is now known to be very small, the SDA of protein in this experiment was about 45%. Rubner starved the dog again on the following day and measured an energy expenditure of 746 kcal. Many studies of the same kind in humans and in animals tend to prove that the magnitude of SDA or diet-induced thermogenesis (DIT) depends not only on the ingested food, but also on other factors, such as the size of the meal, time elapsed since the previous meal, nutritional status, and pathological state. Benedict and Carpenter (2) estimated this "cost of digestion" to be the highest for proteins (15%), between 5% and 10% for carbohydrates, and less then 5% for fat. More recent studies, and reinterpretation of older studies of Rubner, Benedict and others, indicate the DIT of protein to be about 40% to 50%, and that the DIT of carbohydrate is close to 5% when fed below energy requirements but increases to 30% or more when given in great excess (35-37). Benedict, who had a special interest in fatty goose liver, noticed that when he gave three times the measured energy expenditure as food intake to his geese they showed an increase in energy expenditure of about 100%, due to the specific dynamic action of the nutrients (38). More than 10 years ago, Durnin pointed out that when food intake was precisely measured during the same time as energy expenditure, in any group of 20 or more subjects, with similar attributes and activities, food intake can vary as much as 2fold (39). In those studies where both energy intake and energy expenditure are measured, there is often a good agreement for average values of the group, but usually large discrepancies between individual intake and individual expenditure (40-41). Studies in countries with economic problems showed that some people are perfectly healthy and active on energy intakes which, by current standards, would be regarded as inadequate (42). On the other hand studies by Miller, et al. (43,44) showed that subjects can be overfed without presenting any gain of weight. In contrast some obese people, when submitted to severe reducing diets, do not succeed in losing weight. Many obese people ingest no more, and sometimes less food, than those who are not obese.

To the absolutely unsolved question, which is geopolitically most important, posed by Durnin (39): "How much food does man require? " there may be at least a partial answer in major differences in diet-induced thermogenesis in different individuals and in different circumstances, or perhaps resting energy expenditure may vary greatly from one individual to another according to his muscular activity at rest. Although there are great individual variations, the following statements remain valid for long periods of time.

When the weight of a healthy individual remains constant over long periods, it proves that his energy intake equals his energy loss.
When the weight of an individual increases, it proves that his energy intake is greater than his energy loss, and that he increased his fat.
When the weight of an individual decreases, it proves that his energy intake is smaller than his energy loss, and that his fat store decreased.

ACTIVITY ENERGY EXPENDITURE AND TOTAL ENERGY EXPENDITURE

For practical purposes, mainly for prescribing diets for various clinical conditions, including undernutrition, obesity, acute illness, sepsis, or other situations where patients are unable to have a balanced food intake, we have to be able to evaluate total energy expenditure. A severely ill patient at rest in his bed may have an increase in his energy expenditure of 10% to 100%, but one has also to take into account his total energy expenditure. Remember the different components of energy expenditure:

Basal energy expenditure (BEE) or basal metabolic rate (BMR)
Diet induced thermogenesis (DIT) or specific dynamic action (SDA)
Resting energy expenditure (REE) or resting energy metabolism (REM)
Activity energy expenditure (AEE)
Total energy expenditure (TEE)

By definition:

$$REE = BEE + DIT \text{ and } TEE = REE + AEE$$

Since we have previously shown that the use of standards with correction factors for evaluating energy needs is often misleading, measurement of energy expenditure should be performed before prescribing the composition and the quantity of daily food intake. Measurements performed at the bedside of critically ill patients will represent the resting energy expenditure at the moment of measurement.

If we assume that at the start of this century the scientists of nutrition were very strict in the criteria used to define basal metabolic rate, the measured values were remarkably constant, as can be seen from the following data. Zuntz between 1888 and 1917, aged 41 to 70, measured his own basal metabolism several times. Du Bois did the same between 1913 and 1927 when he was between the ages of 30 and 44. Since this is striking information we show some of those values in Table 2.8 taken from Lusk's *The Elements of the Science of Nutrition* (12). These numbers are remarkably constant. Energy expenditure varied no more than 7% above and below the average values. In dogs in whom a constant diet was administered in a cage, where mobility was reduced, the variation of energy expenditure was only 1.9% over a period of 15 months (45).

Table 2.8.
Basal metabolic rate of Zuntz and of Du Bois.[a] To obtain kJ from kcal multiply by 4.184.

Metabolism of Zuntz				Metabolism of Du Bois.			
Year	Age	Weight	EE (kcal/m²/day)	Year	Age	Weight	EE (kcal/m²/day)
1888	41	65.7	804	1913	30	75.5	914
1901	54	67.6	780	1914	31	74.3	921
1903	56	67.6	773	1915	32	74.6	892
1910	63	68.5	792	1916	33	76.5	931
1917	70	59.4	723	1922	39	78.0	855
				1923	41	74.7	880
				1927	44	75.7	871

[a]Adapted from Lusk (12).

Normal men perform all physiological functions at rest at an energy expenditure between 60 and 70 kcal (250 and 293 kJ)/hr. It is of undoubted interest to estimate, even approximately, how various types of physical or intellectual activities will modify this resting value. Table 2.9 gives a few examples of these modifications.

Most of the data presented in Table 2.9 were derived from measurements performed in the twenties (12). If the specific energy required for any of the above activities is to be estimated, one may subtract from the total amount the 70 kcal (293 kJ) hr^{-1} taken as an approximate standard value for resting or basal energy expenditure. If the reader has a special interest in these measurements, he will find endless tables of the caloric cost for all kinds of human and animal activities in different situations

Table 2.9.
Energy expended during different kinds of activities.

Activity	kcal per hour	kJ per hour
Rest (lying)	70	293
Sitting	86	360
Standing	90	377
Walking	180	753
Playing piano		
Beethoven's *Appassionata*	128	536
Chopin's *Etudes*	146	611
Liszt's *Tarentella*	158	661
Playing violin	150	628
Playing cello	114	477
Dancing		
Waltz	280	1172
Fox-trot	335	1402
Polka	529	2213
Mazurka	761	3184
Running, 8.5 km/hr	550	2301
Bicycle riding (race)	600	2510
Swimming, 3.2 km/hr	624	2611
Manual work		
Tailor	114	477
Shoemaker	160	669
Metal worker	211	883
Furniture painting	215	900
Carpenter	334	1397
Wood sawing	458	1916
Housecleaning	227	950
Typing (50 words/min)	94	393

and in different climates (12, 46,47). Although it is our intention to discuss later the different ways of controlling obesity, the reader who has this kind of problem might start with a special dancing course in the mazurka, which seems to be a pleasant but forgotten technique to increase energy expenditure. Since it it not easy to continue this activity for several hours per day, we further suggest a combination of mazurka, polka, or even fox-trot with other techniques for losing weight.

INDIRECT CALORIMETRY-THEORY AND PRACTICE

The method of choice for measuring human energy expenditure has been and remains indirect calorimetry, which is based on measurements of O_2 consumption, CO_2 production, and N excretion.

Indirect calorimetry is based on two major principles:

The first law of thermodynamics, known as the law of conservation of energy, which states: "when the chemical energy content of a system changes, the sum of all forms of energy given off or absorbed by the system must be equal to the magnitude of the change."
This law may be expressed as:

$$dE = dQ + dW + dR \tag{10}$$

where: dE = decrease in chemical energy, dQ = heat given off, dW = mechanical work performed, and dR = other forms of energy given off.

The second principle is that the energy produced by oxidation of foodstuffs in the body is equivalent to that produced by combustion in a bomb calorimeter (46), which measures the heat generated when a foodstuff is combusted in an excess of O_2 (Figure 2.4). This is valid even though in the body oxidation involves a series of enzyme-catalyzed reactions which take place at 37° C, and in a bomb calorimeter oxidation is more direct, at high pressure and temperature. In thermodynamics, the initial and final states are all that is important; the pathway is irrelevant.

For fat and carbohydrate the end products of oxidation, CO_2 and water, are the same for the body as for the bomb calorimeter. This is not true for protein. In the calorimeter, protein is converted to CO_2, H_2O, SO_4, and N_2. In the body, the end product for N is mostly urea together with small amounts of other constituents, while the end products for C, H, and S are the same as in the calorimeter. This means that the energy derived from protein oxidation in the body is less than that derived from the bomb calorimeter. This difference was evaluated by Atwater by measuring the nitrogen and energy (by bomb calorimeter) of urine and determining the ratio of energy to N. He found this to average 7.9 kcal (33 kJ) per g N, equal to 1.25 kcal (5.2 kJ) per g of oxidized protein (48). Therefore, the practice since Atwater is to subtract 1.25 kcal (5.2 kJ) per g from values of energy of oxidation of protein as measured in a bomb calorimeter in order to determine the amount of energy to be expected from the partial oxidation of protein which takes place in the body. This procedure assumes that the N constituents of urine are completely responsible for the energy of combustion of urine. This is very close to true for urine of healthy, fed subjects in whom organic compounds other then those containing N are minimal. It would not be true for urine of fasting subjects, which contains ketone bodies, or of diabetics, which contains glucose. More recently Southgate and Durnin (49) carefully repeated Atwater's measurements to obtain a value of 8.34 kcal per g N, equivalent to 1.34 kcal (5.6 kJ) per g oxidized protein in urine. We have used this figure together with 5.65 kcal (23.6 kJ) for an

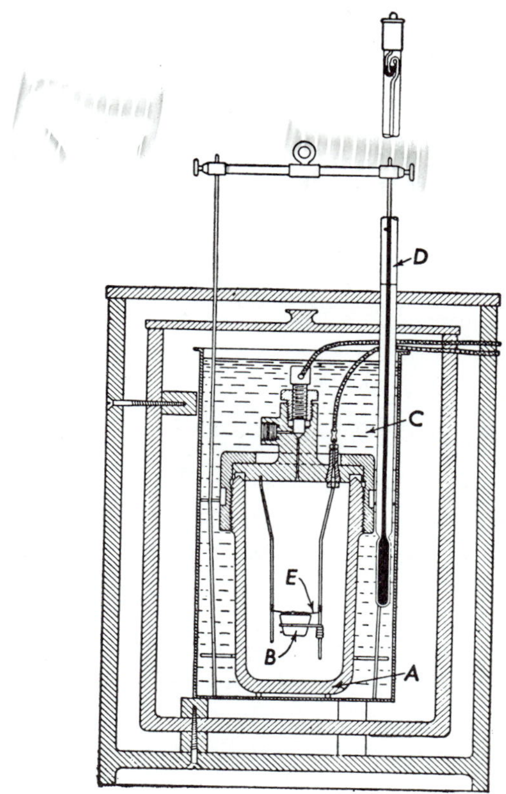

Figure 2.4. The bomb calorimeter. It consists of (**A**) a heavy steel bomb with a platinum or gold-plated copper lining; (**B**) a capsule where a weighed amount of sample is placed; and (**C**) a weighed amount of water where the bomb is placed after having charged it with a pressure of oxygen of at least 20 atmospheres.The water is constantly stirred and its temperature is measured with a differential thermometer (**D**), giving a reading to a thousandth of a degree. An electric fuse (**E**) ignites the sample that will undergo complete combustion because of the large amount of oxygen present. After correction arising from oxidation of the iron wire used as fuse, the number of calories due to the combustion of the sample can be obtained.

average value for protein energy derived from the bomb calorimeter, to give a value, after rounding, of 4.3 kcal (18.0 kJ) per g protein available to the human or mammalian body. This is given in Table 2.12. Since the main end point of protein metabolism in birds is uric acid, rather then urea, different values for the energy of protein available to the bird must be obtained.

Stoichiometric equations for any food component can be derived from these measurements. Equations for a typical carbohydrate, fat, and protein are as shown:
Glucose per g:

$$1\ g\ glucose + 0.747\ liter\ O_2 \rightarrow 0.747\ liter\ CO_2 + 0.60\ g\ H_2O + 3.75\ kcal\ (15.7\ kJ) \quad (11)$$

per mole:

$$\begin{array}{llllll} C_6H_{12}O_6 + & 6\ O_2 \rightarrow & 6CO_2 + & 6H_2O + & E \\ 180\ g & 134.5\ liter & 134.5\ liter & 108\ g & 672\ kcal\ (2812\ kJ) \end{array}$$

Tripalmitin per g:

$$1\ g\ tripalmitin + 2.011\ liters\ O_2 \rightarrow 1.416\ liters\ CO_2 + 1.09g\ H_2O + 9.5\ kcal\ (39.7\ kJ) \quad (12)$$

per mole:

$$\begin{array}{llllll} C_{51}H_{98}O_6 + & 72.5\ O_2 \rightarrow & 51CO_2 + & 49H_2O + & E \\ 807\ g & 1625\ liter & 1143\ liter & 883\ g & 7657\ kcal\ (32{,}036\ kJ) \end{array}$$

Beef protein

$$1\ g\ protein + 0.992\ liter\ O_2 \rightarrow 0.848\ liter CO_2\ 0.38g\ H_2\ O + 0.332\ g\ urea\ (0.166\ g\ N) + 4.4\ kcal\ (18.4\ kJ) \quad (13)$$

This equation assumes that the end product of protein oxidation is urea, which is the main end product for mammals. The respiratory quotient (RQ) for equation 13 is 0.85. In birds the main end product of protein metabolism is uric acid. For birds equation 13A is applicable:

$$1\ g\ protein + 0.893\ liter\ O_2 \rightarrow 0.649\ liter\ CO_2 + 0.49\ g\ H_2O + 0.498\ g\ uric\ acid\ (0.166\ g\ N) + 4.0\ kcal\ (16.7\ kJ) \quad (13a)$$

Note that the amounts of O_2 and CO_2 are different for equations 13 and 13a, the RQ for equation 13a is 0.727. Because of these differences, the equations of indirect calorimetry which are generally derived for mammals need to be modified in order to be used with birds or other animal classes or phyla in which urea is not the main end product of protein oxidation.

Ordinarily we eat mixtures of carbohydrates, proteins, and fats. Each of these have slightly different equations, and yield slightly different amounts of energy. Some examples are shown in Table 2.10, adapted from Merrill and Watt (48) and Southgate and Durnin (49). It is impractical to analyze food intake for each carbohydrate, protein, or fat constituent; therefore we must use average values for purposes of indirect calorimetry. This introduces some errors into our measurements, and the type and magnitude of the errors are different for each of the three groups of nutrients.

Table 2.10.
Caloric values of some foodstuffs.[a]

Nutrients (1 g)	% of Total in Mixed Diet	Bomb Calorimeter kcal	Metabolizable %	Metabolizable kcal
Proteins				
Meats, fish, poultry	31	4.30	97	4.17
Eggs	7	4.40	97	4.26
Dairy products	25	4.30	97	4.17
Total protein of animal origin	63	4.31	97	4.18
Cereals	23	4.45	86	3.81
Legumes, nuts	6	4.35	78	3.37
Vegetables	6	3.65	70	2.52
Fruits	2	3.85	85	3.26
Total protein of plant origin	37	4.27	82	3.48
Carbohydrates				
Of animal origin	8	3.95	98	3.87
Cereals	40	4.20	98	4.12
Legumes, nuts	3	4.20	97	4.07
Vegetables	9	4.19	93	3.90
Fruits	8	4.00	90	3.60
Sugars, syrups	32	3.95	98	3.87
Total carbohydrate of plant origin	92	4.10	97	3.98
Fat				
Meat, fish, poultry, eggs	40	9.50	95	9.02
Dairy products	18	9.25	95	8.79
Total fat of animal origin	77	9.42	95	8.95
Total fat of plant origin	23	9.30	94	8.74

[a]For proteins, 1.34 kcal g^{-1} has been subtracted from the values actually measured in the bomb calorimeter, representing the difference between oxidation in the body and in the calorimeter (see text). To obtain kJ from kcal multiply by 4.184.

Carbohydrates

Energies of oxidation for several sugars and for starch, as measured by Rubner in 1885 (50), are shown in Table 2.11. Energy yields per gram vary by 22%, going from dextrose, which is the monohydrate of glucose, to starch. When measured per mole of hexose residue, the differences are less than 2% and within the experimental error of the method. Almost all carbohydrates used for food are composed of glucose, and to a lesser extent of other hexoses, as fructose and galactose, either in the form of the free sugar, or as di- or polysaccharides formed by elimination of water between free sugars. There are negligible differences in energy of oxidation between the different hexoses, and the energy of hydrolysis of the glycoside linkage may also be neglected. Therefore, per mole of hexose residue, the energy of oxidation of all carbohydrates is the same. It follows also that the respiratory quotient and the caloric value of O_2 consumed are the same for all carbohydrates. Thus, use of an average value for all carbohydrates introduces no appreciable error into indirect calorimetry. However, it is important to keep in mind that the energy per gram will vary depending on the degree of hydration of the compound involved.

Table 2.11.
Heats of combustion of carbohydrates.[a]

		Heat of Combustion			
		per gram		per mole	
Compounds	Residue Weights	kcal	kJ	kcal	kJ
Glucose	180	3.692	15.45	665	2782
Lactose	171	3.877	16.22	663	2774
Sucrose	171	3.959	16.56	677	2833
Starch	162	4.116	17.22	667	2791
Dextrose (glucose monohydrate)	198	3.356	14.04	665	2782

[a]Adapted from Rubner (50).

A specific of glucose and of carbohydrate metabolism in general is that the amounts of oxygen consumed (VO_2) and carbon dioxide produced (VCO_2) are the same. In this case the volume of expired air is also equal to the volume of inspired air; the RQ = VCO_2/VO_2 or 0.746/0.746 for 1 g sugar, or 0.829/0.829 for 1 g starch, is then equal to 1.

Fats

The composition of fats is more variable than that of carbohydrates. Fats consist of triglycerides that contain 3 molecules of fatty acid joined to 1 molecule of glycerol. There are many different fatty acids in fats, most commonly palmitic, stearic, oleic, and linoleic acids, and each has somewhat different values for energy of oxidation, for RQ, and for the caloric value of the O_2 consumed. The most common fatty acids in the human body fat stores are approximately in the following proportions:

Palmitic acid ($C_{16}H_{32}O_2$): 29.2%
Stearic acid ($C_{18}H_{36}O_2$): 16.3%
Oleic acid ($C_{18}H_{34}O_2$): 40.5%
Linoleic acid ($C_{18}H_{32}O_2$): 8.0%

Therefore, when the actual composition of fat varies from the average value used for calculation, some error is introduced, although as can be seen from Table 2.10, these errors are not very large. Rubner (50) evaluated the caloric values of some fats in 1885.

	Heat of Combustion	
Type of Fat	kcal g^{-1}	kJ g^{-1}
Olive oil	9.384	39.26
Animal fat	9.372	39.21
Butter	9.179	38.40

He suggested 9.3 as a mean factor to express the amount of heat produced by the combustion of 1 g of fat, and subsequent investigations confirm that this is probably the best value (48,49). The RQ for fat oxidation will be 1.427/2.019 = 0.707

Proteins

Differences in the composition of proteins are much larger than for other foods, and this is particularly true for the artificial amino acid mixtures used for intravenous feeding (Table 2.17) (51). This means that the actual values for energy per g protein, N per g protein, and O_2 consumed or CO_2 produced per g protein may differ markedly from the average values used for indirect calorimetric calculations. For proteins the RQ will be 0.781/0.965 = 0.809.

These errors, due to the use of average values for energy of oxidation, caloric value of O_2, and N per g protein, can introduce substantial errors into the calculation of the amount of protein, fat, and carbohydrate oxidized. In studies of fuel utilization it is important to keep the possibility of such errors in mind, and if necessary to use values based on the actual foods consumed. Fortunately, these errors are not important in calculating energy expenditure, which is the sum of the energy expenditures calculated for the three food constituents. This is because the caloric equivalent of the O_2 consumed varies little between the three foods. From equations 11, 12, and 13 we can calculate the caloric equivalent of O_2 by dividing E in kilocalories by the liters of O_2 consumed. These are for glucose, 5.03; for tripalmitin, 4.71; and for beef protein, 4.44 kcal liter^{-1}. These correspond respectively to 21.0, 19.7, and 18.6 kJ liter^{-1}. Even if we have considerable error in assigning how much of the O_2 consumed is due to each food, as long as the measurement of total O_2 consumption is accurate there will be little error in the calculation of energy expenditure.

Furthermore, the caloric equivalents of O_2 for other food components, such as nucleic acids, phospholipids, and alcohol are very similar to those for carbohydrate, fat, and protein. Therefore, although we completely ignore these components in deriving our standard equations, this contributes a negligible error to the calculation of energy expenditure.

Traditional Calculations of Indirect Calorimetry

There are a number of different sets of standard equations presently used. These are derived from those developed by Zuntz (52) and Cathcart and Cuthbertson (53). None differ from each other by more than 2%. This has been clearly demonstrated in a recent article by Westenkow, et al. (54). As long as any one set is used consistently, it does not matter which is used. The standard constants used here, taken in part from Ben Porat, et al. (55), in part from Merrill and Watt (48), and from Southgate and Durnin (49), are shown in Table 2.12. A general value for RQ that is usually reported in the textbooks is 0.84 resulting from the arithmetic mean of the RQ of the three foodstuffs: 1 for carbohydrate, 0.809 for protein, and 0.707 for fat, so that

$$\frac{1 + 0.809 + 0.707}{3} = 0.84.$$

Very recently an important paper by Livesey and Elia has appeared (56) concerning heats of combustion, N content, RQ, and caloric equivelents of O_2 and CO_2 for 171 food proteins, 161 food fats, and a variety of carbohydrates.

This is by far the most exhaustive treatment of this subject ever to appear. The authors detail the effects of fatty acid chain length and degree of unsaturation, amino acid composition, and use of polyols such as glycerol, xylitol, and sorbitol on RQ, heat of combustion, and caloric equivalent of O_2 and CO_2. They also present the errors introduced by use of standard conversion factors when they are not applicable, with particular attention to the use of artificial nutrients containing polyols, medium chain fatty acids, and unusual amino acid composition. The standard conversion factors which they obtain differ slightly from most previous values and from those given in Table 2.12. The most important difference is for protein, since they calculate heat of combustion in the body by subtracting, from bomb calorimeter values, the heat of combustion of estimated end products (90% urea, 5% ammonia, and 5% creatinine) instead of that of urine. This gives a standard value of 4.7 kcal (19.7 kJ)per g protein instead of 4.3 kcal (18.0 kJ) as given in Table 2.12. Livesey and Elia note that errors in conversion factors have little effect on calculation of energy expenditure, of the order of 1% to 2%, but have a very much bigger effect on calculation of fuel utilization. Their paper is an essential resource

Table 2.12.
Standard conversion factors for protein, fat and carbohydrate metabolized in the body.[a]

Items	Protein		Fat	Starch or		
	As Protein	As Nitrogen		Glycogen	Glucose	Dextrose
Oxygen liter/g	0.965	6.030	2.019	0.829	0.746	0.678
Carbon dioxide liter/g	0.781	4.880	1.427	0.829	0.746	0.678
Respiratory quotient	0.809	0.809	0.707	1.000	1.000	1.000
Gross energy, kcal/g	4.3	26.9	9.3	4.17	3.75	3.41
kJ/g	18.0	112.5	38.9	17.4	15.7	14.3
Metabolizable energy kcal/g	4.0	25.0	9.1	4.10	3.75	3.41
kJ/g	16.7	104.6	38.0	17.2	15.7	14.3
Caloric equivalent of O_2 kcal/liter	4.46	4.46	4.61	5.03	5.03	5.03
kJ/liter	18.7	18.7	19.3	21.0	21.0	21.0
Caloric equivalent of CO_2 kcal/liter	5.51	5.51	6.52	5.03	5.03	5.03
kJ/liter	23.1	23.1	27.3	21.0	21.0	21.0
Water of oxidation g/g	0.41	2.56	1.07	0.56	0.60	0.64
Nitrogen content g/g	0.16	1.00	0	0	0	0

[a]Data adapted from Merrill and Watt, Southgate and Durnin, and Ben Porat et al. (48,49,55).

for anyone who wishes to measure carbohydrate, fat, or protein oxidation by indirect calorimetry.

Traditionally, the calculations of fuel utilization and energy expenditure from O_2 consumption, CO_2 production, and urinary nitrogen excretion (Nu) have been performed as follows.
Symbols used are:

Nu = urinary nitrogen, g
VO_2 = oxygen consumption, liters
VCO_2 = carbon dioxide production, liters

Subscripts f, c, p, and np when used with VO_2, VCO_2, and RQ refer to the values associated with fat (f), carbohydrate (c), protein (p), or nonprotein (np) oxidation; as VO_{2np} = nonprotein O_2 consumption, or RQ_f = the RQ for fat oxidation,

EE = energy expenditure, kcal or kJ
H_2OM = water of oxidation, g
F = fat oxidized, g
C = carbohydrate oxidized, g (starch or glycogen)
P = protein oxidized, g
Fe, Ce, Pe = fat, protein and carbohydrate oxidized in kcal or kJ

1. The first step is to calculate P, Pe, VO_{2p}, and VCO_{2p} from Nu, using the conversion factors shown in Table 2.12.
2. Next, VO_{2p} and VCO_{2p} are subtracted from VO_2 and VCO_2 respectively, to give VO_{2np} and VCO_{2np}, the nonprotein values for O_2 consumption and CO_2 production.
3. RQ_{np} is calculated from VO_{2np} and VCO_{2np}, and the caloric value of VO_2 is looked up in Table 2.13, taken from Lusk (57).
4. Nonprotein energy expenditure is calculated by multiplying this caloric value by VO_{2np}.
5. Total energy expenditure, E, is obtained as the sum of nonprotein energy expenditure and protein energy expenditure Pe, obtained in step 1.
6. The fraction of nonprotein energy due to fat or carbohydrate is then determined from Table 2.13, using the values for percentage of total heat produced by carbohydrate or fat at any given RQ. An alternate procedure is as follows: The volume of O_2 used for fat (VO_{2f}) and for carbohydrate (VO_{2c}) can be obtained from VO_{2np} and VCO_{2np} because the RQs of each are different. These relationships can be expressed as in equations 14 and 15, where 1 represents the RQ for pure carbohydrate, 0.707 the RQ for pure fat, and 0.293 the difference between them:

$$VO_{2c} = VO_{2np} \frac{RQ - 0.707}{0.293} \tag{14}$$

$$VO_{2f} = VO_{2np} \frac{1 - RQ}{0.293} \tag{15}$$

The energies of carbohydrate (Ce) and fat (Fe) oxidation can be calculated from the appropriate VO_2 by multiplying by the caloric equivalent of O_2 for the two pure substances (Table 2.12):

$$Ce\ (kcal) = 5.03 \times VO_{2c} \quad Ce\ (kJ) = 21.0 \times VO_{2c} \tag{16}$$

$$Fe\ (kcal) = 4.61 \times VO_{2f} \quad Fe\ (kJ) = 19.3 \times VO_{2f} \tag{17}$$

Calculating Ce and Fe by equations 14-17 can be used with RQ_{np} above 1 when Fe is negative, indicating the amount of fat which is synthesized. This is an advantage over the method of using Table 2.13, since that table does not give values for RQ_{np} above 1.

Current Methods of Calculation of Indirect Calorimetry

Weir (58) and subsequently Consolazio et al. (46) pointed out that the traditional procedure is unnecessarily cumbersome, and that simple regression equations can be derived for each desired quantity. Equations

Table 2.13.
Analysis of the oxidation of mixtures of carbohydrate and fat.[a]

	Percentage of Total Oxygen Consumed		Percentage of Total Heat Produced		Calories per Liter	
RQ	Carbohydrate (1)	Fat (2)	Carbohydrate (3)	Fat (4)	O_2 (5)	CO_2 (6)
0.707	0	100.0	0	100.0	4.686	6.629
0.71	1.02	99.0	1.10	98.9	4.690	6.605
0.72	4.44	95.6	4.76	95.2	4.702	6.533
0.73	7.85	92.2	8.40	91.6	4.714	6.459
0.74	11.3	88.7	12.0	88.0	4.727	6.388
0.75	14.7	85.3	15.6	84.4	4.739	6.320
0.76	18.1	81.9	19.2	80.8	4.751	6.252
0.77	21.5	78.5	22.8	77.2	4.764	6.186
0.78	24.9	75.1	26.3	73.7	4.776	6.122
0.79	28.3	71.7	29.9	70.1	4.788	6.062
0.80	31.7	68.3	33.4	66.6	4.801	6.002
0.81	35.2	64.8	36.9	63.1	4.813	5.942
0.82	38.6	61.4	40.3	59.7	4.825	5.883
0.83	42.0	58.0	43.8	56.2	4.838	5.829
0.84	45.4	54.6	47.2	52.8	4.850	5.775
0.85	48.8	51.2	50.7	49.3	4.862	5.722
0.86	52.2	47.8	54.1	45.9	4.875	5.668
0.87	55.6	44.4	57.5	42.5	4.887	5.616
0.88	59.0	41.0	60.8	39.2	4.899	5.566
0.89	62.5	37.5	64.2	35.8	4.911	5.518
0.90	65.9	34.1	67.5	32.5	4.924	5.471
0.91	69.3	30.7	70.8	29.2	4.936	5.423
0.92	72.7	27.3	74.1	25.9	4.948	5.378
0.93	76.1	23.9	77.4	22.6	4.961	5.333
0.94	79.5	20.5	80.7	19.3	4.973	5.288
0.95	82.9	17.1	84.0	16.0	4.985	5.243
0.96	86.3	13.7	87.2	12.8	4.998	5.202
0.97	89.8	10.2	90.4	9.58	5.010	5.163
0.98	93.2	6.83	93.6	6.37	5.022	5.124
0.99	96.6	3.41	96.8	3.18	5.035	5.085
1.00	100.0	0	100.0	0	5.047	5.047

[a]From Lusk G: Animal Calorimetry. XXIV. Analysis of the oxidation of mixtures of carbohydrate and fat. A correction. *Metabolism* 31:1234-1240, 1924. To obtain kJ from calories multiply by 4.184.

11, 12, and 13 were designed for the specific nutrients, glucose, tripalmitin, and beef protein. If we adopt the constants of Merrill and Watt, Southgate and Durnin, and of Ben Porat et al. given in Table 2.12, we may write the more general equations 18, 19 and 20:

$$1\ g\ C + 0.829\ liter\ O_2 \rightarrow 0.829\ liter\ CO_2 + 0.56\ g\ H_2O + 4.17\ kcal\ (17.4\ kJ) \tag{18}$$

$$1\ g\ P + 0.965\ liter\ O_2 \rightarrow 0.781\ liter\ CO_2 + 0.41\ g\ H_2O + 0.16 g\ Nu + 4.3\ kcal\ (18.0\ kJ) \quad (19)$$

$$1\ g\ F + 2.019\ liter\ O_2 \rightarrow 1.427\ liter\ CO_2 + 1.07\ g\ H_2O + 9.3\ kcal\ (38.9\ kJ) \quad (20)$$

Equations 18, 19, and 20 have a practical implication, and we may assume that in the body, the three nutrients are metabolized simultaneously, in varying proportions, according to numerous factors, many of which are not yet very well known. The oxygen consumed in a certain period of time will be the amount of oxygen that was used for oxidizing given quantities of carbohydrate, protein, and fat, each of these nutrients consuming 0.829 liter, 0.965 liter, and 2.019 liter of oxygen, respectively, per g metabolized (Table 2.12). This statement may also be written as:

$$VO_2\ (liter) = 0.829\ C\ (g) + 0.965\ P\ (g) + 2.019\ F\ (g) \quad (21)$$

where VO_2 is the amount of oxygen consumed in 1 minute by the metabolism of the three nutrients C, P, and F, and 0.829, 0.966, and 2.019 are the amounts of oxygen expressed in liters consumed by 1 g of C, P, and F, respectively (Table 2.12). At the same time carbon dioxide is produced in the amounts of 0.829 liter, 0.781 liter and 1.427 liter per g, of carbohydrate, protein, and fat, respectively. This may be expressed by the next equation:

$$VCO_2\ (liter) = 0.829\ C\ (g) + 0.781\ P\ (g) + 1.427\ F\ (g) \quad (22)$$

where VCO_2 is the amount of carbon dioxide produced by the metabolism of the three nutrients C, P, and F, and 0.829, 0.781, and 1.427 are the amounts of CO_2, expressed in liters, produced by the metabolism of 1 g of C, P, and F, respectively (Table 2.12). During metabolism of these amounts of carbohydrate, protein, and fat, a certain amount of energy or of heat is produced and this can be expressed by the following equation:

$$\begin{aligned} EE\ (kcal) &= 4.17\ C + 4.3\ P + 9.3\ F \\ EE\ (kJ) &= 17.4\ C + 18.0\ P + 38.9\ F \end{aligned} \quad (23)$$

where EE is the amount of energy or of heat produced by the metabolism of the three nutrients C, P, and F and 4.17, 4.3, and 9.3 are the quantities of energy or of heat, expressed in kcal or kJ, produced by one g of C, P, and F respectively (Table 2.12). Equations 21, 22, and 23 represent events happening at the same time and can be considered as a system of three equations, in which unfortunately there are 4 unknowns (C, P, F, and EE). In order to enable us to solve this system, one has to find a way to evaluate one of the 4 unknowns. The classic method for solving this problem is to measure the total nitrogen in a 24-hour urinary collection or to derive the nitrogen excretion from the urea excreted in the 24-hour urinary output. Since 1 g of metabolized nitrogen (Nu) is considered to have been produced by 6.25 g of protein, the system of 3 equations with 4 unknowns becomes a system of 4 equations with 4 unknowns that can be solved for C, P, F, and EE:

$$VO_2\,(liter) = 0.829\,C\,(g) + 0.965\,P\,(g) + 2.019\,F\,(g) \qquad (21)$$

$$VCO_2\,(liter) = 0.829\,C\,(g) + 0.781\,P\,(g) + 1.427\,F\,(g) \qquad (22)$$

$$EE\,(kcal) = 4.17\,C + 4.3\,P + 9.3\,F$$

$$EE\,(kJ) = 17.4\,C + 18.0\,P + 38.9\,F \qquad (23)$$

$$P\,(g) = 6.25\,Nu \qquad (24)$$

The resolution of this system will allow the calculation of EE, C, and F as a function of VO_2, VCO_2 and Nu, since P is already known from the measured nitogen or urea in the urine, as shown in equation 24.

$$EE\,(kcal) = 3.581\,VO_2 + 1.448\,VCO_2 - 1.773\,Nu$$

$$EE\,(kJ) = 14.98\,VO_2 + 6.06\,VCO_2 - 7.42\,Nu \qquad (25)$$

$$C = 4.114\,VCO_2 - 2.908\,VO2 - 2.543\,Nu \qquad (26)$$

$$F = 1.689\,(VO_2 - VCO_2) - 1.943\,Nu \qquad (27)$$

Equations 18 and 26 are designed for polymeric carbohydrate, i.e., starch or glycogen. When glucose or dextrose is used, the following equations should be used:

$$C\,(glucose) = 4.571\,VCO_2 - 3.231\,VO_2 - 2.826\,Nu \qquad (28)$$

$$C\,(dextrose) = 5.028\,VCO_2 - 3.554\,VO_2 - 3.108\,Nu \qquad (29)$$

For practical purposes, mainly in prescribing diets for all kinds of patients, it is convenient to calculate the respective amounts of foodstuffs in caloric equivalents, as in the following formulas:

$$Ce\,(kcal) = 17.16\,VCO_2 - 12.13\,VO_2 - 10.60\,Nu$$

$$Ce\,(kJ) = 71.8\ VCO_2 - 50.8\ VO_2 - 44.4\ Nu \tag{30}$$

$$Fe(kcal) = 15.71\ (VO_2\text{-}VCO_2) - 18.07\ Nu$$

$$Fe(kJ) = 65.7\ (VO_2\text{-}VCO_2) - 75.6\ Nu \tag{31}$$

For carbohydrate, only one equation is used since the caloric equivalents of O_2 and CO_2 are the same for all carbohydrates, regardless of the state of hydration. The energy from protein oxidation is calculated directly from Nu, using the constant of Table 2.12.

$$Pe\,(kcal) = 26.9\ Nu$$

$$Pe\,(kJ) = 112.5\ Nu \tag{32}$$

When C, P, and F are known the amount of water of oxidation (H_2OM) produced by the metabolism of foodstuffs can also be calculated, since oxidation of 1 g of C, P, and F forms during their oxidation 0.56, 0.41, and 1.07 g of water, respectively (Table 2.12, see equations 18, 19, and 20),

$$H_2OM\,(g) = 0.67\ C\,(g) + 0.41\ P\,(g) + 1.07\ F\,(g)$$

$$H_2OM\,(g) = 0.497\ VCO_2(liter) - 0.179\ VO_2(liter) - 0.943\ Nu\,(g) \tag{33}$$

Some Problems in Applying Indirect Calorimetry Techniques

The three values VO_2, VCO_2, and Nu can be measured by totally noninvasive methods (Chapters 3 and 5). By applying the above equations, energy expenditure (EE), substrate utilization (C, P, F), and water of oxidation (H_2OM) can be calculated. Some imperfections in this attractive method have to be emphasized at this point of the presentation.

Accurate measurement of VO_2 is not easy at the bedside of critically ill patients, particularly if they require oxygen enrichment of inspired air or when they are mechanically ventilated (59).

If the measurement of VCO_2 seems to be technically easier and more reliable than the measurement of VO_2, VCO_2 is much more sensitive to any modification in the patient's respiratory pattern. Indeed, it has to be kept in mind that the metabolic evaluation over a given period of time makes sense only if the amount of exhaled CO_2 corresponds to the amount produced metabolically during the same time. Alveolar ventilation may increase or decrease during the measurement, for psychological or other reasons, and the measured VCO_2 will then be different from that produced by metabolism. This inconvenience may be avoided if measurements are performed during a prolonged period of time (at least 20 to 30 minutes).

While VO_2 and VCO_2 are instantaneous measurements, corresponding directly to the oxygen consumed and carbon dioxide produced by metabolism of foodstuffs during the measurement, in real time, the nitrogen measured in the urine does not correspond in the same way. This is because there is a large and variable urea pool in the body, of the order of 5 g of N, which can vary between 2 and 50 g or more depending on diet or disease. Variations of 2 fold or more may occur in individuals during a single day. Average excretion of urea N in 1 hour, about 0.5 g N, represents only 10% of this pool which could easily change in magnitude by 5% during the same period. Therefore, accurate measurements of net protein breakdown by determining the N content of urine can only be performed over much longer periods, usually one day. In contrast to urea, body pools of CO_2 and O_2 are much smaller with respect to rate of excretion (Table 2.14). VO_2 in 1 hour is 25 times the size of the body pool, and VCO_2 is 0.6 times, while urea N is only 0.1 times. Furthermore variations in the sizes of O_2 and CO_2 pools are proportionally much smaller than for urea.

Table 2.14.
Body content and rate of excretion of O_2, CO_2, and urea N.

	Body Pool	Excretory Rate	Excretory Rate as Ratio to Body Pool		
			Per Min	Per Hour	Per Day
O_2	0.6 liter	0.25 liter/min	0.42	25	600
CO_2	20 liter	0.20 liter/min	0.01	0.6	14.4
Urea N	5 g	0.0085 g/min	0.0017	0.1	2.4

The inability to make accurate estimates of urea production from urea excretion over short time periods is not important for nutritional purposes, since daily values of energy expenditure and fuel utilization are the significant factor. However, it does severely limit the accuracy of indirect calorimetry for measuring rates of fuel utilization over periods of minutes or even hours. Fortunately, as discussed in the next section, errors in measurement of N excretion have a negligible effect on calculation of energy expenditure, and urinary N measurements are not necessary for measuring energy expenditure (46,58,60,61).

Energy Expenditure Determined from VO_2 and VCO_2 or from VO_2 Alone

From equation 25 it can be seen that the most important measurement of energy expenditure is VO_2. Typical values for this equation might be 0.250 liter min^{-1} for VO_2, 0.225 liter min^{-1} for VCO_2, and 0.01

g min^{-1} for Nu, yielding 1.233 kcal (5.16 kJ) min^{-1} for EE. A 10% error in VO_2 (25 ml min^{-1}) causes a 7% error in EE (0.090 kcal [0.38 kJ] min^{-1}), a 10% error in VCO_2 (22.5 ml min^{-1}) causes a 3% error in EE (0.026 kcal [0.11 kJ] min^{-1}), and a 100% error in Nu causes only a 1% error in EE (0.011 kcal [0.05 kJ] min^{-1}). It is clear that an estimate of N excretion, even if in error by twice the amount used here, will cause an error of only 2% in EE, approximately equal to technical errors in measurements. Bursztein et al. (62) used an average value for N excretion to develop an equation suitable for acutely ill patients in the intensive care unit (ICU). They found that the median for N excretion in 180 patients was 18.25 g day^{-1}, with 97% of the values falling between 1.5 and 35 g day^{-1}. They derived an equation for calculating EE based only on VO_2 and VCO_2 by substituting 18.25 for Nu in the general equation for EE. Thus if we substitute 18.25 g day^{-1} for Nu in equation 25 we get equations 34 and 35.

$$EE(kcal\ day^{-1}) = 3.581\ VO_2\ (liter\ day^{-1}) + 1.448\ VCO_2(liter\ day^{-1}) - 32.4$$

$$EE(kJ\ day^{-1}) = 14.98\ VO_2\ (liter\ day^{-1}) + 6.06\ VCO_2(liter\ day^{-1}) - 136 \tag{34}$$

$$EE(kcal\ min^{-1}) = 3.581\ VO_2(liter\ min^{-1}) + 1.448\ VCO_2(liter\ min^{-1}) - 0.022$$

$$EE(kJ\ min^{-1}) = 14.98\ VO_2(liter\ min^{-1}) + 6.06\ VCO_2(liter\ min^{-1}) - 0.092 \tag{35}$$

The Bursztein equation differs from these only by the original choice of constants, which were slightly different from those given in Table 2.12. Bursztein et al. compared the results of using the equation without N to the complete equation, in 26 critically ill patients. The average error was 27 kcal (113 kJ) day^{-1} or 1.8%, and the largest error was 49 kcal (205 kJ) day^{-1} or 4.9%. This clearly demonstrates that determination of N excretion is not necessary for estimating energy expenditure, even in critically ill patients whose N excretion is very large and very variable. The Bursztein equation or equations 34 or 35 are entirely satisfactory. While this eliminates the need to measure N excretion in order to estimate energy expenditure, it does not mean that N excretion may not be useful in estimating N requirements. This will be discussed in more detail in Chapters 3 and 7.

In many circumstances it is feasible to neglect VCO_2 as well as N measurements. As noted above, a 10% error in VCO_2 results in only a

3% error in EE. This means that if the RQ can be estimated within 10%, then VCO_2 can be calculated from VO_2 within 10%. In general, in the normal population, RQs rarely vary by more than 10% from a value of 0.9 except for fasting conditions, which makes it possible to neglect VCO_2 measurements. For ill patients, RQs are much more variable ranging from 0.7 to 1.2, and it is therefore desirable to measure both VCO_2 and VO_2. This is not a problem since any equipment available to measure VO_2 in patients also has the capability of measuring VCO_2.

Calculation of energy expenditure solely from VO_2 measurements is widely used in exercise and respiratory physiology. A number of approaches have been used, the most important of which is the Weir equation, as shown in equation 36 (58)

$$EE(kcal) = \frac{1.0548 - 0.0504\ FEO_2}{1 + 0.082p} \times VE \qquad (36)$$

$$EE(kJ) = \frac{4.413 - 0.211\ FEO_2}{1 + 0.34p} \times VE$$

where VE = ventilatory rate, FEO_2 = concentration of O_2 in expired air, and p = fraction of total dietary energy from protein.
Equation 36 may be rearranged as follows:

$$EE\ (kcal) = \frac{5.04}{1 + 0.082p} \times (0.2093 - FEO_2) \times VE \qquad (37)$$

The value (0.2093 - FEO_2) represents the difference in O_2 content of inspired and expired air. When multiplied by VE this equals VO_2. The constant 5.04 is the caloric value of O_2 with no protein in the diet, and the term (1 + 0.082p) corrects this value for protein intake. If intake were entirely protein, the caloric equivalent of O_2 would become 4.66 kcal liter^{-1}, similar to the value shown in Table 2.12. The constant, 5.04 kcal liter^{-1}, is that for carbohydrate (Table 2.12), and the Weir equation assumes a nonprotein RQ of 1.0. A comparison of the Weir equation to traditional methods of indirect calorimetry, in several subjects performing a variety of activities, showed it consistently to overestimate EE by about 1% (46). This is very satisfactory and well within the technical errors of measurement. A more flexible procedure than either the Weir or Bursztein equation is to estimate both N excretion and RQ for the particular purposes at hand and to modify Equation 25 accordingly. Since

$$VCO_2 = VO_2 \times RQ$$

$$EE\ (kcal) = 3.581\ VO_2 + 1.448\ RQ \times VO_2 - 1.773\ Nu. \quad (38)$$

$$EE\ (kJ) = 14.98\ VO_2 + 6.06\ RQ \times VO_2 - 7.418\ Nu$$

It is simple then to substitute estimates for either or both Nu and RQ to derive an appropriate equation.

Energy Expenditure Estimated from Standard Formulas

An alternate to measuring energy expenditure is to estimate it from standard formulas such as those of Harris and Benedict, and others, (7,9,18) suitably adjusted for degree of malnutrition or stress (14,63). While these procedures are reasonably useful for estimates of normal subjects or even for mean values in ill patients, they are not adequate for determining nutritional requirements of individual critically ill patients. This is because variability in such patients is very great as illustrated in Table 2.15, and can vary as much as 50% above or below predicted (15).

Table 2.15.
Measured versus estimated values for EE.

	Measured	Estimated	Estimated + Correction Kinney	Rutten
kcal				
Mean	1551	1002	1562	1753
±SD	359	272	473	476
kJ				
Mean	6489	4192	6535	7335
±SD	1502	1138	1979	1992

Errors in Measuring Fuel Utilization

As discussed above, errors in measuring or estimating urinary urea or VCO_2 have little effect on calculation of energy expenditure. This is because the caloric equivalents of O_2 are very similar for carbohydrate, 5.03, fat, 4.61, and protein, 4.46 kcal liter^{-1} (21.0, 19.3 and 18.7 kJ liter^{-1}) (Table 2.12). This is also true for other foods; for instance, the value for alcohol is 4.84 kcal (20.3 kJ). The range of values from 4.46 to 5.03 kcal (18.7 to 21.0 kJ) is only 12%. No matter how different the actual composition of the food oxidized is from that estimated, the error in EE is unlikely to be more than 2% to 4%. Obviously this cannot be true for calculating utilization of individual fuels. An error of 100% in estimating Nu, which leads to only a 1% error in EE, gives a 100% error in the amount of protein oxidized, and to errors of the same magnitude for fat and carbohydrate. An error of 10% in VCO_2 gives an error of only 3% in EE, but errors in fat and carbohydrate oxidation are of the order of 50% to 100%. The effect of errors in N estimation was demonstrated in the experiment of Bursztein et al. cited above (62). Use of a standard value for Nu, which caused an error of only 1.8% in EE, caused errors of 89% in fat oxidation and 22% in carbohydrate oxidation.

Furthermore, when considering fuel utilization, the average constants listed in Table 2.12 may not be adequate (56). This will be particularly true if the diet does not consist only of fat, carbohydrate, and protein. As an extreme example, study of a man consuming 50% of calories as alcohol would find that 100% of energy expenditure would be accounted for by oxidation of fat, carbohydrate, and protein if the standard calorimetric coefficients were used.

Metabolizable Energy

Two entries for energy coefficients of protein, fat, and carbohydrate are shown in Table 2.12, under gross and metabolizable energy. Gross energy represents the values calculated from bomb calorimetry for oxidation of protein, carbohydrate, and fat as they occur in the body. When the food is eaten, however, not all of it is absorbed; some passes through the intestine and is excreted in the feces. Metabolizable energy represents the fraction of each component that is absorbed from the intestine: 0.93 for protein (4.0/4.3), 0.98 for starch (4.10/4.17), and 0.98 for fat (9.1/9.3) (48, 49, 51). These digestibility factors are average values that are used to estimate the available or metabolizable energy of foods.

The metabolizable constants, multiplied by total intake, will give the energy actually obtained by the body. Alternatively, one could first calculate the amount of food actually absorbed and metabolizable, by multiplying total intake by the digestibility factors given above, 0.93 for protein and 0.98 for fat and carbohydrate, to give net intake. Net intake is then multiplied by the gross energy factors to give the energy actually obtained. The constants for converting grams of food to liters of O_2 and CO_2 and for the caloric equivalent of a liter of O_2 or CO_2 (Table 2.12) have been derived from stoichiometric equations for food oxidation and are, therefore, associated with the gross energy constants, not the metabolizable energy constants. Therefore, when we calculate the amounts of food oxidized and the derived energy from values of VO_2, VCO_2, and Nu, we must use the gross energy constants that will give us the amount of net food intake that is actually metabolized, and not total intake. Therefore, in calculating the amounts of carbohydrate, fat and protein oxidized, from measurements of VO_2, VCO_2 and Nu, we have used the gross energy values rather than the metabolizable energy values. Others (46, 55) have used the metabolizable energy values, yielding slightly smaller values for energy expenditure. In principle, we believe this to be incorrect; in practice, the differences are too small to be of practical importance.

There are important differences in the metabolizable energy of the foodstuffs depending on whether they are from animal or vegetable origin, as shown by data reported in 1900 by Atwater and Bryant (Table 2.16). They studied diets of 185 families and concluded that in the average American diet, 61% of the protein, 92% of the fat, and 5% of the carbohydrate came from animal sources and the remainder from vegetable sources (64). These values have probably changed in the last 20 years because of the publicity concerning the dangers of ingesting fat of animal origin which is thought to be responsible for increasing the levels of cholesterol, and so favoring onset of cardiovascular disease. Since it is difficult to avoid animal fat and still eat animal protein, both of these important elements of culinary pleasure are being reduced or eliminated from modern diets.

Table 2.16.
Caloric value of foodstuffs from animal and vegetal origin.

	Caloric Value			
	Bomb Calorimeter		Metabolized in the Body	
Nutrient	(kcal g^{-1})	(kJ^{-1})	(kcal g^{-1})	(kJ^{-1})
Protein				
Animal	5.65	23.6	4.25	17.8
Vegetal	5.65	23.6	3.55	14.9
Fat				
Animal	9.40	39.3	8.95	37.4
Vegetal	9.30	38.9	8.35	34.9
Carbohydrate				
Animal	3.90	16.3	3.80	15.9
Vegetal	4.15	17.4	4.00	16.7

While gross rather than metabolizable energy should be used as a basis for estimating energy expenditure by indirect calorimetry, the opposite is true for estimating energy intake. The difference between gross and metabolizable energy represents that part of intake which is not converted to O_2, CO_2, and Nu, but rather lost in the stool because it is not absorbed or to a less extent from the breath, as in the case of alcohol, or as glucose or ketone bodies in diabetic urine. Therefore, when intake of energy is to be estimated, one must use the metabolizable energy values. This is usually done using predetermined constants for various foods as discussed in detail by Merrill and Watt (48). For accurate balance work in research the most satisfactory procedure is to analyze all intake and excreta by bomb calorimetry. The difference represents the metabolizable energy.

Lipogenesis

In their book on clinical chemistry, Peters and Van Slyke (61) were not yet aware of Krebs work on the tricarboxylic acid cycle and at this time the conversion of glucose into fat was considered as a simple chemical reaction of the type:

$$3\,(C_6H_{12}O_6) \rightarrow C_{18}H_{36}O_2 + 8\,O_2 \qquad (39)$$

where 3 molecules of glucose are converted into one molecule of stearic acid with the liberation of 8 molecules of oxygen. This kind of "endogenic oxygen production" related to the conversion of a substance relatively rich in oxygen (glucose) to one relatively poor in oxygen (stearic acid or other fat) could explain why during the process of fat synthesis from glucose there was a discrepancy between the increase in CO_2 production and the relatively stable value of VO_2 (57). This also explains the fact that an RQ above 1.0 is characteristic of lipogenesis; indeed, if VCO_2 increases sufficiently and VO_2 remains stable this ratio must increase above 1.

Indirect calorimetry measures net fat oxidation (nonprotein RQ below 1.0) or net lipogenesis (nonprotein RQ above 1.0), but this does not mean that both may not occur simultaneously. Lipogenesis in some tissues may be appreciable when the RQ is below 1.0, if fat oxidation occurring elsewhere is greater (35).

It is possible to derive a variety of equations for lipogenesis, each of which gives different values for VO_2, VCO_2, and RQ associated with lipogenesis. For instance we may assume that the lipid produced consists of triglycerides containing equimolar amounts of palmitic, stearic, and oleic acids represented by a compound $C_{55}H_{105}O_6$ and called palmitylstearyloleyltriglyceride. The conversion of glucose to this fat may be represented by the following equation (65).

$$\begin{array}{llll} 13.5\,C_6H_{12}O_6 + 3\,O_2 \rightarrow & C_{55}H_{104}O_6 + 26\,CO_2 + & 29\,H_2O & (40) \\ 2432\,g \quad 67.2\,liter \rightarrow & 861.5\,g \quad 582.4\,liter & 522.3\,g & \end{array}$$

This equation assumes that all of the acetyl coenzyme A that can be produced from 13 moles of glucose is converted to fatty acid. The additional 0.5 mole of glucose is converted to glycerol. This gives a calculated RQ of 8.7. However, such a value will never be obtained in any subject, since no living creature can derive all its energy from fat synthesis. The highest values for RQ are those reported for the overstuffed goose, which reached 1.40.

Other equations have been written for the conversion of carbohydrate to fat. These equations take into account that glucose oxidation mainly produces NADH, while fatty acid synthesis requires NADPH, and there are limitations in adipose tissue as to the extent of interconvertibility of NADH to NADPH (66). Therefore additional glucose may have to be oxidized via 6-phosphogluconic acid, to provide extra NADPH. This gives different values for VO_2 and VCO_2 and much lower values of RQ associated with lipogenesis. None of this need be of concern to indirect calorimetry, which, like its progenitor, thermodynamics, deals only with initial and final states and sheds no light on the intermediate mechanisms involved in achieving these states. These initial and final states include F, C, P, O_2, CO_2, Nu, and H_2O, whether in the diet, in the air, stored as fat, as protein, or glycogen in the body or as excreted in the urine. Therefore the equations that we have derived for their interconversion are valid in all circumstances. This question has been examined in detail by Elia and Livesey (67). On a hypercaloric diet containing little or no fat, more fat will be synthesized than oxidized and there will be storage of such synthesized fat in the body. This storage or lipogenesis or positive fat balance appears in the calculations as negative fat oxidation. From measurements of VO_2, VCO_2, and Nu it is impossible to determine how much of this fat synthesis comes from protein or from carbohydrate. Therefore, we cannot assign how much carbohydrate is oxidized and how much is converted to fat. All we can arrive at is the total amount of carbohydrate utilized, the total amount of protein utilized, and the total amount of fat utilized or synthesized.

Gluconeogenesis, Ketogenesis and RQs below 0.7

There are two processes, which we have not yet considered that tend to lower the RQ perhaps below 0.707, which is the RQ of fat. These are net production of glucose or ketone bodies. Ordinarily the RQ never drops as low as 0.707, for even if no carbohydrate is being oxidized, there is always some protein oxidation and the overall RQ will be between that of fat, 0.707, and that of protein, 0.809. If for instance an individual is oxidizing no carbohydrate but expending 2,500 kcal (10,460 kJ) day^{-1} and excreting 4 g N day^{-1}, the RQ will be 0.711, and he will be oxidizing 257 g of fat and 25 g of protein.

Gluconeogenesis involves conversion of fat and protein, both O_2 poor substances, to glucose, which is O_2 rich, and therefore it has a lowering effect on RQ. Although gluconeogenesis occurs often, it is generally under conditions in which the glucose formed is subsequently oxidized and there is no net accumulation of glucose. The only condition in which there is likely to be net accumulation is in a human or animal on a meat diet which is high in protein, and carbohydrate-free. After a meal there will be gluconeogenesis and storage of glucose as glycogen. Subsequently, in the postabsorptive state the glycogen will be oxidized (68). In an extreme case, a subject consuming 1000 kcal (4180 kJ) protein and 2000 kcal (9360 kJ) fat in a single meal and depositing 100 g glycogen in a 12-hour absorptiveperiod, the RQ would be low, 0.701, but not appreciably below that offat. Nevertheless, equation 26 would give a negative value for carbohydrate, indicating glycogen storage at the rate of 200 g day^{-1}.

Ketogenesis also represents conversion of an O_2-poor substance (fat), to O_2-rich substances (betahydroxybutyrate, acetoacetate and acetone). Again if they are subsequently oxidized they do not enter into the equations of indirect calorimetry. However, if they accumulate in sufficient quantity in urine, they must be taken into consideration. (Accumulation in body water is too small to be of practical importance). Unlike lipogenesis and gluconeogenesis, in which the end products are included, the end products of ketogenesis are not included in the equations of indirect calorimetry. Therefore, the amounts in urine must be measured and used to correct the values for O_2 and CO_2 to be used in equations 25-31. Also the energy derived from ketogenesis must be added to that calculated from equation 25. A stoichiometric equation for ketogenesis assuming a mixture, in molar terms, of 5 parts of betahydroxybutyrate, 5 parts of acetoacetate and 3 parts of acetone is given in equation 41.

$$0.716\ g\ fat + 0.437\ liter\ O_2 \rightarrow 1\ g\ ketones + 0.111\ liter\ CO_2 + 0.129\ g\ H_2O + 2.039\ kcal\ (8.53\ kJ) \qquad (41)$$

Differences in composition of the ketone bodies produced will have only a small effect on this equation. From equation 41 we can calculate that excretion of 1 g of ketones requires 0.716 g fat and 0.437 liter O_2, and is accompanied by production of 0.111 liter CO_2, 0.129 g H_2O, and 2.039 kcal (8.53 kJ) of energy. The RQ is 0.255. The amounts of O_2 and CO_2 due to ketogenesis must be substracted from VO_2 and VCO_2 before the general equations (equations 25-27) of indirect calorimetry are used. In an extreme case we may assume that a subject will oxidize 129 g fat, convert another 43 g of fat to 60 g of urinary ketones (in long-term fasting, discussed in Chapter 4, about 10 g of ketones appear in urine) and oxidize 25 g protein. Twenty-four-hour energy expenditure will be 1425 kcal (5960 kJ), of which 120 are derived from ketogenesis. The RQ will be 0.68, whereas if the same amount of energy was produced without ketogenesis it would have been 0.72. We may note that the caloric equivalent of O_2 for ketogenesis, 4.67 kcal (19.5 kJ)/liter, is similar to that of fat oxidation; therefore, for calculation of energy expenditure only, ketogenesis may be ignored. This is not true for fuel utilization.

Thus indirect calorimetry can detect net gluconeogenesis and accommodate ketogenesis, in the latter case with the aid of additional equations. Although both of these processes in themselves have low RQs, it is unlikely that gluconeogenesis can lower the RQ below 0.70, or that ketogenesis could lower it below 0.68. Nevertheless, most investigators who use indirect calorimetry will occasionally observe RQs below 0.68 and some of these values have been reported in the literature. It seems likely that most of these observations are due to hypoventilation or artifacts of measurement. Nevertheless some of us have observed RQs below 0.68 which do not seem to be measurement errors, but as yet we know of no biological process which can account for such low values.

ENERGY BALANCE

The concept of energy balance is very simple:

$$\textit{Energy balance} = \textit{energy in minus energy out} \qquad (42)$$

If *energy in* equals *energy out*, the subject is in zero energy balance, or just in balance. If energy in is greater than energy out, the subject is in positive balance and is storing energy as fat, carbohydrate, or protein. If energy out is greater than energy in, the subject is in negative energy balance and must be oxidizing endogenous stores of energy, again as either fat, carbohydrate, or protein.

Measurement of energy balance according to equation 42, that is by measuring input and output, is almost invariably performed by indirect calorimetry. In principle, direct calorimetry could also be used. However, equipment for direct calorimetry is not generally available. When the two are performed simultaneously there is good agreement (69). It is also possible to measure energy balance without measuring input or output, but by measuring changes in weight of the whole body or of various body components, such as fat, lean body mass, or body cell mass. These body composition methods are more accurate than balance methods over periods of months to years, whereas balance methods are more precise over shorter periods, days to weeks. For instance, body weight is a simple and good method for estimating changes in body fat as people become obese or in weight reduction programs. However, balance methods are not accurate enough to measure a positive energy balance of 100 kcal (418 kJ) per day, which, if continued for a year, will produce a weight gain of 5.5 kg. On the other hand, weight changes give little information about changes in energy stores in acutely ill or malnourished hospitalized patients over periods of a few days to a few weeks, since large changes in body fluids, of the order of 5 to 10 kg, may completely mask changes in fat, carbohydrate, and protein.

Body composition measurements and a general consideration of balance measurements will be discussed in detail in the chapter on nitrogen balance. In this section we will deal with the use of indirect calorimetry for measuring energy balance and two of its components, fat and carbohydrate balances.

Measurement of energy balance has been and remains an important research tool for understanding the interrelations among the composition and quantity of dietary intake, the rate of energy expenditure, and rates of loss and gain of fat and protein in malnutrition, obesity and various disease states. Clinically, measurement of energy balance by indirect calorimetry has its greatest application in monitoring the dietary needs of critically ill or malnourished, hospitalized patients who require artificial nutrition, either enteral or parenteral.

Energy Out

As described in previous sections, accurate values for energy expenditure require measurement only of VO_2 and VCO_2, and under manyconditions, even VCO_2 may be neglected. However, except in a very few research centers, it is not possible to get continuous measurements of energy expenditure. Estimates of daily energy expenditure are required for nutritional purposes; these must be extrapolated from one or more measurements made over short time periods of several minutes to an hour. Reliable estimates of 24-hour resting energy expenditure (95% confidence limits of ±5%) may be derived from 3 to 5 accurate measurements of gas exchange, of 20 to 30 min duration, evenly spaced throughout the 24 hours (70). For patients on mechanical ventilation, equal accuracy can be obtained with two 15-minute measurements approximately 12 hours apart (71) (Chapter 5). In bedridden patients REE is almost identical with total energy expenditure. In ambulatory patients or normal subjects, energy due to physical activity must also be estimated. Several research centers throughout the world have indirect calorimetry chambers. These are small rooms furnished with bed, chair, toilet facilities, etc., in which the subject can eat, sleep, and exercise for many days at a time. Webb (69) designed a suit that can be worn for days at a time, which measures energy expenditure by direct and indirect calorimetry simultaneously. With these facilities AEE and TEE can be measured as accurately as REE. For normal subjects, apparatus such as the Kofranyi-Michaelis meter may be used during physical activity (46). This weighs about 3 kg and can be strapped to the subject's back (Chapter 1). It measures VE and collects samples of expired air for subsequent off-line analysis in a Pauling oxygen meter or Haldane gas analyzer. A noseclip and a mouthpiece must be used. The Kofranyi-Michaelis meter or similar apparatus has been used extensively to derive EE for various types of physical activities, as illustrated in Table 2.9. Although it is relatively inexpensive, it is not suitable for continuous measurement of 24-hour EE. Its main use has been in exercise and respiratory physiology and for the derivation of values of EE for various activities. These values, together with a log of the subject's activities, can be used to calculate 24-hour total energy expenditure. However, this is very time-consuming, and much less accurate than 24-hour measurements in a calorimeter chamber or in Webb's suit. The procedure is much too tedious and time-consuming to be used on a routine basis with hospitalized patients.

An alternate procedure for indirect measurement of AEE has been used with hospitalized patients (65,72). This is restricted to use with patients receiving continuously infused high-carbohydrate diets for at least 4 days. For the first day or two after increasing carbohydrate, a major part of this intake will go to increasing glycogen stores in liver and muscle. By day 3 or 4, glycogen stores will plateau at a level appropriate to the new level of intake and no further storage will occur. This will be indicated by a corresponding plateau in resting RQ and resting carbohydrate balance, which is shown in Figure 4.5. For bedridden patients, this steady-state carbohydrate balance is zero; for ambulatory patients it is positive, even for intakes substantially below energy expenditure. Since glycogen stores are not changing from one day to the next, this positive carbohydrate balance at rest, representing glycogen storage at rest, must be balanced by an equal utilization of glycogen during physical activity. Therefore the amount of glycogen deposition at rest, as measured over each 24 hours, is exactly equal to the amount of glycogen consumed during physical activity during the same 24-hour period. If we assume further that, when resting RQs are above 1, there is no contribution of fat or protein to the added energy expenditure due to exercise, then 24-hour glycogen storage at rest is equal to 24-hour AEE. The assumption of no change in protein oxidation during light exercise is supported by studies measuring muscle output of N (73). The assumption that changes in rates of fat oxidation or lipogenesis do not occur with exercise when the RQ is above 1 has not been experimentally tested. However, we can assume that such changes would be relatively small, and that use of resting carbohydrate balance to estimate AEE gives reasonable values. Certainly such values are better than we can obtain by any other method. Using this technique, average values for ambulatory, malnourished hospitalized patients receiving TPN have been found to be in the range of 6 to 7 kcal (25 to 30 kJ) per kg per day, about 25% of REE or 20% of TEE. Standard deviations were about 4 to 5 kcal (16 to 21 kJ) per kg per day (70,72). These values can be used as a rough estimate of AEE for evaluating energy requirements of patients.

While we can measure REE in hospitalized patients to within ± 5%, estimates of AEE are much less precise, except for bedridden patients in whom it is close to zero. However, AEE averages only about 20% of TEE in these patients, so that even an error of 50% in estimating AEE contributes only a 10% error to TEE.

Energy In

Energy intake is equal to the sum of the caloric intakes of fat, carbohydrate, and protein and, when applicable, alcohol. It should be pointed out that many investigators report energy intake as equal only to the caloric intakes of carbohydrate and fat, neglecting protein. This is particularly true in the clinical literature. This is also incorrect. Energy derived from protein is used to generate ATP to roughly the same extent as energy derived from fat or carbohydrate. If protein intake is reduced, it is necessary to increase either fat or carbohydrate intake in order to maintain energy balance. It is true that DIT is greater for protein than for the other nutrients, so that somewhat fewer calories of carbohydrate or fat are needed to replace the lost protein calories; nevertheless, they are needed.

The most accurate method for measuring energy intake is to determine the energy of the food eaten and of all excreta in a bomb calorimeter. The difference between the two is the amount of metabolizable foods absorbed by the subject. Even with this procedure there is an important problem. It is simple to combust all the excreta, or suitably measured aliquots thereof, since we have no further use for it. But food cannot be eaten after combustion in a bomb calorimeter. Therefore we must take representative samples of all foods eaten and combust them, and hope that the composition of each sample in the bomb is the same as that eaten by the person. For ordinary everyday foods this is very difficult, and for accurate studies it is necessary to restrict the diet to a few specially prepared, homogeneous (and very boring) foods which are easy to sample. Most investigators do not have, or for good reason prefer not to use, a bomb calorimeter. In this case, the quantities of each food eaten must be measured, and estimates of the energy content made from published values for these foods as illustrated in Table 2.10. In addition, since we are not using a bomb calorimeter to measure the energy content of the excreta, we must use the metabolizable energy values, not the gross energy values, as discussed above under "Metabolizable Energy." Extensive tabulations of the nutrient composition of foods, including the energy content, are available, such as the one from the U. S. Department of Agriculture (74), and are widely used for preparing diets for many purposes.

Use of chemically defined diets for tube-feeding, or of dextrose and amino acid solutions, and lipid emulsions for parenteral nutrition, greatly simplifies and improves estimates of intake. The normal procedure is to weigh each bottle or bag with its associated tubing before and after infusion. The weight is then multiplied by the content of each constituent as listed by the manufacturer. While this procedure is much simpler and more accurate than procedures for measuring oral intake, there are nevertheless a number of problems to keep in mind:

1. Weight measurements are more accurate than volume measurements for estimating intake. This means that the composition, usually given by the manufacturer per unit volume, must be converted to unit weight.
2. It must be remembered that the caloric content of dextrose, which is the monohydrate of glucose, of 3.41 kcal (14.3 kJ) g^{-1}, is not the same as that of glucose, 3.75 kcal (15.7 kJ) g^{-1}, or of starch which is 4.17 kcal (17.4 kJ) g^{-1} (Table 2.12). Thus the energy content of 1 liter of 5% dextrose solution is 170 kcal (711 kJ), not 200 kcal (837 kJ)which is often used in the clinical literature.
3. The energy constants to be used with parenteral solutions are the gross energy constants (Table 2.12), not the metabolizable constants, since there is no intestinal loss of these nutrients. Infusions of alcohol, which is now rarely used, constitute an exception, since 2%, however administered, is lost via the breath. With enteral infusions there may be losses due to lack of absorption. Nevertheless, since these nutrients are often highly refined, average digestibility factors or metabolizable energy constants are usually not appropriate.
4. The contents as listed by the manufacturer may not be correct. For instance, one study using amino acid solutions found them to be 5 $\pm$ 3% (mean $\pm$SD) higher in N content than listed (70). By contrast,

50% dextrose solutions were within 1% of listed values. Such variations are not important for clinical monitoring, but analysis of solutions may be necessary for accurate research studies.

5. The composition of intravenous amino acid solutions may vary greatly from typical protein composition as shown in Table 2.17 (51). In particular, energy values may differ widely from that of 4.3 kcal (18.0 kJ) g^{-1} protein, or 26.9 kcal (112.5 kJ) g^{-1} N, listed in Table 2.12.

Table 2.17.
Protein-to-nitrogen ratios and caloric values of some enteral preparations and intravenous amino acid mixtures.[a]

	True Protein: Nitrogen Ratio	Bomb Calorimetric Values (per g protein)		Corrected Values for Energy Produced in the Body (per g protein)	
		kcal	kJ	kcal	kJ
Enteral					
Albumaid XP	6.44	5.8	24.3	4.5	18.8
Amin-aid	7.33	6.7	28.0	5.4	22.6
Vivonex S	5.40	5.6	23.4	4.3	18.0
Vivonex HN	5.89	5.6	23.4	4.3	18.0
Parenteral					
Aminosol	6.66	5.7	23.8	4.4	18.4
Freeamin II	5.62	6.0	25.1	4.7	19.7
Nephramine	7.13	5.2	21.8	3.9	16.3
Travenol BCAA mix	7.76	7.4	31.0	6.1	25.5
Vamine 9	6.39	5.8	24.3	4.5	18.8
Vamine 14	5.39	6.0	25.1	4.7	19.7

[a]Adapted from Livesey G and Elias M (51).

We may conclude that, without very careful measurements requiring equipment not available to the average therapist or investigator, there may be substantial errors in measuring food intake. While it is difficult to generalize, we may guess that errors of 5% to 10% or even higher are probably the norm.

Energy In Minus Energy Out

Although with standard equipment now available in many institutions, it is possible to measure REE with an accuracy of 2%, extrapolation to 24-hour values increases the error to about 5%. An additional 5% or more will be added from estimates of AEE. If we take 2000 kcal (8,370 kJ) day^{-1} as a representative total energy expenditure, the errors in estimating TEE will range from about 100 kcal (418 kJ) day^{-1} in bedridden patients (no AEE) to about 200 kcal (837 kJ) day^{-1} in ambulatory patients. Measurements of intake are, if anything, less precise than measurements of expenditure. Therefore, errors of the order of 100 to 200 kcal (418 to 837 kJ) day^{-1} should be expected as normal in measurement of one day's energy balance in an individual. Fortunately, many or most of these errors are random in nature; therefore, they will tend to cancel out as many daily measurements are made in a single individual, or when a number of subjects are used. However, some of these errors are tendentious, as discussed in more detail in Chapter 3. These tendentious errors, even if small, can severely limit the usefulness of energy balance measurements in long-term studies.

Carbohydrate and Fat Balances

Errors in measuring carbohydrate and fat oxidation are substantially greater than errors in measuring energy expenditure. The amount of work and expense involved in order to make accurate determinations are too great for use in clinical monitoring. Fortunately, these parameters are not needed, since the major point of interest is energy expenditure. The amount of total energy intake should preferably be based on measurements of energy expenditure in the particular individual. However, the optimal amount of each component—fat, carbohydrate, or protein—should not be determined from individual measurement, but from entirely different considerations, as discussed in Chapters 3-5 and 7. Carbohydrate and fat balances can be very useful for research purposes, but extreme care is needed in order to obtain accurate data. The burden is on the individual investigator to prove that his or her methodology is adequate to provide meaningful information.

Energy Balance and Obesity

L'obésité ne se trouve jamais ni chez les sauvages, ni dans les classes de la société ou on travaille pour manger et ou ne mange que pour vivre. Les principales causes de l'obésité sont:

la premiere est la disposition naturelle de l'individu
la seconde est dans les farines et les fecules dont l'homme fait la base de sa nourriture journalière
la troisième est une double cause de l'obésité resultant de la prolongation du sommeil et du defaut d'exercice
la derniere cause d'obésité consiste dans l'exces du boire et du manger. (Brillat-Savarin: 1756–1826).

There are two important conditions, or perhaps diseases, relating to energy balance: protein calorie malnutrition and obesity. There are two general causes of malnutrition: inadequate food supply, which affects large sections of the world's population in the less affluent countries; and inability to digest or absorb food which is common to a variety of disease states related to the intestinal tract, and which occur among both the less and the more affluent. These causes are easy to understand, and from the scientific point of view, the first is easy to treat.

If more food is made available, hungry people will eat it and in time cease to be malnourished. As to the second, if the intestinal problems are cured the patient can eat and recover. If the disease is incurable, or if malnourished subjects from either category are too ill to depend on oral diets, then they will need artificial nutrition, either enteral or parenteral, until they can return to oral diets or for the rest of their lives. These solutions are conceptually simple, although many scientific and medical questions are raised in searching for the optimal methods of preventing the occurrence of malnutrition and repleting the depleted patient. Some of these points will be discussed in Chapters 3 and 7.

Obesity is very different. It is true of course that it is a disease of overeating, and the cure is to stop eating too much. But how to do that is not simple, either from a scientific or practical view.

As Brillat-Savarin observed 200 years ago, obesity is a disease of affluence; it occurs neither among savages, nor among those who must work to eat and eat only to survive. As the world has become more affluent, the incidence of obesity has spread greatly and is highest in the most affluent country of our present time—the United States of America. However, despite the wide concern about (diet books are outsold only by cookbooks in the U. S.), and extensive investigation of, obesity, we do not really understand why some people become obese and others do not, and have little idea of how to control or manage obesity on a long-term basis. Indeed, if we modify his second cause, to add fat to the grains and other starchy foods, Brillat-Savarin's principal causes of obesity are essentially those we would list today.

There is no question that obesity is consistent with the first law of thermodynamics—that energy can neither be created or destroyed. This means that obesity can only occur if energy in is greater than energy out and energy balance is, therefore, positive. But this positive balance may be surprisingly small. The weight increase during the development of obesity is about 2/3 fat and 1/3 lean body mass (LBM). The energy content of fat is 9300 kcal (38,900 kJ) kg^{-1}, that of LBM about 900 kcal (3766 kJ) kg^{-1}. Therefore the energy content of the weight gained averages 6500 kcal (27,200 kJ) kg^{-1}. Someone who eats, on the average, 100 kcal

(418 kJ) extra per day above requirements, equivalent to a small piece of lightly buttered toast, will gain 1 kg in 65 days, 5.5 kg. in a year, and 55 kg in a decade. Yet this amount extra, 100 kcal, is less than 5% of daily requirements and is too small to be determined accurately by energy balance techniques. It can only be measured by observing changes in weight or of body fat content over long periods. Some who have measured energy balance in obese individuals have concluded that they get fat without a positive energy balance and thus defy the first law of thermodynamics. It seems more reasonable to conclude that their techniques for measuring energy balance were inadequate for the job.

What is perhaps more surprising than that some people become obese, is that many people go through adult life barely changing weight from year to year or from decade to decade. A weight change of 2 kg in 10 years corresponds to an average daily energy balance of + 4 kcal (16 kJ). Thus the ordinary non-obese adult maintains energy in to within ± 4 kcal (16 kJ) per day of energy out. This is despite very large variation in daily rates of food intake for one individual and between individuals. Widdowson observed daily food intake ranging from 1772 to 4955 kcal (7400 to 20,700 kJ) day^{-1} in normal healthy men and from 1453 to 3110 kcal (6100 to 13,000 kJ) day^{-1} in women. The variation was even greater in children(75,76). What makes possible these enormous differences in diet intake which do not lead either to starvation or to obesity?

One factor of course is differences in physical activity. A laborer will expend more energy than an office worker. A restless person who fidgets a lot may consume 80% more oxygen sitting down than someone who does not. The energy expenditure of two individuals walking down the same road may differ up to 100% (43).

A second factor is related to diet-induced thermogenesis. As discussed earlier, DIT of carbohydrate is only about 5% when given below requirement, but rises to 30% or higher when given above requirement. That weight gain was much less than to be expected from excess food was observed in 1888 by Voit(77) and in 1902 by Neuman (78), who termed it "Luxuskonsumption". Furthermore the effect of exercise is to increase the DIT even more (43,79). Even food ingestion on the previous day will influence the interaction between exercise and food intake (80,81).

A third factor is reduced digestibility of foods. But this accounts for only 3% to 6% of caloric intake and does not seem to be an important factor (40,43)

A fourth factor is variability in body composition. BMR or REE are closely correlated with body cell mass (BCM). If BCM is a high or low fraction of body weight than REE and BMR should be correspondingly high or low. However, observed differences in BCM can account for only a small fraction of the differences in total energy expenditure.

Elucidating factors that explain differences in EE among individuals, does not explain why some people become obese and others do not. It may be that obese people do not fidget much, but there are also non-obese people who do not fidget. Obese people, on the whole, exercise less than their lean counterparts, but is this what causes obesity or does obesity cause the reduction in exercise? One parameter that does seem to be related to obesity is diet-induced thermogenesis. After a meal of 1000 kcal (4180 kJ), 10 lean and 14 obese subjects had similar increases in O_2 consumption ranging from 12% to 17%. With exercise, O_2 consumption in the lean group increased an additional 17%, the obese group by only 1% (82). A reduced DIT has also been observed in obese women (83). Differences in energy expenditure alone cannot explain the differences between obese and lean individuals. Differences in appetitive behaviour are equally if not more important. While differences have been shown in eating behavior they are outside the scope of this treatise.

It is still not known to what extent genetic or environmental factors modulate the onset and maintenance of obesity. But there is a recognition that once increases in body weight occur, the nature of the newly formed adipose tissue itself may resist loss of this weight. Fat is stored as droplets in adipocytes, one droplet to each adipocyte. The size of the adipocyte or amounts of fat per adipocyte are very uniform in the lean individual. Fat stores are increased by increasing the size of droplets but mainly by increasing the number of adipocytes. Once formed, these new adipocytes are here to stay. Reduction of fat stores reduces the size of the droplets below normal values but not the number of adipocytes. One thesis is that these adipocytes with smaller than normal droplets are "hungry." They would prefer a normal size droplet and signal the brain in some way to increase energy intake in order to restore their lost fat.

There are many succesful ways to treat obesity and particularly morbid obesity in the short run. All of them of necessity involve reducing energy in below energy out. This can be done by reducing intake, increasing expenditure, or both. There is some evidence that an exercise program not only increases energy expenditure but also makes it easier to reduce intake. While these methods can successfully remove fat, the experience of most therapists, who treat the morbidly obese is that it is extremely difficult for their patients not to become obese once again after they have finished with the program. Even those of us, including at least three of the authors of this book, who are only moderately overweight, know how easy it is to put on weight and how hard to take it off, and look with envy on our spouses and friends who eat all they want whenever they want and never gain an ounce.

REFERENCES

1. Pawan GLS: Metabolism of alcohol (ethanol) in man. *Proc Nutr Soc* 31: 83–89, 1972.
2. Kleiber M: *The Fire of Life.* New York, John Wiley and Sons, 1961.
3. Goldman RF: Effect of environment on metabolism. In Kinney JM (ed): *Assessment of Energy Metabolism in Health and Disease*, Columbus, Ross Laboratories, pp 117–121, 1980.
4. Du Bois D, Du Bois EF: Clinical calorimetry. A formula to estimate the approximate surface area if height and weight be known. *Arch Intern Med* 17:863-871,1916.
5. Takahira H: Report from the Metabolic Laboratory, Imperial Government Institute of Nutrition. Tokyo,1,1925.
6. Meeh K: Oberflaechenmessungen des menschlichen Koerpers *Z Biol* 15:425-458, 1879.
7. Harris JA, Benedict FG: *A Biometric Study of Basal Metabolism in Man.* Washington, Carnegie Institute, 1919, Publ 279, p 266.
8. Boothby WM , Berkson J, Dunn HL: Studies of the energy metabolism of normal individuals. *Am J Physiol* 116:468-484, 1936.
9. Fleisch A: Le metabolisme basal standard et sa determination au moyen du "Metabocalculator." *Helv Med Acta* 18:23-44, 1951.
10. Du Bois EF: Energy metabolism. *Ann Rev Physiol* 16:125-134, 1954.
11. Spencer JL, Zikria AB, Kinney JM, Broell JR, et al.: A system for the continuous measurement of gas exchange and respiratory functions. *J Appl Physiol* 33:523-528, 1972.
12. Lusk G: *The Elements of the Science of Nutrition*, ed 4. Philadelphia, WB Saunders Company, 1928.
13. Mann S, Westenskow DR, Hautchens BA: Measured and predicted caloric expenditure in acutely ill. *Crit Care Med* 13:173-177, 1985.
14. Rutten P, Blackburn GL, Flatt JP, et al.: Determination of optimal hyperalimentation infusion rate. *J Surg Res* 18:477-483, 1975.
15. Weissman C, Kemper M, Askanazi, J, et al.: Resting metabolic rate of the critically ill patient: measured versus predicted. *Anesthesiol* 64:673-679, 1986.
16. Sherman HC: *Chemistry of Food and Nutrition, ed 8.* The MacMillan Company, New York, 1952, pp 154–176.
17. Sherman HC: *Chemistry of Food and Nutrition, ed 8.* The MacMillan Company, New York, 1952, p 168.
18. Aub JC, Du Bois EF: Clinical calorimetry. The basal metabolism of old men. *Arch Intern Med* 19:823-831, 1917.
19. Grande F: Energy expenditure of organs and tissues. In Kinney JM (ed): *Assessment of Energy Metabolism in Health and Disease.* Columbus, Ross Laboratories, 1980, pp 88–92.
20. Sokoloff L, Fitzgerald GG, Kaufman EE: Cerebral nutrition and energy metabolism. In Wurtman RJ and Wurtman JJ (eds): *Nutrition and the Brain.* New York, Raven Press, 1977, pp 87.
21. Blaxter KL: Methods of measuring the energy of animals and the interpretation of the results obtained. *Fed Proc* 30:1436-1443, 1971.
22. Kien CL, Rohrbaugh DK, Burke JF, et al.: Whole body protein synthesis in relation

to basal energy expenditure in healthy children and in children recovering from burn injury. *Pediatr Res* 12:211-216, 1978.

23. Enright L, Cole VV, Hitchcock FA: Basal metabolism and iodine excretion during pregnancy. *Am J Physiol* 113:221-228, 1935.
24. Benedict FG, Emmens LE: A comparison of the basal metabolism of normal men and women. *J Biol Chem* 20:253-262, 1915.
25. Fuhrman FA, Hollinger JM, Crismon JM, et al.: Metabolism of the excised brain of the large mouthed bass Huro Salmonides at graded temperature levels. *Physiol Zool* 17:42-50, 1944.
26. Kinney JM, Roe CF: Caloric equivalent of fever. 1. Pattern of postoperative response. *Ann Surg* 156:610-622, 1962.
27. Roe CF, Kinney JM: The caloric equivalent of fever. 2. Influence of major trauma. *Ann Surg* 161:140-147, 1965.
28. Rodriguez JL, Weissman C, Damask MC, et al.: Morphine and postoperative rewarming in critically ill patients. *Circulation* 68:1238-1246, 1983.
29. Elwyn DH, Kinney JM, Askanazi J: Energy expenditure in surgical patients. *Surg Clin N Am* 61:545-556, 1981.
30. Aulick LH: Studies in heat transport and heat loss in thermally injured patients. In Kinney JM(ed): *Assessment of Energy Metabolism in Health and Disease.* Columbus, Ross Laboratories, pp 141–144, 1980.
31. Wilmore DW, Mason AD, Johnson DW, Pruitt BA: Effect of ambient temperature on heat production and heat loss in burn patients. *J Appl Physiol* 38:593-597, 1975.
32. Himms-Hagen J: Current status of nonshivering thermogenesis In Kinney JM(ed): *Assessment of Energy Metabolism in Health and Disease.* Columbus, Ross Laboratories, 1980, pp 92–102.
33. Hemingway A, Hataway SR: An investigation of chemical temperature regulation. *Am J. Physiol* 134:596-602, 1941.
34. Werner AY, Dawson D, Hardenbergh E: Spontaneous rewarming of the hypothermic curarised dog. *Science* 124:1145-1147, 1956.
35. Acheson KJ, Schutz Y, Bessard T, et al.: Nutritional influence on lipogenesis and thermogenesis after a carbohydrate meal. *Am J Physiol* 246:E62-E70, 1984.
36. Jéquier E: Influence of nutrient administration on energy expenditure in man. *Clin Nutr* 5:181-186, 1986.
37. Shaw SN, Elwyn DH, Askanazi J, et al.: Effects of increasing nitrogen intake on nitrogen balance and energy expenditure in nutritionally depleted adult patients receiving parenteral nutrition. *Am J Clin Nutr* 37:930-940, 1983.
38. Benedict FG, Lee RC: *Lipogenesis in the Animal Body with Special Reference to the Physiology of the Goose.* Washington DC, Carnegie Institute, Publ. 489, 1937.
39. Durnin JVGA, Edholm OG, Miller DS, Waterlow JC: How much food does man require? *Nature* 242:418, 1972.
40. Widdowson EM: Nutritional individuality. *Proc Nutr Soc* 21:121-128, 1962.
41. Rose GA, Williams RT: Metabolic studies on large and small eaters. *Br J Nutr* 15:1-9, 1961.
42. Ashworth A: An investigation of very low caloric intakes reported in Jamaica. *Br J Nutr* 22:341-355, 1968.
43. Miller DS, Mumford PM: Gluttony, I. An experimental study of overeating low or high protein diets. *Am J Clin Nutr* 20:1212-1222, 1967.
44. Miller DS, Mumford PM, Stock MJ: Gluttony, II. Thermogenesis in overeating man. *Am J Clin Nutr* 20:1223-1229, 1967.

45. Rapport D: The relative specific dynamic action of various proteins. *J Biol Chem* 60:497-511, 1924.
46. Consolazio CF, Johnson RE, Pecora LJ: *Physiologic Measurements of Metabolic Functions in Man.* New York, McGraw-Hill, 1963, pp 313–339.
47. Altman PL, Dittmer DS: *Metabolism. Biological Handbooks*, Washington DC, Federation of American Societies for Experimental Biology, 1968.
48. Merrill AL, Watt BK: *Energy Value of Foods.* Agriculture Handbook, No 74, U. S. Government Printing Office, Washington 25, DC, 1955.
49. Southgate DAT, Durnin JVGA: Calorie conversion factors. An experimental reassessment of the factors used in the energy value of human diets. *Br J Nutr* 24:517-535, 1970.
50. Rubner M: Calorimetrische Untersuchungen, I. Einleitung. *Z Biol* 21:250, 1885.
51. Livesey G, Elia M: Food energy value of artificial feeds for man. *Clin Nutr* 4:99-111, 1985.
52. Zuntz N, Schumburg H: *Studien zur einer Physiologie des Marsches,* Berlin, Berlin Publishers, 1901.
53. Cathcart EP, Cuthbertson DP: The composition and distribution of the fatty substances of the human subject. *J Physiol* 72:349-360, 1931.
54. Westenkow DR, Schipke CA, Raymond JL, et al.: Calculation of metabolic expenditure and substrate utilization from gas exchange measurements. *JPEN* 12:20-24, 1988.
55. Ben Porat M, Sideman S, Bursztein S: Energy metabolism rate equation for fasting and for postabsorptive subjects. *Am J Physiol* 244:R764-R769, 1983.
56. Livesey G, M: Estimation of energy expenditure, net carbohydrate utilization and net fat oxidation and synthesis by indirect calorimetry: evaluation of errors with special reference to the detailed composition of fuels. *Am J Clin Nutr* 47:608-628, 1988.
57. Lusk G: Animal calorimetry. XXIV. Analysis of the oxidation of mixtures of carbohydrate and fat. A correction. *Metabolism* 31: 1234-1240,1924.
58. Weir JB De V: New methods for calculating metabolic rate with special reference to protein metabolism. *J Physiol* 109:1- 9, 1949.
59. Ultman JS, Bursztein S: Analysis of error in the determination of respiratory gas exchange at varying FIO_2. *J Appl Physiol* 50:210-216,1981.
60. Bursztein S, Saphar P, Glaser P et al: Determination of energy metabolism from respiratory function alone. *J Appl Physiol* 42:117-119, 1977.
61. Peters P, Van Slyke DD: *Quantitative Chemistry, Interpretation,* Baltimore, Williams and Wilkins, 1946, Vol 1, pp 3–93.
62. Bursztein S, Elwyn DH, Saphar P, Singer P: Critical analysis of indirect calorimetry measurements. *Am J Clin Nutr,* in press 1988.
63. Kinney JM: The application of indirect calorimetry to clinical studies. In Kinney JM(ed): *Assessment of Energy Metabolism in Health and Disease.* Columbus, Ross Laboratories,1980, pp 42–48.
64. Widdowson EM: Assessment of the energy value of human foods. *Proc Nutr Soc* 14:142-154, 1955.
65. Elwyn DH, Kinney JM; A unique approach to measuring total energy expenditure by indirect calorimetry. In Kinney JM (ed): *Assessment of Energy Metabolism in Health and Disease.* Columbus, Ross Laboratories,1980, pp 54–61.
66. Flatt JP: The biochemistry of energy expenditure. In Bray GA (ed): *Recent Advances in Obesity Research* 12, London, Newman, 1978, pp 54–63.

67. Elia M, Livesey G: Theory and validity of indirect calorimetry during net lipid synthesis. *Am J Clin Nutr* 47:591-607, 1988.
68. Elwyn DH, Parikh HC, Shoemaker WC, Amino acid movements between gut, liver and periphery in unanesthetized dogs. *Am J Physiol* 215:1260-1275,1968.
69. Webb P: Energy balance over a 45 hour period with a suit calorimeter. In Kinney JM(ed): Assessment of Energy Metabolism in Health and Disease. Columbus, Ross Laboratories, 1980, pp 24–31.
70. Chikenji T, Elwyn DH, Gil KM, et al.: Effects of increasing glucose intake on nitrogen balance and energy expenditure in malnourished adult patients receiving parenteral nutrition. *Clin Sci* 72:489-501, 1987.
71. van Lanschot JJB, Feensta BWA, Vermeij CG, Bruining HA: Extrapolation accuracy of intermittent metabolic gas exchange recordings and its relation to the diurnal variation of critically ill patients. *Crit Care Med* 16:737-742,1988.
72. Elwyn DH, Gump FE, Munro HN, et al.: Changes in nitrogen balance of depleted patients with increasing infusions of glucose. *Am J Clin Nutr* 32:1597-1611, 1979.
73. Felig P, Wahren J: Amino acid metabolism in exercising man. *J Clin Invest* 50:2703-2714, 1971.
74. Adams CF: *Nutritive values of foods. Agriculture Handbook*, No 456, U. S. Government Printing Office, 1975.
75. Widdowson EM, McCance RA: Iron in human nutrition. *J Hyg Camb* 36:13-23,1947.
76. Widdowson EM: *A study of individual children's diets.* Med Res Council, Special Report Soc 257, London, HM Stationery Office, 1947.
77. Voit C: *Physiologie des Stoffwechsels. Hermansons Handbuch der Physiologie* 6:209-213,1881.
78. Neuman RO: Experimentelle Beitraege zur Lehre von des Taeglischen Nahrunsbedarf des Menschen unter besondere Beruecksichtigung der notwendigen Eiweissmenge. *Arch Hyg* 45:1-87,1902.
79. Reinhold D: Behaviour of some values for gaseous metabolism as affected by time of day and food intake. *Z Ges Inn Med Ihre Grenzgebiete* 19:609-615, 1964.
80. Bray GA, Whipp BJ, Koyal SN: The acute effects of food intake on energy expenditure during cycle ergometry. *Am J Clin Nutr* 27:254-259, 1974.
81. Stock MJ: Effects of fasting and refeeding on the metabolic response to a standard meal in man. *Eur J Appl Physiol* 43:35-40, 1980.
82. Zahorska-Markiewicz B: Thermic effect of food and exercise in obesity. *Eur J Appl Physiol* 44:231-235, 1980.
83. Bessard T, Schutz Y, Jéquier E: Energy expenditure and postprandial thermogenesis in obese women before and after weight loss. *Am J Clin Nutr* 38:680-694, 1983.

CHAPTER

3

Nitrogen Balance

Methods of Measuring Changes in and Absolute Values of Body Composition
- Critique of Balance Methods
- Direct Measurements of Body Composition

Interpretation of Body Composition Measurements
- Deviations from Normal
- Body Composition Changes

Interrelation Between Nitrogen Balance and Nitrogen and Energy Intake
- Adults
- Minimum and Recommended Requirements of Protein
- Maintenance and Repletion of Body Cell Mass in Hospital Patients
- Interrelation between N Balance and Dietary Intake in Children

For about 150 years (1) measurement of nitrogen balance has been the method of choice for determining changes in fat-free body weight or lean body mass (LBM). Approximately 95% of total body N is found in protein. In turn, protein, after water, is the major constituent of all cells except adipocytes, comprising 15% to 20% of most mammalian tissues. Nitrogen contents of different proteins vary somewhat, but on the average are close to 16%, and the standard factor for converting N to protein is 6.25, as discussed under "Indirect Calorimetry," in Chapter 2. Approximately two-thirds of body protein is intracellular, comprising the major functional elements of the cell, including enzymes, transport proteins, and contractile and structural elements. The other third is extracellular, mainly collagen and elastin, which serve as structural components of bone, cartilage, tendons, ligaments and connective tissue, and, in addition, hair and plasma proteins. During childhood, N balance measures growth of the entire lean body mass, including both intra- and extracellular elements, while changes in total body weight reflect the sum of changes in both LBM and fat. Independent estimates of fat may be obtained by several methods, including underwater weighing, anthropomorphic measurements, and electrical conductance, which are described in more detail below.

In human adults, N balance mainly measures changes in the intracellular protein content, since during starvation or nutritional depletion, there are minimal changes in extracellular structures (2). The intracellular component of LBM has been termed body cell mass (BCM) and is defined by Moore et al. (3), as "that component of body composition containing the oxygen-exchanging, potassium rich, glucose-oxidizing, work performing tissue . . . with which one is primarily concerned in the consideration of the working, energy metabolizing portion of the human body . . . . In any anthropomorphic consideration of the energy conversion of foodstuffs, oxygen requirement, carbon dioxide production or work performance, the body cell mass is the basic reference entity."

Nitrogen balance is the most important, but only one of many balances which measure changes in body composition. Measurements are also made of Na, K, Ca, P, and as we have seen in Chapter 2, of fat, carbohydrate, and total energy balances. A limitation of balance methods is that while they measure changes in the amounts of various body components, they cannot measure the absolute amounts of these components. There are other methods which do measure absolute amounts of body components. These include anthropomorphic measurements, indicator dilution techniques, neutron activation analysis, and more recently, nuclear magnetic resonance. Since interpretation of N and energy balances are often aided by measurements of other constituents, we will briefly describe the methods and assess the merits of various techniques for measuring body composition in the next section.

METHODS OF MEASURING CHANGES IN AND ABSOLUTE VALUES OF BODY COMPOSITION

Balance measurements are very simple in principle; for any component, one measures intake and excretion, the difference is the amount retained or lost by the body. If intake is greater than excretion there is retention or positive balance; if intake is less than excretion, there is loss or negative balance; if intake and excretion are equal, the subject is in zero balance or just "in balance."

In practice, accurate balance measurements are difficult to achieve. All intake must be analyzed and measured. This is very difficult for normal oral diets. It requires maintenance of a stock of reasonably uniform foods, such as meats, bread, vegetables, cereals, desserts, milk and fats. Portions must be weighed before and after cooking and uneaten parts must be reweighed. Spillage and loss of food in dirty containers must be minimized and estimated. For N balance, analysis of both food and excretion is traditionally performed by the Kjeldahl procedure, which involves digestion to ammonia with concentrated sulfuric acid together with a catalyst such as selenium or mercury, and subsequent determination of the NH_3 by distillation and titration, or by colorimetric methods. A procedure which is frequently used is that of the Association of Official Agricultural Chemists (4). This gives very accurate values for N and is relatively simple to perform. Chemical luminescence techniques for measuring total N have recently been introduced (5). They are much faster than and as reliable as Kjeldahl procedures. By contrast to N analysis, methods of analysis of foods for carbohydrate and fat are more tedious and less accurate. Because of the difficulty of working with a large variety of foods, many investigators simplify the diet to only a few uniform constituents. This is reasonable for studies using subjects who are motivated, by pay or otherwise, to accept the discomfort of a monotonous diet, but is not suitable for study of the general population, or in particular of hospitalized patients. Nitrogen balance measurements in patients are greatly simplified by use of parenteral or commercially prepared, chemically defined enteral diets. For many purposes the values listed by the manufacturer are sufficiently accurate. Where greater accuracy is required, analysis of several samples from each lot number is sufficient. In our experience, analysis of amino acid solutions gives values somewhat higher but within 5% of reported values, while analysis of dextrose solutions was within 1% (6).

Quantitative collection of all excreta is also necessary for accurate balance measurements. For N, these include urine, stool, drainages, and integumental and miscellaneous losses (blood, semen, saliva, tears, etc.). Collection of excreta usually requires a specialized research setting with adequate personnel. Even collection of 24-hour urines is surprisingly difficult in a clinical setting. While accurate urine samples may be obtained in specialized units, such as the ICU, this is only possible if all personnel, from the director down, are thoroughly convinced of the importance of such collections.

Complete collection of integumental losses has been performed in only a few laboratories and is not feasible with sick patients, even under the best of conditions. For sedentary individuals on normal diets these losses are about 0.5 g N per day (7). They may increase to 1 g N or more with very high N intakes (8), and even higher with sweating. For most clinical purposes use of a constant value of 0.5 g N for integumental and miscellaneous losses (other than blood) is satisfactory. A very widespread practice for monitoring patients is to measure 24-hour urinary urea excretion, and to add a constant, or multiply by a constant, in order to account for all other excreted N (9–12). As pointed out above, it is essential, for this procedure to be useful, that accurate collection of 24-hour urine is ensured. If this is not possible, the results are meaningless. Even with accurate urine collections, use of a single factor limits the usefulness of the method. A recent report based on a retrospective review of 260 patients and 37 normal subjects, fed intravenously, gives values for nitrogen other than urinary urea N for different disease states, normal, malnourished, postoperative, septic, and accidentally injured, and for the added effects of diarrhea and drainages (13). With this addition, limited to subjects receiving intravenous nutrition, this procedure is satisfactory for clinical monitoring of severely ill patients who require nutritional support. It also may be useful in some types of research studies where N balance is not the major subject of investigation.

For most research purposes, particularly when N balance is central to the study, it is essential to measure the N content of all excreta except for integumental losses for which a reasonable estimate can be provided. It is also important to measure creatinine excretion as a check that urinary collections are complete. In normal subjects creatinine excretion is very constant and closely related to muscle mass. Therefore variation in measured creatinine excretion indicates inadequate urine collection. In sick patients creatinine excretion is more variable. This is particularly true for critically ill patients with extensive muscle damage. Nevertheless, for most sick patients, daily measurement of creatinine is still useful. Moreover, urinary creatinine excretion expressed as the creatinine height index (CHI), which is the ratio (as %) of observed to predicted value based on sex and height, is an excellent index of the extent of nutritional depletion (14). In addition, urinary urea should be determined as a check on urine sample handling and the value for total urinary N. Normally urea accounts for 60% to 95% of urinary N. Values much outside this range indicate errors in sample handling or analysis. Blood urea N should also be measured every day or every second day, since large changes in body urea will require a correction for accumulation or loss of urea (6). This is because N balance is assumed to indicate changes in body protein only. While accurate determination of N excretion would be useful for clinical monitoring, it is very expensive and results are not usually available for many days or weeks; therefore, it is not recommended.

Daily balance of Na and K are potentially useful both for clinical monitoring and for research. Sodium balance represents changes in volume of extracellular fluid; K balance represents changes in intracellular fluid or in body cell mass. As with N balance, accurate determination of electrolyte balances depends on accurate measurements of intake and of all forms of excretion. Substantial amounts of Na and K are excreted in stool and drainages. For research purposes these must be measured. If only urinary measurements are made, for clinical purposes, the amount expected in stool and drainages needs to be kept in mind. As with N there are substantial integumental losses of Na and K. Indirect estimates, made by comparing water balance to electrolyte balance, suggest that integumental electrolyte losses in hospitalized patients average in the neighborhood of 25-40 mEq per day (15-17).

Critique of Balance Methods

There is a general tendency of balance methods to give too positive results. Intake is usually overestimated, since all that is measured may not be eaten, some being lost in dirty containers, or spilled. Errors in measuring excreta tend to underestimate output due to sample losses and failure to collect some types of excreta. As a result there is a tendency in all balance measurements toward overly positive values. One study of adult subjects over 5- to 7-month periods found an average positive N balance of approximately 1 g per day although weight remained stable (18). It seems highly improbable that over a 7-month period, there could be an increment of 210 g N, equivalent to an 18% increase in body cell mass, with no change in body weight. Even so, errors of this magnitude, as long as they are reasonably constant, do not render the N balance method useless, although the possibility of such errors must be kept in mind in experimental design and in interpretation of results. More disturbing have been suggestions that the size of error in N balance is proportional to N intake. If this is true to an appreciable extent, it would be impossible to measure the effect of increasing N intake on N retention using the N balance method. Hegsted (19) compared a number of studies in normal adults. He found as to be expected that below minimal N requirements there was a good correlation between N intake and N balance and that about 80% of any increase in N intake was retained (Figure 3.1). However, above minimal requirements, there was also a good correlation between balance and intake with positive N balance accounting for 20% of the increase in N intake. It is generally accepted that normal adults who neither gain or lose weight must be in zero N balance; therefore, this positive N balance comprising 20% of additional N intake was interpreted as due to unknown errors of the N balance method. Analysis of the individual studies shows this interpretation to be at best only partially true. One key study (20) showed an average N balance of 2 g per day in young men with a daily N intake of 13 g who did not gain weight over several months. However, integumental losses were not measured or estimated. Since the men spent about one hour per day in active physical exercise, their integumental losses, including sweat, could easily have accounted for this 2 g discrepancy. More recently, Oddoye and Margen (8) using very careful techniques, including measurements of integumental losses, found zero N balance over 57 days in young men in weight balance who received 12 g N per day, but that N balance increased by 1.7 g per day when intake was raised to 36 g N per day. Thus 7% of the added N intake appeared to be retained over a 53-day period. This is less than the 20% of Hegsted, but still appreciable. With the advent of neutron activation equipment, which can measure total body N content with an accuracy of about 2%, it should be possible to repeat the experiment of Oddoye and Margen, and determine whether this apparent accumulation of N is real or represents an unknown error in N balance methodology.

A possible source of such an error might be conversion of amino N to nitrogen gas (N_2) in the body and expiration via the lungs. That this may occur has been repeatedly suggested since 1839 or earlier (1). Krogh (21), in 1906, concluded from careful experiments that if there was any net expiration of N_2 in mice it was within experimental error and less than 0.01 percent of the volume of absorbed O_2. Extrapolated to humans, this would account at most for 40 mg N per day, well below the limits of accuracy of the best N balance techniques. Reports of substantial excretion of N_2 by the lungs, as measured by the difference in

D. M. HEGSTED

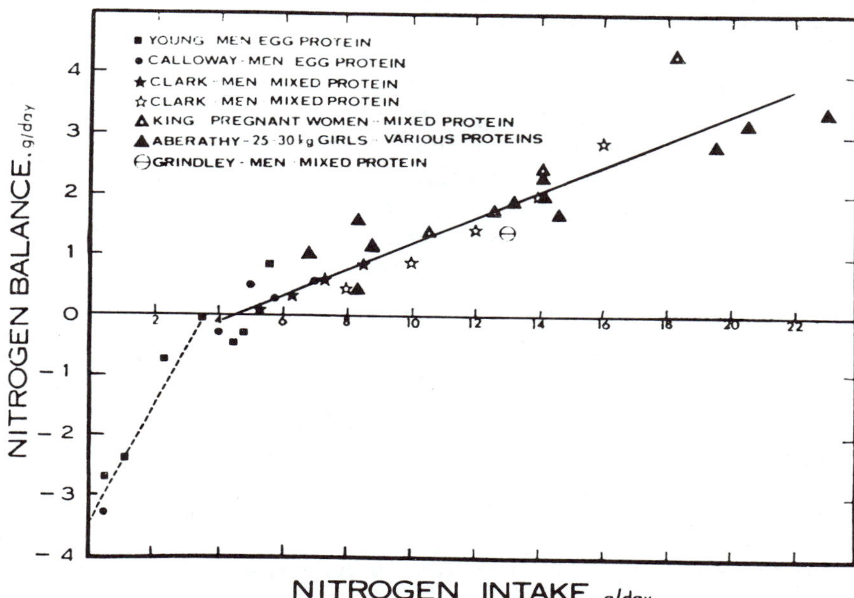

Figure 3.1. Reproduced from Hegsted M: Balance studies. *J Nutr* 106:307-361, 1976, with permission from the *Journal of Nutrition*. Relation between N balance and N intake in adults. Data compiled from various sources.

N_2 contents of expired and inspired air, have continued to appear since Krogh's studies. Rates as high as 128 ml N_2 per min, corresponding to 160 mg N per minute or 230 g N per day, have been claimed (22). Leaving such apparently preposterous results aside, there does appear to be evidence of net expiration of N_2 by the lungs. But if so, the major source appears to be N_2 absorbed through the skin. Muysers et al. (23) placed human subjects in a nitrogen-free atmosphere for 24 hours, reducing N_2 expiration from 2.5 to 0.5 ml per minute. However, even 0.5 ml N_2 per min, if it truly represents endogenous N_2 production, is an appreciable amount, corresponding to 0.9 g N per day. Rosenberg (24) measured arterial-venous concentration differences of N_2 across the lungs in unanesthetized dogs either fasting or after protein meals, and found very small differences, less than 1 microliter N_2 per liter of blood. Extrapolated to a human subject with a cardiac output of 5 liters per min, this corresponds to less than 0.005 ml N_2 per min, less than 1% of the 0.5 ml found by Muysers. To some extent these differences may be due to methodology, measurement of respiratory as opposed to blood gases. Furthermore it is possible that if Muysers experiment in a N_2-free atmosphere had been continued another 24 hours the value for N_2 may have decreased further. Although there are some questions still unresolved, it does not seem likely that conversion of amino N to N_2 in the body accounts for more than a negligible fraction of total N excretion. This is important not only to N balance studies, but also to respiratory measurements since almost all methods for measuring O_2 consumption and CO_2 production assume, based originally on Krogh's experiments, that the amounts of N_2 in contents of inspired and expired air are equal.

Direct Measurements of Body Composition

A variety of techniques are available for measuring absolute values of various body components. These include anthropomorphic measurements, underwater weighing, electrical conductance, indicator dilution methods, whole body counting of ^{40}K, and neutron activation.

Anthropomorphic Measurements

Measurements of weight and height are essential for interpretation of other body composition measurements. In addition, measurements of skin-fold thickness and limb circumference at various locations can be used to estimate the amount of body fat and lean body mass. (25-28). The normal range of values for LBM, for given height, age, and sex, is about ± 10%. The accuracy of estimates of LBM from anthropomorphic measurements is also about ± 10%. Loss of BCM or LBM is the most important indicator of protein calorie malnutrition. However, unless anthropomorphic measurements were made prior to the onset of malnutrition, estimates of the extent of loss may easily be off by 15% of total LBM. A recent 15% loss of LBM indicates moderately severe malnutrition. However, anthropomorphic measurements might indicate as little as no loss or as much as 30%, constituting severe malnutrition. Anthropomorphic measurements are much more useful in following changes in a single subject, since the errors of distribution and many of the errors of measurement cancel out in repeated measures.

Density and Electrical Conductance

The assumptions of underwater weighing are that fat and lean body mass have invariant densities, and that residual lung air volume can be accurately estimated. The subject is weighed in air and underwater to determine density; the weight and density are corrected for residual air volume, and the amounts of fat and LBM are calculated based on assumed invariant densities (2, 29). This method is quite useful and accurate for normal subjects, but because of the underwater weighing, cannot be used with sick patients.

Electrical conductance is widely used in the meat industry to determine fat and LBM. Recently apparatus has been introduced to make similar measurements in people (30). This is readily applicable to sick patients, and is probably more precise and reproducible than the density method.

Indicator Dilution Methods

Indicator dilution methods have been the most widely used methods for measuring body composition and have been extensively reviewed (3, 31). The principle is very simple. A known amount of indicator is administered, usually as a single bolus given intravenously or orally. Time is allowed for equilibration, the amount of excreted material during this time is measured, and the concentration of indicator is then measured, usually in blood, but sometimes in other fluids such as saliva. The amount of indicator in the body, dose (D) minus that excreted (E), is divided by the concentration (C) to give the space (S) of distribution:

$$S = (D - E) / C \tag{1}$$

In practice, the measurements and calculations may be more complicated. Some indicators may equilibrate with one pool or compartment and more slowly with a second. An example is the use of dyes which bind to serum albumin, or of radioiodinated serum albumin (RISA), to measure plasma volume. Equilibration within the vascular bed is rapid, less than 5 minutes. But serum albumin equilibrates slowly between intra- and extravascular spaces. Therefore concentration measurements are made at 5, 10, and 20 minutes and extrapolated to zero time to obtain the plasma volume (32). Similar considerations are involved when radioactive sulfate is used to measure extracellular water (ECW). Although concentrations of free $^{35}SO_4^{=}$ in intracellular fluid are negligible, $^{35}SO_4^{=}$ is metabolized. Therefore, repeated measurements of concentration must be made and extrapolated to zero time. Values for ECW measured with $^{35}SO_4^{=}$ in this way are different from those obtained with indicators such as $^{22}Na^{+}$ or $^{82}Br^{-}$ which are not metabolized. The $^{35}SO_4^{=}$ space, which has been termed the "functional" extracellular space, was found to contract postoperatively (33), whereas, measured with other indicators, ECW is found to expand postoperatively. Corrections for Donnan equilibrium must be made when using ionized indicators.

Frequently, equilibration of the indicator may take longer in sick patients than in normal subjects. It may be necessary, in such instances, to demonstrate that equilibration has been achieved by taking multiple samples.

Some Frequently Used Indicators

Properties for an indicator are: (*a*) that it distributes itself approximately within a definable compartment, such as plasma, ECW, or total body water (TBW); (*b*) that it not be a normal constituent of that space, otherwise the total amount in the space is not known; and (*c*) its concentration in blood or other fluid samples should be readily determinable. Before the discovery of isotopes, substances with these properties were few. Thiocyanate, which is nontoxic and not present in appreciable amounts, was used for ECW, the drug antipyrine was used for total body water, and the dye Evans blue was used for plasma volume. The discovery of isotopes provided a variety of new indicators since the isotopic forms of normal body constituents could be used. Deuterium- and tritium-labeled water have been extensively used for measuring total body water (3, 32, 34). The anions $^{82}Br^-$, and $^{35}SO_4^=$ have been used for ECW (3, 32, 33). The cations $^{22}Na^+$ and $^{42}K^+$ have been used to measure extracellular and intracellular spaces, respectively (3, 29, 34). Bone contains Na^+ and K^+; however, these cations in bone exchange only slowly with the aqueous phase. It is possible, therefore, to measure the exchangeable sodium (Na^+_e) and potassium (K^+_e) which are in solution, without appreciable error due to bone cations. While $^{42}K^+$ gives good results in normal subjects, it takes longer to equilibrate in sick patients, and since its half-life is very short, 12.4 hours, by the time it has equilibrated in 3 days, the amount of radioactivity may be too low to measure (32, 34). Shizgal and colleagues (34) have devised an ingenious method to measure K^+_e indirectly through measurements of Na^+_e, total body water and the Na^+ and K^+ concentrations in plasma. Since all tissues are in osmotic equilibrium, and since Na^+ and K^+ provide the bulk of the cation components, the whole body content of the sum of K^+ and Na^+ is obtained by multiplying their concentrations in plasma (meq/liter H_2O) by total body water (liters) measured with ^3H_2O. Exchangeable sodium is measured with $^{22}Na^+$ and K^+_e is obtained by difference.

Neutron Activation, ^{40}K and Whole Body Counting

There are two methods for determining body constituents involving whole body counting. One takes advantage of the natural occurrence of a radioactive isotope of potassium, ^{40}K. Since the specific activity of ^{40}K is constant, measuring the total body radioactivity gives a direct measurement of whole body potassium. A more general method involves prior irradiation with neutrons obtained from a cyclotron or in more available form from a portable plutonium beryllium source. The latter instrument can be installed at an approximate cost of $25,000. The neutrons can activate a number of elements, including Na, Cl, Ca, P and N. Each of these has a characteristic gamma ray spectrum which can be measured. Reproducibility of the method is of the order of 2% or less, which compares favorably with isotope dilution methods which have a reproducibility of the order of 5% or more (32).

INTERPRETATION OF BODY COMPOSITION MEASUREMENTS

Deviations from Normal

Normal tables and regression equations for body composition have been compiled by Moore et al. (3). However, one of the problems in comparing observed values to these tables is the great variability within the normal population. The coefficient of variation for most measurements is about 10%, which means that about one-third of normal subjects will differ from mean values by more than this. Therefore, measurements in patients are not necessarily abnormal unless they differ from the predicted value by substantially more than 10%. Where the patient's own normal or usual value is known, as is usually the case with weight or height, a difference of 10% may be very significant. However, it is rare that normal values of other parameters, such as ECW, TBW, intracellular water (ICW), blood volume (BV), LBM, or BCM have been measured in any one individual. One measurement, ECW/ICW, shows little variation in the normal population (32, 35) and is very useful in diagnosing changes in extracellular fluid which occur with malnutrition or inflammatory disease.

Body Composition Changes

Changes in body composition are often of greater interest than the absolute values. These can be obtained by balance procedures, or by serial direct measurements. With the latter, it is important to keep in mind that small errors in absolute values are greatly magnified by taking the difference in successive measurements. Thus, if there is a 5% error in measuring K_e, and K_e increases by 7% in two weeks, there will be a 100% error in estimating that 7% increase. For changes of less than 10% in body compartments, balance methods are probably more suitable (36). Nevertheless, these measurement errors tend to cancel out, and with reasonable numbers of subjects, accurate mean values may be obtained in studies of short duration. An important advantage of neutron activation analysis is that the reproducibility is better, of the order of 1% to 2%, than with isotope dilution procedures. Furthermore, the analytical procedures, once the apparatus is installed, are much quicker and simpler. Thus neutron activation analysis, although initially expensive, has great promise for clinical studies of body composition changes, and may be suitable for following short-term changes in individuals.

Another problem in interpretation of body composition changes occurs in extrapolating from the actual measurements to conceptual compartments, such as body cell mass, extracellular water, body fat, blood volume, and total body water. What is actually measured is a space of distribution of an indicator, a total amount of an element, skin-fold thickness, and the like. Many assumptions and approximations are involved in converting these measurements to estimates of the size or change in size of body compartments. Furthermore, many of the assumptions are unique to specific methods and differ between methods. Thus, as noted above, the functional ECW measured with $^{35}SO_4^{=}$ contracts during critical illness, whereas the total ECW measured with $^{22}Na^+$ or $^{82}Br^-$ expands under the same conditions. Changes in N, K^+, or intracellular water (measured as the difference between TBW and ECW) all indicate changes in body cell mass. However, the composition of body cell mass changes in illness. In particular, K^+ tends to be lost more rapidly than N under a variety of circumstances (37-40), and as a corollary, during nutritional repletion, K^+ is often gained more rapidly than N (16). Under some circumstances there may be a simultaneous gain in N and loss in K^+, or vice versa. Under other conditions, K^+ and N are lost or gained in constant proportions (41-43). Therefore, if these measurements are interpreted simplistically, the quantity of BCM gained or lost will depend on the method used. Interpreted properly, simultaneous measurements of several components of BCM can provide important information as to the changes in composition of BCM during critical illness, nutritional depletion, or nutritional repletion.

INTERRELATION BETWEEN NITROGEN BALANCE AND NITROGEN AND ENERGY INTAKE

To a first approximation, N balance is dependent on both N and energy intake. If either is insufficient there will be net loss of N or negative N balance. Excess energy intake causes a positive N balance. These statements presuppose an adequate supply of all other essential nutrients, particularly those which are important intracellular constituents. This is illustrated by a study of Rudman et al. (43) of malnourished patients given TPN (Figure 3.2). On a complete diet they were in marked positive balance of both N and K. Complete removal of N, K, or P from the diet, all intracellular constituents, caused negative N and K balances on the first day. Removal of Na, an extracellular constituent, also decreased N and K balances, which nevertheless remained slightly positive. We may note the very similar changes in K and N balance under these conditions, both of which serve as indices of body cell mass.

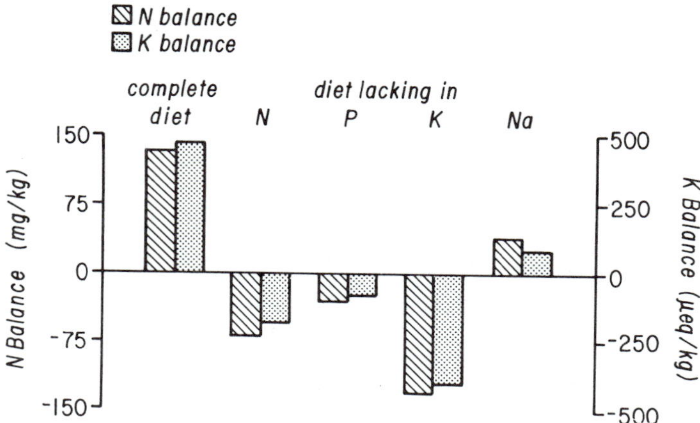

Figure 3.2. Data of Rudman et al. (43). Reproduced from Elwyn DH: Nutritional requirements of adult surgical patients. *Crit Care Med*8:9-20, 1980, with permission of *Critical Care Medicine.* Effects on N and K balances of eliminating essential nutrients from intravenous diets of malnourished patients.

Adults

Interrelations of N and energy intake and N balance in normal subjects, from a number of studies (Figures 3.3 and 3.4), have been summarized by Calloway and Spector (44). The data in Figure 3.3 show N balance as a function of energy intake at constant values of N intake; the same data are presented in Figure 3.4, showing N balance as a function of N intake at constant values of energy intake. Increasing either N or energy intake increases N balance until the other factor becomes limiting. Thus, at an N intake of zero, increasing energy intake from zero to 700 kcal day^{-1} increases N balance from -12 to -7 g day^{-1}; but further increases in energy intake, up to 3000 kcal per day, have no additional effect (Figure 3.3). If N intake is increased to 1.1 g per day, N balance can be further increased by raising energy intake to 1000 kcal day^{-1}. When both energy and N intake reach minimal requirements, N balance reaches zero.

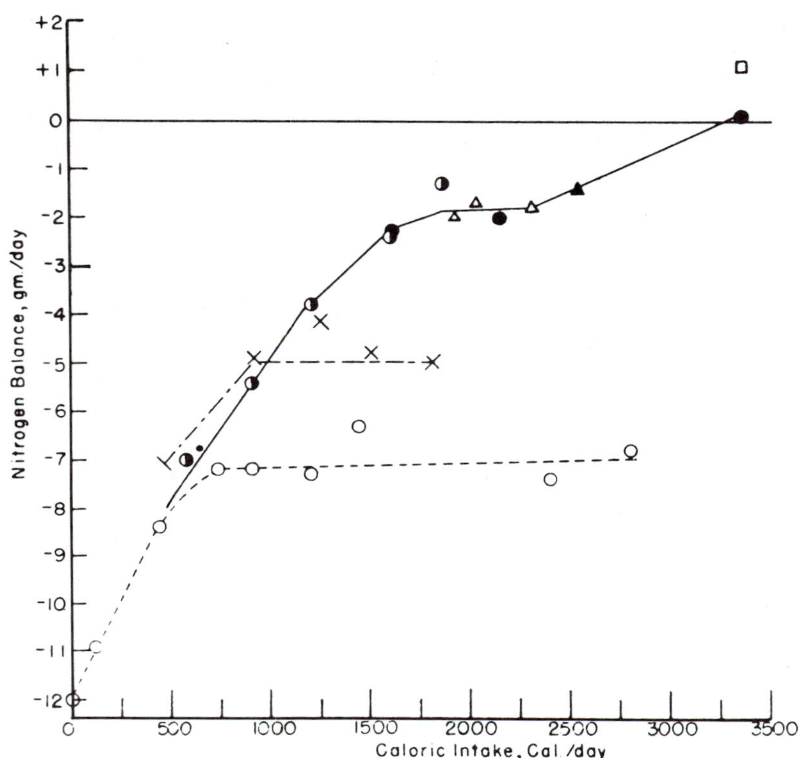

Figure 3.3. Reproduced from Calloway DH and Spector N: Nitrogen balance as related to caloric and protein intake in young men. *Am J Clin Nutr* 2:405-412, 1959, with permission from the *American Journal of Clinical Nutrition.* N balance at various levels of energy intake in normal young men. ○ protein-free, followed by N intake, g day^{-1}: / 1.0-1.9, **X** 2.4-5.0, ◐ 5.4-7.7, ● 8.1-9.7, △ 10.4-11.7, ▲ 12.4, □ 15.4.

When energy intakes exceed energy requirements and energy balance is positive, N balance continues to increase with increasing intake. However, at zero energy balance further increases in N intake will cause only a transient positive N balance in well-nourished adults, and after 3 or 4 days N balance will return to zero. This transient positive N balance results in retention of what has been called "labile protein," which is lost when N intake is returned to the previous level (45, 46). This transient deposition of protein occurs because changes in urinary excretion of N lag behind changes in intake. When N intake is abruptly increased in subjects who are at zero N balance, urinary N excretion rises grad-

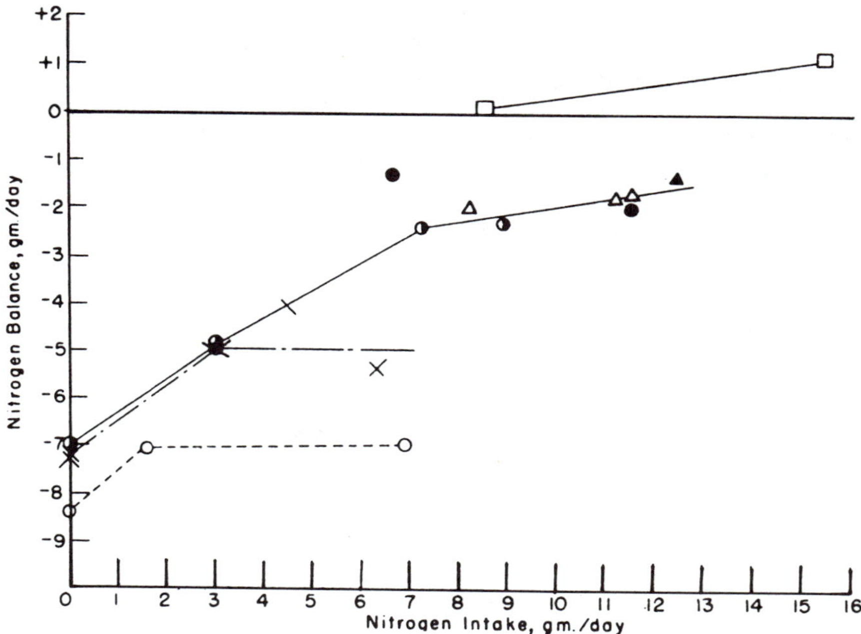

Figure 3.4. Reproduced from Calloway DH and Spector N: Nitrogen balance as related to caloric and protein intake in young men. *Am J Clin Nutr* 2:405-412, 1959, with permission from the *American Journal of Clinical Nutrition.* N balance at various levels of N intake in normal young men. Energy intake, kcal day^{-1}: ○400-575, **X** 750-1100, \ 1200-1430, ◑1400-1650, ● 1800-1975, △ 2025-2350, ▲ 2530, □ 3350.

ually so that there is a temporary positive N balance (Figure 3.5). After 4 days, excretion catches up to intake and the subject returns to zero balance. With an abrupt decrease in N intake, the reverse occurs, there is a transient period of negative N balance, and if N intake is still above minimum requirements, a return to zero N balance after 4 days (Figure 3.5). Except for these transient increases or decreases, it is generally accepted that adult human subjects, who are in zero energy balance and therefore in zero weight balance, must necessarily be in zero N balance, irrespective of the level of N intake. If this were not true, and if N balance were positive at high N intakes, then we would have the situation in which there would be no change in the size of body compartments, no change in weight, but a continuous increase in the N content of lean body mass. At a positive N balance of 1 g per day, the N content of LBM would double in 5 years. Since N represents protein, this corresponds to an increase in the protein content of LBM from 20% to 40% and is patently absurd. The careful studies of Oddoye and Margen (8) confirm this concept for normal protein intakes up to 12 g per day. However, when they fed 36 g N per day they found a small positive balance of 1.3 g/day. As discussed above, this appears to be due to unknown errors in N balance methods, although it is not inconceivable that a positive balance might persist for the 57 days of their experiment. It is inconceivable that this could continue indefinitely.

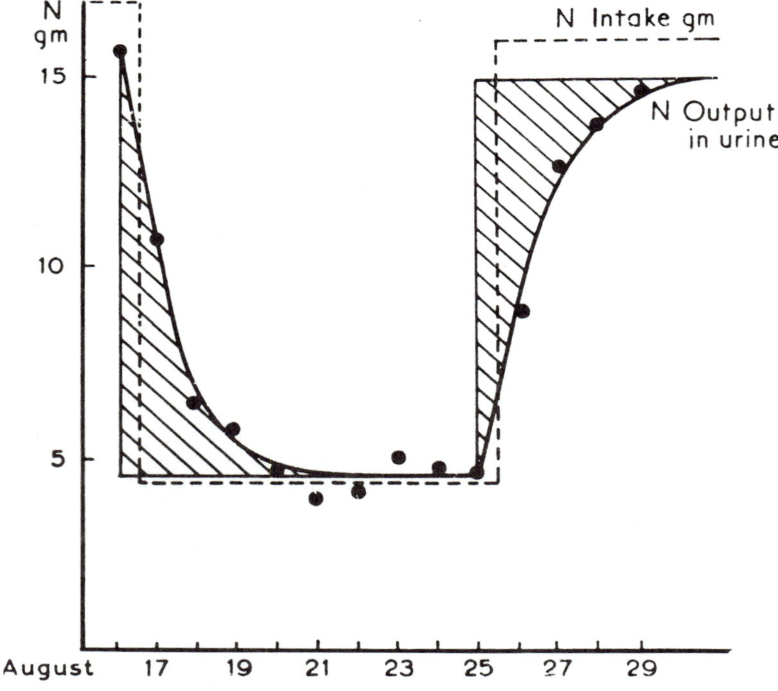

Figure 3.5. Data of Martin and Robison (45). Reproduced from Munro HN: General aspects of the regulation of protein metabolism by diet and hormones. In Munro HN, Allison JB (eds): *Mammalian Protein Metabolism.* New York, Academic Press, 1964, Vol.1, pp 382–482, with permission of Academic Press. Relations between N intake, urea excretion, and N balance after an abrupt decrease or increase in N intake.

Minimum and Recommended Requirements of Protein

Requirements of protein can be measured by varying protein intake with a constant energy intake equal to expenditure. Below N requirements the subject will be in negative balance; at or above N requirements

PM

Fri Mar 21 1997

PAGING SLIP - The item/s listed below has been requested. Go to the stacks and pull it.

Ogg Science Library
Math/Science Bldg, Room 308
BGSU
Bowling Green, Ohio 43403

Science Stacks
CALL NO: QP176.E541989
AUTHOR:
Energy metabolism, indirect calorim
BARCODE: A11309582291
REC NO: i18839198
PICKUP AT: Health Sci

JOSEPH BURTON WILLIAMS
ZOOLOGY
OVALWOOD
1680 UNIVERSITY DR
MANSFIELD CAMPUS
INSTITUTION: Ohio State University
PATRON TYPE: ohlnk faculty

the subject will be in zero N balance. The minimum requirement is that which first brings the subject into N balance. This will vary with weight, sex, energy expenditure, and source of dietary protein. In addition, there is substantial individual variability. Minimum requirements of 18 mg protein per kcal of basal metabolism for women and 19 for men have been estimated for the U. S. population, based on a protein intake with a biological value of 100% (47). The National Research Council has used a value of 20 mg protein per kcal basal metabolic rate for both men and women (48). To this they add 30% for individual variability, and divide by 0.7 assuming the average biological value of dietary protein to be 70%. This gives a recommended value of 37 mg protein per basal kcal. For a 70-kg reference man with a basal energy expenditure of 1750 kcal (7300 kJ) per day, the average minimum requirement is 35 g protein per day (5.6 g N), or 0.05 g protein per kg per day (80 mg N). In order to ensure that all individuals with higher than average minimum requirements receive enough, the recommended minimum intake is 65 g protein per day (10.4 g N), or 0.93 g protein per kg per day (148 mg N). Thus for most individuals, recommended intakes are substantially higher than minimum requirements would be if they were measured in that individual.

It is not generally appreciated that the minimum requirement is also affected by the nonprotein composition of the diet, and by other factors as well. The normal U. S. diet contains substantial amounts of both carbohydrate and fat. By contrast, a meat diet, as eaten by some peoples including the Eskimo, contains essentially no carbohydrate. Minimum requirements on a carbohydrate-free diet, discussed in more detail below, have been estimated as lying between 85 and 155 g protein, or 13.6-24.8 g N per day (49), more than twice the minimum requirements on a normal Western diet.

It seems probable that adaptation to lower intakes reduces requirements of protein as well as other essential nutrients. While the requirements in other affluent countries may be very similar to those in the U. S., requirements in less affluent societies may be substantially smaller. The World Health Organization's recommended protein requirements are 0.57 g per kg per day (91 mg N) for men and 0.53 g per kg per day (84 mg N) for women, about 45% below the U. S. recommendation (50). Injury, sepsis, and probably other diseases appear to cause an increase in minimal N requirements. These will be discussed in more detail below.

EFFECTS OF UNDER AND OVER NUTRITION.

Increasing energy intake above expenditure causes deposition of fat in adipose tissue which can lead, in time, to obesity. Protein deposition resulting in an increase in lean body mass is associated with this fat in the rough proportion of 1/2 part LBM to 1 part of fat (Table 3.1). This protein is probably not deposited in adipose tissue to any appreciable extent, but rather in other tissues, including blood vessels and muscle to support the extra weight. While LBM contributes a significant part of the weight gain, it accounts for only a negligible portion of the stored energy (Table 3.1). The ratio of LBM: fat, lost or gained, is very similar for normal men with energy intakes just below or just above requirements, or for malnourished surgical patients during repletion with hypercaloric TPN. Thus, energy intakes above requirements, unlike the effect of high N intakes, will cause a positive N balance which continues indefinitely. Furthermore, with energy intakes ranging from about 20% below energy expenditure to greatly in excess of energy expenditure the ratio of LBM: fat is fairly constant and close to 0.5, although it will vary depending on the ratio of energy to N in the diet. Thus the major component gained in obesity, or lost during starvation at marginally low intakes, is fat. When energy intake is much lower than expenditure, the ratio of LBM to fat lost increases markedly. Keys et al. (2) studied physically active young men

Table 3.1.
Effects of Various Dietary Conditions on the Ratio of Gain or Loss of Body Cell Mass to Fat.

Dietary Condition	Ratio of Loss or Gain of BCM	Ratio of Loss or Gain of Fat	Energy Loss due to BCM Loss	Reference
	kg:kg	kcal:kcal kJ:kJ	% of total	
Normal men-gross overfeeding	0.59	0.05	5	51
Normal men—close to energy balance	0.35-0.51	0.03-0.04	3-4	52
Depleted patients—hypercaloric TPN	0.54	0.04	4	53
Normal men—intake = 1/2 requirement				
first 12 weeks	1.8	0.14	12	2
second 12 weeks	1.3	0.10	9	2
Fasting 31 days—normal man	2.6	0.21	17	41
Elective operation				
-men	2.6	0.21	17	54
-women	1.7	0.13	12	54
Major injury—men	4.5	0.36	26	55

who were fed for 24 weeks at a mean energy intake of 1570 kcal (6570 kJ) day^{-1}, 45% of their initial energy expenditure (Figure 3.6). Weight loss was 12.6 kg in the first 12 weeks, comprising 8.0 kg of body cell mass and 4.6 kg fat, a ratio of 1.8:1 (Table 3.1). With loss of weight, and particularly BCM, energy expenditure decreased and during the second 12 weeks, weight loss was only 4.3 kg, 2.4 kg BCM and 1.9 kg fat, for a ratio of 1.3 to 1. By 24 weeks energy expenditure had been reduced to 45% of initial and, therefore, was now equal to intake. As a result there was no further loss of weight. Over the 24 weeks there was a 25% reduction in weight and a 26% reduction in BCM, so that BCM as a percentage of body weight remained almost constant. For fat there was a 67% loss in 24 weeks, proportionally much more than for BCM. The 55% loss in energy expenditure was due to two main components: (*a*) a reduction in BCM, which would account for a decrease of 26%, less than one-half the reduction in total energy expenditure; and (*b*) a larger reduction in energy expenditure for activity, reflecting a great decrease in the capacity of these men to perform physical work. While, in a sense, these men were able to adapt to this reduced intake, it was only at the expense of substantial loss of functional ability.

It is noteworthy that there were no appreciable changes in extracellular space or in bone solids. This is characteristic of fasting or starvation in the absence of disease. Nevertheless, the relative size of these components increased, so that by the end of 24 weeks extracellular space comprised 34% of body weight, and all subjects manifested pitting edema. An increased ratio of extracellular space to body weight or to BCM is characteristic of protein calorie malnutrition, as well as of disease states such as injury and sepsis (31). However, with sepsis or injury there is an absolute as well as a relative expansion of extracellular space.

For the next 12 weeks the men were restricted to 2900 kcal (12,100 kJ) day^{-1} and were then allowed to eat ad libitum. By 20 weeks, weight had returned to prestarvation levels, due mainly to excess fat deposition, but BCM was still low. It was not until 58 weeks that BCM was completely restored and that body composition had completely returned to normal. This illustrates how much quicker and easier it is to deplete BCM than it is to restore it. Just the opposite to fat which is easier to gain than to lose. Complete fasting is similar to severe partial starvation; however, the ratio of BCM to fat lost is slightly higher (Table 3.1).

Injury and Sepsis

The effects of injury or sepsis, superimposed on starvation, are to increase further the rate of N loss. After elective operation N losses are similar to those during fasting, but these patients are receiving 5% dex-

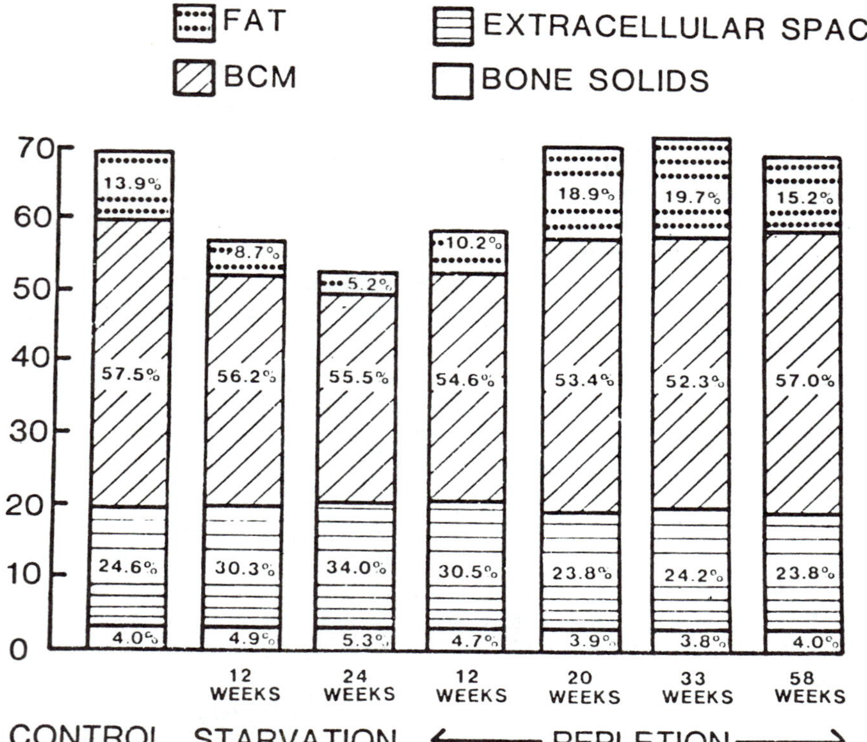

Figure 3.6. Reproduced from Insel J, and Elwyn DH: Body Composition. In Askanazi J, Starker PM, Weissman C (eds): *Fluid and Electrolyte Management in Critical Care.* Boston, Butterworths, 1986, pp 3–37, with permission of Butterworths. Effect of 24 weeks of starvation (45% of energy requirements) followed by 58 weeks of repletion on body composition of active young men. Data adapted from Keyes et al. (2). Control energy requirements were estimated at 3490 kcal (14,600 kJ) day^{-1}. Energy intake was restricted to an average of 2900 kcal (12,130 kJ) day^{-1} for the first 12 weeks of repletion; subsequently the subjects were fed ad libitum.

trose by vein which has a marked N-sparing effect. After accidental injury, N losses can be much greater even with 5% dextrose infusions. Even so, protein losses account for only 26% of energy derived from body stores; fat accounts for 74% (Table 3.1). Since both disease and dietary intake affect N excretion, any comparison of the catabolic effect of different disease states should be done under the same dietary conditions. Such a comparison, for patients receiving 5% dextrose as sole energy source, is shown in Figure 3.7. These data are instances taken from the literature for N excretion of subjects in various conditions; they are not accurately determined average values for any of these states. Nevertheless, they illustrate the large variation in N excretion which can occur, ranging from 27 g day^{-1} in severely burned patients to 2 g day^{-1} in fasted normal subjects. Nitrogen excretion, in the particular group of malnourished patients shown here, was greater than normal, indicating considerable underlying disease, not unusual in patients requiring TPN. In other studies N excretion in malnourished patients has been shown to be less than normal (13). Effects of surgical operation vary considerably with the type of intervention; cystectomy for instance is much more catabolic than is total hip replacement. It is of interest that sepsis, which in other respects may be more stressful than accidental injury, does not have as big an effect on N excretion.

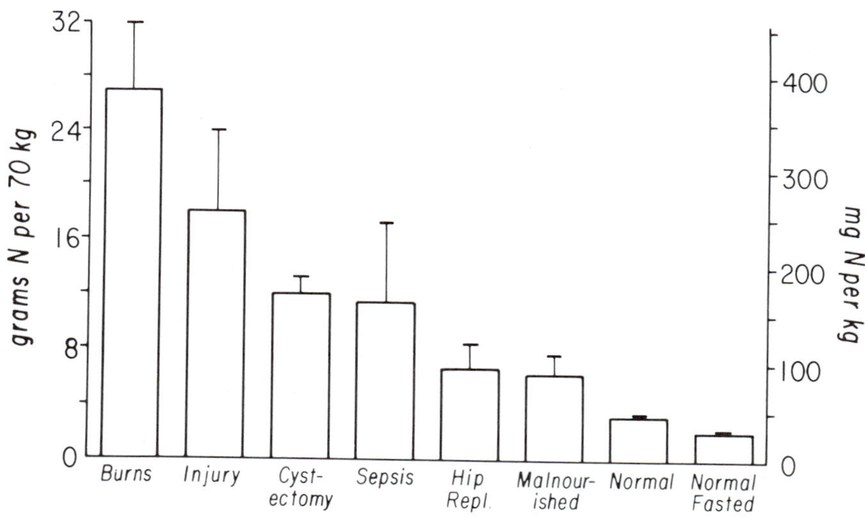

Figure 3.7. Reproduced from Elwyn DH: Protein metabolism and requirements in the critically ill patient. *Crit Care Clin* 3:57-69,1987. With permission of *Critical Care Clinics.* Total N excretion during 5 percent dextrose infusion in burned, injured, septic, or malnourished patients and normal subjects. Mean ± SD. Data compiled from various sources.

Maintenance and Repletion of Body Cell Mass in Hospital Patients

Twenty years ago death from starvation was commonplace in almost all hospitals because the therapeutic tools to prevent it were not available. With development of effective techniques of enteral, and particularly of parenteral, nutrition it is now possible to prevent severe effects of malnutrition in almost all instances. However, compared to oral diets use of enteral and parenteral nutrition places much greater responsibility on the therapist to provide optimum amounts and composition of nutrients. Normal subjects control food intake very accurately through appetite and the physiological functioning of the enteral tract. In parenteral feeding, with complete bypass of the intestine, there are no such controls over nutrient intake and the physician is God. He or she completely controls the amounts of all nutrients, with no feedback from the patient. Enteral feedings by tube or enterostomy lie between. Appetite no longer functions, but intestinal responses, particularly diarrhea, still act to limit intake into the blood if not into the intestine itself. Because the power of the therapist is so complete in enteral and parenteral nutrition, it is important that it be well informed and exercised according to the best available criteria. One of the most important criteria for establishing appropriate amounts to give of carbohydrate, fat, and protein are the quantitative effects of these nutrients on maintenance or repletion of BCM, usually measured in terms of N balance. These effects need to be considered for two types of patients: those with protein calorie malnutrition and those with injury or sepsis.

Malnourished Patients

In malnourished patients, changes in N balance in response to increasing energy intake (Figure 3.8) are similar to those seen in normal subjects (Figure 3.3). At low-carbohydrate intake the response is large, an increase of about 7.5 mg in N balance for each additional kcal of intake (1.8 mg N kJ^{-1}) (Figure 3.8). Above one-half of energy requirements the effect is much smaller, about 1.5 mg N $kcal^{-1}$ (0.36 mg N kJ^{-1}). However, this is the range of intake of interest in treating malnourished patients, since the goals are to restore lost BCM which requires a positive N balance.

A scheme relating N balance in malnourished patients to N intake and energy balance is shown in Figure 3.9, based on data derived from several sources. This scheme illustrates an important difference between malnourished and normal adult subjects in that the former can achieve positive N balance at zero or even negative energy balances. Thus in the range of the experimental values shown, N balance can be increased either by increasing N intake or by increasing energy intake. Furthermore the effects of increasing N and energy intakes are synergistic, increasing both together produces a greater effect than the sum of the effects of increasing each individually. However, the effect on fat

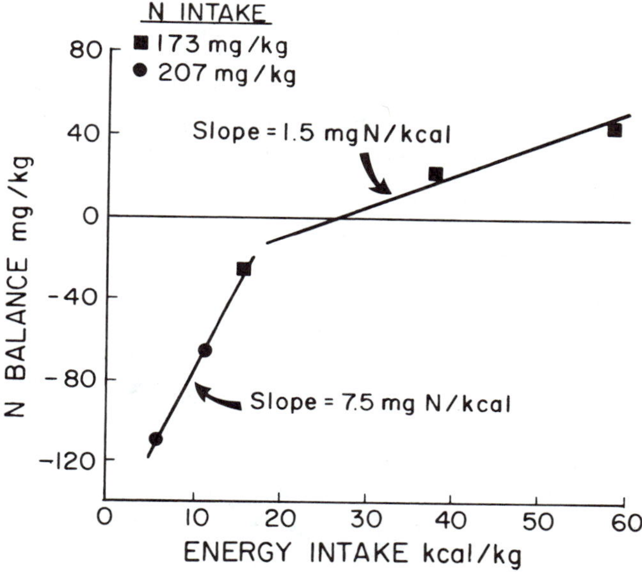

Figure 3.8. Reproduced from Elwyn DH: Nutritional requirements of adult surgical patients. *Crit Care Med* 8:9-20, 1980, with permission of *Critical Care Medicine*. N balance at various levels of energy (glucose) intake in postoperative (●) and depleted (■) patients.

balance and the ratio in which BCM and fat are deposited are very different. Increasing N intake, while maintaining energy balance constant, causes a slight decrease in fat balance. Increasing energy balance, at constant N intake, will markedly increase fat deposition. In principle it is possible to choose energy and N intakes to deposit BCM and fat in any ratio considered desirable. Thus an energy balance of +10 kcal (42 kJ) kg^{-1} (intake of about 40 kcal [167 kJ] kg^{-1}) and N intake of 150 mg kg^{-1}, will deposit new tissue in the ratio of 0.5 parts BCM to 1 part of fat; while an energy balance of +10 kcal kg^{-1} with an N intake of 300 mg kg^{-1} will deposit tissue with a ratio of 2 parts BCM to 1 part of fat. In the first case we have a total calorie to N ratio of 267 to 1; in the second, a ratio of 133 to 1. As discussed above, the composition of acute losses of tissue, taking place over a few weeks to a few months, and often accompanied by injury or sepsis, is in the range of 2-

4 parts BCM to 1 of fat, whereas with chronic losses over many months to years the ratio is closer to 0.5 parts BCM to 1 part of fat (Table 3.1). The amounts of N and energy used to replete malnourished patients should depend, at least in part, on the kind of tissue loss they have experienced. Patients who have undergone chronic starvation, such as those with anorexia nervosa or chronic obstructive pulmonary disease, should be given relatively low N intakes or high calorie to N ratios. Patients with recent acute losses should be given higher N intakes or lower calorie to N ratios. This subject will be discussed in Chapter 7.

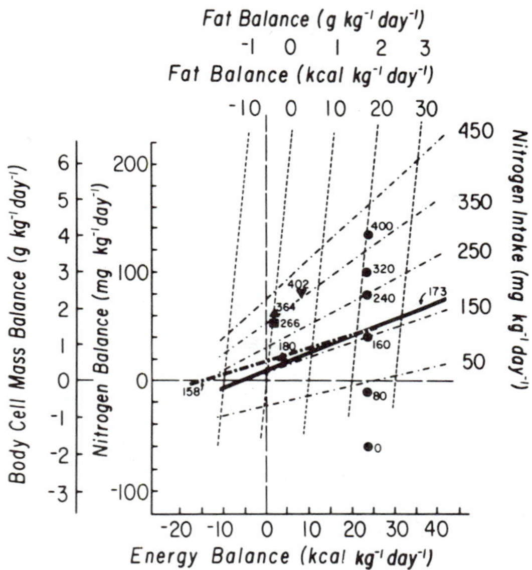

Figure 3.9. The positions of the N intake lines are based on data of Plough et al. (56), Shaw et al. (57), Rudman et al. (43), and Chikenji et al. (6). Solid symbols and heavy lines are experimental data derived from various sources (6,43,53, 57-59). Schematic relations between N balance, or body cell mass balance (y axis), energy balance (x axis), N intake (dotted lines) and fat balance (dashed lines), in malnourished adult patients receiving parenteral nutrition.

Use of this scheme (Figure 3.9) as a guide to amount and composition of diets is greatly facilitated if energy expenditure can be measured rather than estimated from standard equations, since the error in fat deposition will be almost identical to the error in estimating energy expenditure. As discussed in Chapter 5, errors in estimating energy expenditure can be very large in patients who receive artificial nutrition, whether enteral or parenteral. For N balance, errors in estimating energy expenditure are not as important, since the change in N balance with energy balance is relatively small.

A major problem with use of this scheme, as a nutritional guide for malnourished patients, relates to the extreme heterogeneity of malnourished adult patients, many of whom may have substantial underlying disease accompanied by a severe catabolic state, while some may be relatively free of complications. The N requirement for zero N balance at zero energy balance, shown in Figure 3.9, is 120 mg kg^{-1}, whereas for previously fasted normal subjects it is only 40 mg kg^{-1} (Figure 3.7), only one-third as much. On average, this patient population is pretty sick and the variability is very large. The standard deviation for N balance, in the studies from which these data were taken, averaged about 20 mg N $kg^{-1}day^{-1}$. Thus at any given N intake and energy balance, one-sixth of the patients will have an N balance more than 20 mg kg^{-1} less than that shown in Figure 3.9, while another six will be more than 20 mg kg^{-1} higher. Since it is usually not feasible to check the results of nutritional therapy in individual patients by measuring N balance, it may be desirable to increase N intake, above that shown in Figure 3.9, in order to ensure that the sicker patients have a good rate of deposition of BCM.

Nitrogen versus Potassium

Studies in malnourished patients, by Shizgal and Forse (60), of the effects of nutrients on the rate of increase of BCM as measured by changes in exchangeable potassium, show different effects from those obtained with N balance. Increasing N intake from 200 to 400 mg kg^{-1} day^{-1} had a negligible effect in increasing K deposition, in contrast to the marked effects on N balance seen in Figure 3.9. Also, even at high caloric intake, fat had a much smaller effect on K deposition than did carbohydrate. This is in apparent disagreement with a number of studies showing that when carbohydrate comprised 17%-50% of intake, additional fat or carbohydrate had similar effects on N balance (58, 59, 61, 62). In large part these differences can be related to the large amount of K associated with glycogen deposition. When glycogen is deposited in the cell, it is accompanied by 3 g of water for each g of glycogen. This does not change the intracellular concentration of K; therefore, additional K must enter the cell amounting to about 0.5 mEq of K for each g of glycogen. In 8-day studies of the effects of high-carbohydrate TPN (16), it was found that more than 80% of the increase in K balance was associated with glycogen deposition and only 17% with N deposition. In the studies of Shizgal and Forse (60), in which the average period was 2 weeks, the bulk of the increase in K deposition on the low-protein diet would be due to glycogen deposition and, even if it occurred, an increase in K deposition due to increasing N intake might not be statistically significant. Furthermore even if fat and carbohydrate had equal effects on N deposition, glycogen deposition and therefore K deposition would be much greater with carbohydrate than fat.

These differences illustrate the importance of not extrapolating from the effects of nutrients on one component of BCM, such as N, to the effects on any other components, such as K, or vice versa.

Injured and Septic Patients

Injured and septic patients have markedly increased requirements for protein compared to normal subjects, as illustrated in Figure 3.7. However, if not previously malnourished, they respond to increased N intake similarly to normal subjects, in that at zero energy balance they reach a state where additional N intake causes no further increase in N balance. With normal subjects this occurs at zero N balance; with stressed patients it occurs at a negative N balance. This is illustrated for a series of injured and burned patients (63) given energy intakes of 45-50 kcal (188-209 kJ) kg^{-1} day^{-1}.

When N intake was zero they were in very negative balance (Figure 3.10); with increasing N intake up to 200 mg $kg^{-1}day^{-1}$, N balance improved, but further increase in intake had no additional effect. Thus these patients reached a plateau of -3.5 g N per day despite an energy balance well above zero. These data show that minimum requirements for such patients are about 200 mg kg^{-1} day^{-1}, 2-3 times as high as the minimum requirement of 80 for normal subjects, and substantially higher than the 120 for malnourished patients shown in Figure 3.9. However, this minimum does not bring about zero N balance at reasonable energy intakes. In many of these patients it may be possible to achieve zero or positive N balance by increasing energy intakes well above requirements. However this is probably not worthwhile. For previously well-nourished patients who are severely injured or burned, loss of 3 to 4 g N per day for one to two weeks will not cause serious malnutrition. If they have an uncomplicated course, their response to nutrients will improve, and no further N losses will occur. By contrast, if kept on 5% dextrose as sole caloric source, in 10 days they might lose as much as 150 to 250 g N (Figure 3.7), corresponding to 14% to 23% of BCM and become severely malnourished. For such patients the goal should be to minimize losses of BCM; energy should be supplied in amounts equal to or somewhat in excess of expenditure, and N should be given at rates not much in excess of 200 $mg^{-1}day^{-1}$.

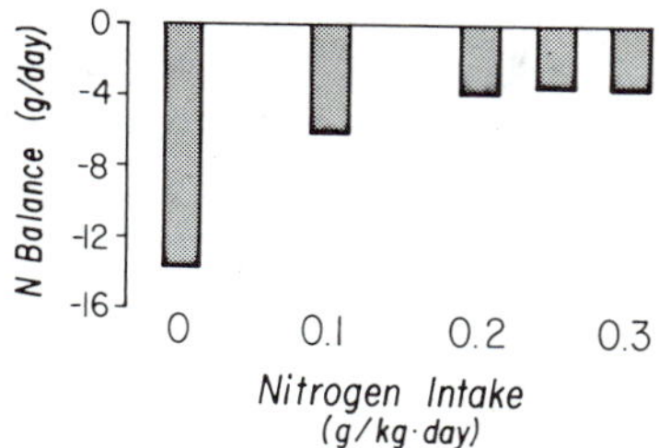

Figure 3.10. Data from Larsson et al. (63). Reproduced from Elwyn DH: Nutritional requirements of stressed patients. In Shoemaker WC (ed): *Textbook of Critical Care Medicine*. In press. With permission of the Society of Critical Care Medicine. Effect of N intake on N balance in patients with severe injury or burns.

Injured or septic patients who are also malnourished differ both in their response to nutrients and in their nutrient requirements. Since they are stressed, their minimum N requirements will be higher than the average for malnourished patients. Since they are malnourished, they will be able to achieve zero or positive N balance by increasing N intake at zero energy balance. If they are not too resistant to nutrition, their energy intake should be enough above expenditure to deposit reasonable amounts of fat, and N intake should be high, up to 400 mg N kg^{-1} day^{-1}, in order to increase BCM at a reasonable rate.

There is a subset of malnourished, stressed patients who are resistant to all nutrients. This includes patients with chronic sepsis and multiple organ failure. These patients remain in negative N balance even though they are severely malnourished and malnutrition severely hampers their treatment. At present we do not have sufficient knowledge to provide adequate nutrition to these patients, and it may be that without improving their acute state, adequate nutrition is not possible.

Carbohydrate and Fat

At low energy intakes the effects of carbohydrate on N balance are much greater than those of fat. Up to about 100 to 150 g the increase in N balance is about 7.5 mg N per kcal (1.8 mg N kJ^{-1} of added carbohydrate, as illustrated in the left-hand portion of Figures 3.3 and 3.8. This effect is not shared by fat. Complete elimination of carbohydrate from the diet increases protein requirements from an average of 35 g protein, 5.6 g N, to somewhere between 85 and 155 g of protein, 14 to 25 g N (49). Above 100 to 150 g, carbohydrate increases N balance by only about 1.5 mg N per added kcal (0.36 mg N kJ^{-1}), and this effect is generally thought to be shared by fat (38). This nitrogen-sparing effect of glucose is related to the metabolism of the brain, which cannot use fat and therefore requires glucose as the almost exclusive source of energy in the fed state. Ketone bodies supplement glucose to a major extent only during starvation. Injured or septic patients may have even higher requirements for carbohydrate for maintenance of protein stores than do normal subjects (64,65).

Other metabolic interrelations of fat and carbohydrate are discussed in Chapter 4.

Amino Acid Composition

Extensive work with animals and humans have shown that optimal amino acid composition not only provides adequate amounts of each essential amino acid but also provides a balanced mixture of nonessential amino acids (66). With oral feeding this is provided by eating proteins of high biological value or mixtures of proteins whose deficiencies cancel out each other. Amino acid composition is also not a problem for enteral feeding since high quality proteins are readily available. Some problems occur with parenteral feeding since:(*a*) two semi-essential amino acids, tyrosine and cystine, are quite insoluble; (*b*) glutamine, which is secreted in large amounts by the intestine into portal blood, is unstable in solution; and (*c*) glutamic and aspartic acids, which are major constituents of proteins, are normally not absorbed as such into portal blood; rather they are converted mainly to alanine and glutamine; furthermore at high blood concentrations they can be toxic. However, none of these potential problems seem to interfere seriously with the ability of intravenous crystalline amino acid preparations to restore lost protein or maintain BCM. While enteral feedings are probably somewhat better than parenteral regimens in terms of N balance, the differences are not for the most part of much physiological importance (67).

There is some evidence to show that protein hydrolyzates are not as good as crystalline amino acid solutions (68,69). This seems to be because of the inability of sick patients, unlike normal subjects, to make effective use of the small peptides which make up a substantial fraction of protein hydrolyzates (70).

One of the most interesting and controversial questions relating to amino acid composition has been the use, in a variety of clinical situations, of amino acid solutions enriched with the branched chain amino acids (BCAA), leucine, isoleucine, and valine. The first application was in hepatic encephalopathy. Most of the essential amino acids are oxidized by the liver. These include methionine, tryptophan, phenylalanine, and tyrosine. In hepatic failure, plasma concentrations of these amino acids increase from 2- to 20-fold. Tyrosine is a precursor of the

neurotransmitter norepinephrine and the false neurotransmitter octopamine. High blood levels of tyrosine increase brain concentration of octopamine more than of norepinephrine. High blood concentrations of tryptophan induce high brain concentrations of its metabolic product, the neurotransmitter serotonin. The BCAA are degraded by muscle, adipose tissue, and brain, and their blood concentrations are low in liver failure. Fischer et al. (71,72) found that administering BCAA-enriched amino acid solutions normalizes the plasma amino acid patterns and can awaken comatose, hepatic encephalopathic patients . However, others have found the BCAA to be less effective (73) and there remains some controversy in their use for hepatic encephalopathy.

Another approach to use of the BCAA stems from the effects of leucine, or its keto acid, to stimulate protein synthesis and decrease protein breakdown in muscle, in vitro (74,75). A number of investigators have found increased N balance with BCAA-enriched solutions in injured or septic patients (76,77), but did not investigate their effects on morbidity. A recent prospective trial has confirmed the improvement in N balance, roughly 1 g N per day for 3 weeks, but has found no improvement in morbidity (78). Administration of BCAA-enriched amino acids to burned guinea pigs had a deleterious effect on morbidity (79). At present, it seems unlikely that BCAA-enriched amino acid solutions will prove useful in nutritional therapy of injury and sepsis.

A third potential use of BCAA stems from their effect to decrease tryptophan entry into the brain by competing for the common transport system for large neutral amino acids. This has the effect of reducing brain levels of serotonin (80). Serotonin has an inhibitory effect on ventilatory drive, gastric-emptying and many other processes. It is possible that BCAA may be used to specifically diminish serotonin inhibition (81) and that this might be useful in specific clinical situations.

Interrelation Between N Balance and Dietary Intake in Infants and Children

Interrelations between N and energy intakes and N balance are quite different in infants and children than in adults. Growth in children involves both body cell mass and extracellular constituents, so that positive N balance represents growth of all lean body mass, unlike repletion of malnourished adults in whom positive N balance represents BCM only.

Nutrient requirements are higher than for adults, highest for low birth weight new born infants, when the rate of growth in proportion to body size is greatest, and decreasing with age and decreasing growth rate. Catzeflis et al. (82) estimate that low birth weight infants require 70 mg N and 40 kcal (167 kJ) of energy kg^{-1} day^{-1} for weight maintenance. These values are not very different from the 80 mg N and 25-30 kcal (105-126 kJ) kg^{-1} day^{-1} required by adults for weight maintenance at rest. A state of weight maintenance, while normal for adults, is not normal for infants. For normal growth, these infants require 100 kcal (418 kJ) and 300-500 mg N kg^{-1} day^{-1} (83), so that roughly two-thirds of energy and 70% to 90% of N intake are used for growing. Newborn infants are much more efficient in utilizing N than are malnourished adults. At intakes of 300-500 mg N and over 80 kcal (335 kJ) kg^{-1} day^{-1}, newborn infants retain 60% to 70% of gross N intake on either oral (82-84) or parenteral (85,86) diets. This corresponds to about 80% of metabolizable intake. By contrast, malnourished adults, even at very high energy intakes, retain less than 30% of metabolizable proteins (Figure 3.9). Even at very high N intake, about 1400 mg kg^{-1} day^{-1}, low birth weight infants retain 44% of the administered N (83). At intakes below 80 kcal (335 kJ) kg^{-1} day^{-1}, energy becomes limiting and N retention is much smaller (86). At these low intakes, 50 to 80 kcal (209-335 kJ) kg^{-1} day^{-1}, increasing energy intake markedly increases N balance, by as much as 6 mg N per kcal (1.4 mg N kJ^{-1}). At higher values Kashyap et al. (84) found no significant effects on N balance of increasing energy intake from 114 to 149 kcal (477-623 kJ) kg^{-1} day^{-1}. If their data are corrected for small differences in N intake, they show an increase of only 0.5 ± 0.3 mg N $kcal^{-1}$ (0.12 ± 0.07 mg N kJ^{-1}), not significantly different from 0, but probably not significantly different from the 1 to 3 mg N $kcal^{-1}$ (0.24 ± 0.72 mg N kJ^{-1}) seen in adult humans and other animals (46, 53).

The most striking difference between the newborn and the adult is the avidity with which the infant retains nitrogen, whereas, if adequately fed, the effect of energy intake is smaller than for the adult, or nonexistent. It is evident that, with increasing age and decreasing rate of growth, children become more like adults and less like the newborn infant. However, a detailing of these changes is outside the range of this treatise.

REFERENCES

1. Boussingault JB: Comparative analysis of the nutrients that are consumed and those excreted by a milk cow: A study undertaken with the aim of examining whether herbiverous animals borrow nitrogen from the atmosphere. *Ann Chim Phys* 71:113-136, 1839.
2. Keys A, Brozek J, Henschel A, et al.: The *Biology of Human Starvation.* Minneapolis, University of Minnesota Press, 1950.
3. Moore FD, Olesen KH, McMurrey JD, et al.: *The Body Cell Mass and its Supporting Environment: Body Composition in Health and Disease.* Philadelphia, WB Saunders, 1963.

4. *Official Methods of Analysis* (9th ed). Washington, D.C., Association of Official Agricultural Chemists, 1963.
5. Ward MWH, Owens CWI, Rennie MJ: Nitrogen estimation in biological samples by use of chemiluminescence. *Clin Chem* 26:1336-1339, 1980.
6. Chikenji T, Elwyn D, Gil KM, et al.: Effects of increasing glucose intake on nitrogen balance and energy expenditure in malnourished adult patients receiving parenteral nutrition. *Clin Sci* 72:489-501, 1987.
7. Calloway DH, Odell ACF, Margen S: Sweat and miscellaneous nitrogen losses in human balance studies. *J Nutr* 101: 775-786, 1971.
8. Oddoye EA, Margen S: Nitrogen balance studies in humans: Long term effects of high nitrogen intake on nitrogen accretion. *J Nutr* 109:336-377, 1979.
9. Lee HA, Hartley TF: A method of determining daily nitrogen requirement. *Postgrad Med* 51:441-445, 1975.
10. Wilmore DW: *The Metabolic Management of the Critically Ill.* New York, Plenum, 1977.
11. Long CL, Schaffel M, Geiger JW, et al.: Metabolic response to injury and illness. Estimation of energy and protein need from indirect calorimetry and nitrogen balance. *JPEN* 3:452-456, 1979.
12. Blackburn GL, Bistrian BR, Maini BS, et al.: Nutritional and metabolic assessment of the hospitalized patient. *JPEN* 1:11-22, 1977.
13. Shaw-Delanty S, Elwyn DH, Jeejeebhoy KN, et al.: Components of nitrogen excretion in hospitalized adult patients on intravenous diets. *Clin Nutr* 6:257-266, 1987.
14. Bistrian BR, Blackburn GL, Sherman M, Scrimshaw N: Therapeutic index of nutritional depletion in hospitalized adults. *Surg Gynecol Obstet* 141:512-516, 1975.
15. Starker PM, Askanazi J, Lasala PA, et al.: The effect of parenteral nutrition repletion on muscle water and electrolytes. *Ann Surg* 198:213-217, 1983.
16. Chikenji T, Elwyn DH, Gil KM, et al.: Short term effects of varying glucose intake on body composition of malnourished adult patients. *Crit Care Med* 15:1086-1091, 1987.
17. Shils ME, Randall HT: Diet and nutrition in the care of the surgical patient. In Goodhart RS, Shils MD (eds): *Modern Nutrition in Health and Disease*, ed 6. Philadelphia, Lea and Febiger, 1980, pp 1103–1104.
18. Mitchell HH: Adult growth in man and its nutrient requirements. *Arch Biochem* 21:335-342, 1949.
19. Hegsted M: Balance studies. *J Nutr* 106:307-311, 1976.
20. Grindley HS: Studies in nutrition. An investigation of the influence of saltpeter on the nutrition and health of men with reference to its occurrence in cured meat. *The Experimental Data of Biochemical Investigation.* Champaign, University of Illinois, 1912, Vol IV.
21. Krogh A: Experimental researches on the expiration of free nitrogen from the body. *Scand Arch Physiol* 18:364-420, 1906.
22. Cissik JH, Johnson RE, Rokosch DK: Production of gaseous nitrogen in human steady state conditions. *J Appl Physiol* 32:155-159, 1972.
23. Muysers K, Smith U, Von Nieding G, et al.: Diffusional and metabolic components of nitrogen elimination through the lungs. *J Appl Physiol* 37:32-37, 1974.
24. Rosenberg E: Nitrogen equality is not a myth. *Life Sciences* 19:61-67, 1976.
25. Committee on Nutritional Anthropometry, Food and Nutrition Board, National Research Council. Recommendations concerning body measurements for the characterizations of nutritional studies. *Hum Biol* 28:115-123, 1956.
26. Krzywicke HJ, Consolazio CF: Body composition methodology in military nutri-

tion surveys. In *Body Composition in Animals and Man.* Washington, D.C., Nat Acad Sci, 1968, pp 492–511.

27. Durnin JVGA, Wormersley J: Body fat assessed from total body density and its estimation from skin fold thickness: Measurements on 481 men and women aged from 16 to 72 years. *Br J Nutr* 32:77-97, 1974.
28. Steinkamp RC, Cohen NL, Gaffey WR, et al:. Measures of body fat and related factors in normal adults. II. A simple clinical method to estimate body fat and lean body mass. *J Chron Dis* 18:1291-1307, 1965.
29. Agriculture Board, Division of Biology and Agriculture, National Research Council. *Body Composition in Animals and Man.* Washington, D.C., Nat Acad Sci, 1968.
30. Presta E, Wang J, Harrison GG, et al.: Measurement of total body electrical conductivity. *Am J Clin Nutr* 37:735-739, 1983.
31. Insel J, Elwyn DH: Body Composition. In Askanazi J, Starker PM, Weissman C (eds): *Fluid and Electrolyte Management in Critical Care.* Boston, Butterworths, 1986, pp 3–37.
32. Elwyn DH, Bryan-Brown CW, Shoemaker WC: Nutritional aspects of body water dislocations in postoperative and depleted patients. *Ann Surg* 182: 76-85, 1975.
33. Shires T, Williams J, Brown F: Acute change in extracellular fluids associated with major surgical procedures. *Ann Surg* 154:803-810, 1961.
34. Shizgal HM, Spanier AH, Humes J, Wood CD: Indirect measurement of total exchangeable potassium. *Am J Physiol* 233:F253-F259, 1977.
35. Shizgal HM: The effect of malnutrition on body composition. *Surg Gynec Obstet* 152:22-26, 1981.
36. Yang MU, Wang J, Pierson RM Jr, Van Itallie TB: Estimation of composition of weight loss in man: A comparison of methods. *J Appl Physiol* 43:331-338, 1977.
37. Hill GL, King RJFG, Smith RC, et al.: Multi-elemental analysis of the living body by neutron activation analysis, application to critically ill patients receiving intravenous nutrition. *Br J Surg* 66:868-872, 1979.
38. Elwyn DH: Repletion of the malnourished patient. In Blackburn GL, Grant JP, Young VR (eds): *Amino Acids: Metabolism and Medical Application.* Boston, Wright PSG, 1983, pp 359–375.
39. McNeil KG, Harrison JE, Mernagh JR, et al.: Changes in body protein, body potassium, and lean body mass during total parenteral nutrition. *JPEN* 6:106-108, 1982.
40. Russell DM, Prendergast PJ, Darby PL, et al.: A comparison between muscle function and body composition in anorexia nervosa: The effect of refeeding. *Am J Clin Nutr* '38:229-237, 1983.
41. Benedict FG: *A Study of Prolonged Fasting.* Washington, D.C., Carnegie Institute, Publication No. 203, 1915.
42. Reifenstein EC Jr, Albright F, Wells SI: The accumulation, interpretation and presentation of data pertaining to metabolic balances, notably those of calcium, phosphorus and nitrogen. *J Clin Endocrinol* 5:367-395, 1945.
43. Rudman D, Millikan WJ, Richardson TJ ,et al.: Elemental balances during intravenous hyperalimentation of underweight adult subjects. *J Clin Invest* 55:94-104, 1975.
44. Calloway DH, Spector N: Nitrogen balance as related to calorie and protein intake in young men. *Am J Clin Nutr* 2:405-412, 1954.
45. Martin CJ, Robison R: The minimum nitrogen expenditure of man and the biological value of various proteins for human nutrition. *Biochem J* 16:407-447, 1922.
46. Munro HN: General aspects of the regulation of protein metabolism by diet and

hormones. In Munro HN, Allison JB (eds): *Mammalian Protein Metabolism.* New York, Academic Press, 1964, Vol I, pp 381–481.

47. Hegsted DM: Protein requirements. In Munro HN, Allison JB (eds): *Mammalian Protein Metabolism.* New York, Academic Press, 1964, Vol II, pp 135–171.
48. National Research Council. *Recommended Dietary Allowances,* ed 7. Washington, D.C., National Academy of Sciences, 1968.
49. Silwer H: Studien uber die N-Ausscheidung im Harn bei einshrankung des Kohlehydrates der Nahrung ohne wesentlische Veranderung des Energienghaltes derselben. *Acta Med Scand* Suppl 79:1-273, 1937.
50. Passmore R, Nicol BM, Rao MN: *Handbook on Human Nutritional Requirements.* Geneva, WHO Monogr. Ser No 61, Table 1, 1974.
51. Keys A, Anderson JT, Brozek J: Weight gain from simple overeating. Character of tissue gained. *Metabolism* 4: 427-432, 1955.
52. Calloway DH: Nitrogen balance of men with marginal intakes of protein and energy. *J Nutr* 105: 914-923, 1975.
53. Elwyn DH, Gump FE, Munro HN, et al.: Changes in nitrogen balance of depleted patients with increasing infusions of glucose. *Am J Clin Nutr* 32:1597-1611, 1979.
54. Kinney JM, Long CL, Gump FE, et al.: Tissue composition of weight loss in surgical patients. *Ann Surg* 168:459-474, 1968.
55. Kinney JM: The tissue composition of surgical weight loss. In Johnston IDA (ed): *Advances in Parenteral Nutrition*, Lancaster, MTP Press, 1977 pp 511–519.
56. Plough IC, Iber FL, Shipman ME, Chalmers T: The effects of supplementary calories on nitrogen storage at high intakes of protein in patients with chronic liver disease. *Am J Clin Nutr* 4:224-230, 1956.
57. Shaw SN, Elwyn DH, Askanazi J, et al.: Effects of increasing nitrogen intake on nitrogen balance and energy expenditure in nutritionally depleted adult patients receiving parenteral nutrition. *Am J Clin Nutr* 37:930-940, 1983.
58. Elwyn DH, Kinney JM, Gump FE, et al.: Some metabolic effects of fat infusions in depleted patients. *Metabolism* 29:125-132, 1980.
59. Nordenström J, Askanazi J, Elwyn DH, et al.: Nitrogen balance during total parenteral nutrition. *Ann Surg* 197:27-33, 1983.
60. Shizgal HM, Forse RA: Protein and caloric requirements with total parenteral nutrition. *Ann Surg* 192: 562-569, 1980.
61. Jeejeebhoy KN, Anderson GH, Nakhooda AF, et al.: Metabolic studies in total parenteral nutrition with lipid in man. Comparison with glucose. *J Clin Invest* 57:125-136, 1976.
62. Bark S, Holm I, Håkansson I, Wretlind A: Nitrogen sparing effect of fat emulsion compared with glucose in the post operative period. *Acta Chir Scand* 142:423-427, 1976.
63. Larsson J, Martenson J, Vinnars E: Nitrogen requirements in hypercatabolic patients. *Clin Nutr* (Special Suppl) 4:O.4, 1984.
64. Long JM, Wilmore DW, Mason AD Jr, Pruitt BA Jr: Effect of carbohydrate and fat intake on nitrogen excretion during total intravenous nutrition. *Ann Surg* 185: 417-422, 1977.
65. Woolfson AMB, Heatley RV, Allison SP: Insulin to inhibit protein catabolism. *N Engl J Med* 300:14-17, 1979.
66. Harper AE, Benevenga NJ, Wohlhueter RM: Effects of ingestion of disproportionate amounts of amino acids. *Physiol Rev* 50:428-558, 1970.
67. Grote AE, Elwyn DH, Takala J, et al.: Nutritional and metabolic effects of enteral and parenteral feeding in severely injured patients. *Clin Nutr* 6:161-167, 1987.

68. Long CL, Zikria BH, Kinney JM, Geiger JW: Comparison of fibrin hydrolyzates and crystalline amino acid solutions in parenteral nutrition. *Am J Clin Nutr* 27:163-174, 1974.
69. Andersen GH, Patel DG, Jeejeebhoy KN: Design and evaluation by nitrogen balance and blood aminograms of an amino acid mixture for total parenteral nutrition of adults with gastrointestinal disease. *J Clin Invest* 53:904-912, 1974.
70. Vinnars E, Fürst P, Hermansson IL, et al.: Protein catabolism in the postoperative state and its treatment with amino acid solution. *Acta Chirurg Scand* 136:95-109, 1970.
71. Fischer JE, Rosen HM, Ebeid AM, et al.: The effect of normalization of plasma amino acids on hepatic encephalopathy in man. *Surgery* 80:77-91, 1976.
72. Cerra FB, Cheung NK, Fischer JE, et al.; Disease-specific amino acid infusion (FO80) in hepatic encephalopathy: A prospective randomized, double blind, controlled trial. *JPEN* 9:288-295, 1985.
73. Eriksson LS, Persson A, Wahren J: Branched chain amino acids in the treatment of chronic hepatic encephalopathy. *Gut* 23:801-806, 1982.
74. Buse MG, Reid SS: Leucine. A possible regulator of protein turnover in muscle. *J Clin Invest* 56:1250-1261, 1975.
75. Fulks RM, Li JB, Goldberg AL: Effects of insulin, glucose and amino acids on protein turnover in rat diaphragm. *J Biol Chem* 250:290-298, 1975.
76. Freund HR, Hoover HC Jr, Atamanian S, Fischer JE: Infusions of branched chain amino acids in postoperative patients. *Ann Surg* 190:18-23, 1979.
77. Cerra FB, Mazushi JE, Chute E, et al.: Branched chain metabolic support. A randomized, double blind trial in surgical stress. *Ann Surg* 199:286-291, 1984.
78. Van Berlo CLH, von Meyenfledt MF, Rouflart M, et al.: Do BCAA enriched TPN solutions improve nitrogen balance, morbidity or mortality in mildly stressed patients? *Clin Nutr* 9 (Special Suppl): 65, 1986 (abstract).
79. Mochizuki H, Trocki O, Dominioni L, Alexander JW: Effect of a diet rich in branched chain amino acids on severely burned guinea pigs. *J Trauma* 26:1077-1085, 1986
80. Fernstrom JP: Effect of protein and carbohydrate ingestion on brain tryptophan levels and serotonin synthesis: putative relationship to appetite for specific nutrients. In Kane MR, Brand JG (eds): *Interaction of the Chemical Senses with Nutrition.* New York, Academic Press, 1981, pp 395–414.
81. Takala J, Askanazi J, Weissman C, et al.: Changes in respiratory control induced by amino acid infusion. *Crit Care Med* 16:465-469, 1988
82. Catzeflis C, Schutz Y, Micheli JL, et al.: Whole body synthesis and energy expenditure in very low birth weight infants. *Pediatr Res* 19:679-687, 1987.
83. Snyderman SE, Boyer A, Kogut M, Holt EM Jr: The protein requirement of the premature infant. 1. The effect of protein intake on the retention of nitrogen. *J Pediatr* 74: 872-880, 1969.
84. Kashyap S, Forsyth M, Zucker C, et al.: Effect of varying protein and energy intakes on growth and metabolic response in low birth weight infants. *J Pediatr* 108:955-963, 1986.
85. Meurling S, Grotte G: Complete parenteral nutrition in the surgery of the newborn infant. *Acta Chirurg Scand* 147:465-473, 1981.
86. Zlotkin SH, Bryan MH, Anderson GH: Intravenous nitrogen and energy intakes required to duplicate in utero nitrogen accretion in prematurely born human infants. *J Pediatr* 99:115-120, 1981.

CHAPTER

4

Fuel Utilization in Normal, Starving, and Pathological States

Life is essentially an energy-utilizing process. Living organisms maintain their identity and integrity only by a continuing process of consumption of energy and nutrients and excretion of waste products. The forms in which energy and nutrients appear are different for different organisms. For plants, energy must be supplied in a very pure form, as light or photons, and the nutrients are simple inorganic compounds which include CO_2, H_2O, nitrate as a source of N, sulfate as a source of S, and a variety of inorganic salts. Chlorophyll catalyzes the combination of photons with water resulting in the transfer of 2 H atoms to reduce organic carbonyl (C = O) groups to hydroxyl (CH - OH) groups while the O forms gaseous O_2, which is excreted (1). The end result is the formation of glucose and O_2 from CO_2, H_2O, and photons. Plants can also reduce nitrate to ammonia or its derivatives, and have the enzymatic capability of producing, from these simple starting materials, all the many organic compounds required by both plants and animals with one notable exception, vitamin B_{12}.

By contrast to plants, animals require energy in the form of organic compounds, energy which is realized by the oxidation of these compounds to CO_2, H_2O, sulfate and various N containing compounds.

Furthermore, although they can synthesize most of the thousands of organic compounds they require, there are approximately twenty basic building blocks, amino acids, vitamins, and a few others which they cannot synthesize.

It is these two nutritional differences between plants and animals which largely explain the entirely diffrent direction in which the two major forms of life have developed, since these differences exist even for unicellular plants and animals which in many other ways are very similar. In plant development, since sunlight, water, and inorganic salts are more or less evenly distributed on land as well as in the ocean, there has been little pressure to develop locomotion, but rather to develop large surfaces to collect sunlight and long roots to increase the region available for collecting water and salts. Thus the tree represents, perhaps, the highest form of plant life, with its widely branching limbs covered with leaves and its extensive root system. Animals, on the other hand, require a variety of organic compounds and can make no use of sunlight as a source of energy. A billion or so years ago, when life on this planet was in its infancy, and the sea was a rich solution of organic compounds produced abiotically, nutrients for animals were as widely distributed as those for plants and there was little pressure for animals to develop in new directions. However, as living organisms ate up all the nutrients in the organic soup, the situation changed. At that time, as today, organic compounds were to be found only in living organisms or their dead bodies. Thus success in the animal kingdom went to those who moved to their prey, whether animal or vegetable, and who could successfully engulf and absorb their constituents. With the appearance of multicellular organisms, this need to prey on others led to specialized tissues and organs devoted to locomotion, attack, ingestion and digestion, and to specialized tissues to coordinate these organs and their functions into an effective whole. This led also to a system for transporting nutrients and waste products to and from organs, and organs for the excretion of the complex waste products they produced. Except for a vascular system for transport, none of these specialized functions have developed in the plant world, except in rare instances such as insect-eating plants. In time, as these specialized functions matured and were refined, the nervous system, mainly responsible for coordination of movement, attack, ingestion, transport, and excretion, developed a brain capable of cognitive thought so that to date, the highest expression of animal development is the human species. Thus these two highest representatives of the animal and plant kingdom, humans and trees, differ so completely anatomically and physiologically because of the differences in their nutritional requirements.

ENERGY CONSUMPTION

Energy consumption by humans and other animals is: *(a)* converted to mechanical energy by muscle for locomotion, pumping blood, breathing, eating food, moving eyes, and so forth; *(b)* used to pump ions and organic molecules across membranes against a chemical gradient; maintenance of ion gradients produces an electrical potential of approximately -86 millivolts across the membranes of almost all cells, and provides the energy for electrical conductance in nervous tissue; *(c)* used for synthesis of the organic constituents which are the structural and functional components of cells and their extracellular appendages, and which undergo continual degradation and renewal, even in the adult organism; and (d) for homeotherms, such as mammals and birds, used to provide the heat necessary to maintain body temperature when environmental temperature is below 37° C.

In order to serve these many functions, the organic compounds we ingest as food cannot be oxidized all at once, as occurs in a bomb calorimeter. Rather they must be oxidized step by step, in a series of enzymatically controlled reactions in which energy is released in small packets which can be readily utilized by the cell. The most important compounds involved in utilizing energy in these small packets are ADP and ATP. They contain what are called high energy phosphate bonds, represented by $\sim$P, a concept which is very useful if somewhat over simplified (1). The hydrolysis of the terminal phosphate anhydride bond of ATP to give ADP, inorganic phosphate (P_i) and H^+, is shown in equation 1.

$$\underset{\textbf{ATP}}{Ad\text{-}O\text{-}\overset{\overset{O}{\|}}{\underset{\underset{O^-}{|}}{P}}\text{-}O\text{-}\overset{\overset{O}{\|}}{\underset{\underset{O^-}{|}}{P}}\text{-}O\text{-}\overset{\overset{O}{\|}}{\underset{\underset{O^-}{|}}{P}}\text{-}O^-} + H_2O \leftrightarrow \underset{\textbf{ADP}}{Ad\text{-}O\text{-}\overset{\overset{O}{\|}}{\underset{\underset{O^-}{|}}{P}}\text{-}O\text{-}\overset{\overset{O}{\|}}{\underset{\underset{O^-}{|}}{P}}\text{-}O^-} + \underset{\mathbf{P_i}}{HO\text{-}\overset{\overset{O}{\|}}{\underset{\underset{O^-}{|}}{P}}\text{-}O^-} + H^+$$

Under intracellular conditions, the energy released by hydrolysis of the terminal ~P bond of ATP yields 12.5 kcal (52.3 kJ) of energy per mole. If ATP is simply hydrolyzed this energy is given off as heat. If it is coupled with some other reaction, then the chemical energy stored in ATP can be transferred to other chemical compounds, or transformed into mechanical or electrical energy. ATP is the source of energy for: *(a)* muscle contraction; *(b)* maintaining ion gradients and therefore electrical gradients across the cell membrane, most notably by means of the sodium pump; and *(c)* electrical conductance, mainly in brain and nerves, but also in other tissues. Together with its sister nucleotides, guanosine triphosphate (GTP), uridine triphosphate (UTP), and cytidine triphosphate (CTP), it is involved in all synthetic reactions in the cell, including synthesis of proteins, glycogen, fatty acids, phospholipids, and mucopolysaccharides.

Most of the ATP produced in the cell is derived from oxidation, in the mitochondria, of the Coenzyme A derivative of acetic acid, acetyl-CoA. But acetyl-CoA cannot be directly oxidized; rather it must undergo a series of reactions known collectively as the Krebs tricarboxylic acid cycle or the citric acid cycle (Figure 4.1). The initial reaction is between acetyl-CoA and oxalacetate to form citrate. Citrate undergoes a rearrangement to isocitrate, which can be dehydrogenated (oxidized) to yield oxalosuccinate and 2 H atoms which are transferred to NAD^+ (not shown in Figure 4.1) to form NADH and an H^+ ion. Oxalosuccinate is decarboxylated to give CO_2 and α-ketoglutarate. This is dehydrogenated and decarboxylated to succinate, yielding another 2 H atoms, another CO_2, and in the process converting 1 ADP to ATP. Succinate is dehydrogenated to fumarate, yielding another 2 H, which this time are transferred to a flavoprotein (FP) to form FPH_2. Fumarate is hydrated to form malate; malate is dehydrogenated to oxalacetate and another 2 H are released. In this way we recover the starting oxalacetate, and the net result has been the consumption of the acetyl group of acetyl-CoA, the production of 2 CO_2, and transfer of 8 H atoms to form 3 NADH and 1 FPH_2. In addition we have formed one, but only one, ATP from ADP.

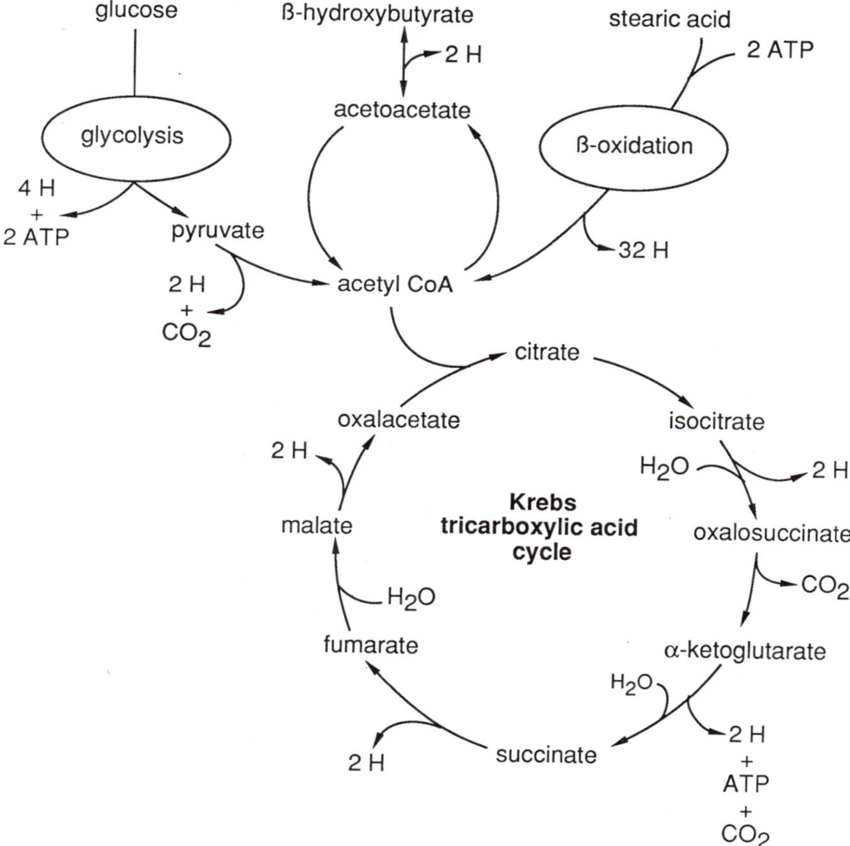

Figure 4.1. Relationships between glycolysis, beta-oxidation, ketogenesis and the Krebs tricarboxylic acid cycle.

Most of the ATP is formed in the process termed oxidative phosphorylation:

$$NADH + H^+ + 1/2\ O_2 + 3ADP + 3P_i \rightarrow NAD^+ + H_2O + 3ATP \quad (2)$$

in which 2 H from NADH and H^+ are combined with oxygen to form H_2O in a coupled reaction in which 3 ADP + 3 P_i form 3 ATP. A similar reaction can be written for FPH_2 except that only 2 ATP are produced.

In these two closely coordinated but separate processes, the reduction of O_2 by H atoms to form H_2O is completely separated from the formation of CO_2.

The net result of the two processes is that 1 mole of acetyl-CoA is oxidized to CO_2 and H_2O to yield 12 moles of ATP, 1 during operation of the Krebs cycle, and 11 from oxidation of NADH and FPH_2 by the oxidative phosphorylation pathway.

The organic compounds we eat as food can all be converted to acetyl-CoA by various pathways which also yield ATP. Glucose is converted by the glycolytic pathway (Figure 4.1) to 2 pyruvates, giving a net production of 2 ATP and 4 H which, by oxidative phosphorylation, yield an additional 6 ATP. The 2 pyruvates in going to acetyl-CoA give another 4 H, which yield 6 more ATP. One glucose produces 2 acetyl-CoA which, in the Krebs cycle and oxidative phosphorylation pathway, yield 24 ATP. Altogether, oxidation of one glucose yields 38 ATP, 14 up to the formation of acetyl-CoA and 24 from oxidation of acetyl-CoA. One mole (180 g) of glucose gives up 675 kcal (2824 kJ) of heat or energy on oxidation (3.75 kcal or 15.7 kJ per g). Of this 12.5×38, or 475 kcal (1987 kJ), is converted to the terminal ~ P of ATP, an efficiency of 70%. The rest is converted to heat.

Stearic acid contains 18 carbons. One mole of stearic acid gives rise to 9 moles of acetyl-CoA by the process of β-oxidation. This generates 32 H, which yield 40 ATP by oxidative phosphorylation. From this we need to substract 2 ATP, required to initially activate stearic acid to stearyl-CoA, leaving 38. The 9 acetyl-CoA give rise to 108 ATP for a total of 146. One mole of stearic acid (285 g) yields about 2650 kcal (11,088 kJ) on oxidation (9.3 kcal or 38.9 kJ per g), of which 146×12.5, or 1825 kcal (7636 kJ), are converted to the terminal ~ P of ATP, an efficiency of 69% very similar to that for glucose.

Amino acids are converted to acetyl-CoA by a variety of pathways. Alanine, glycine, serine, cysteine, and threonine are first converted to pyruvate. Pyruvate is then oxidized to acetyl-CoA, as shown in Figure 7.1. Glutamate, ornithine, arginine, histidine and proline go first to α- ketoglutarate, which proceeds around the cycle to oxalacetate, which can be converted to pyruvate by a pathway not shown in Figure 7.1, and then to acetyl-CoA. Aspartate is transaminated to give oxalacetate directly. Isoleucine, valine, and methionine enter at succinate. Phenylalanine, tyrosine, leucine, lysine, and tryptophan enter at acetoacetate. In addition tyrosine and phenylalanine give rise to fumarate; and isoleucine, leucine, and tryptophan give rise to acetyl-CoA directly. The efficiency of the conversion of amino acids to ATP is about the same as for fat and glucose.

In addition to being oxidized directly, acetyl-CoA, in the liver, is converted to acetoacetate, which can be reduced to β-hydroxybutyrate (Figure 7.1) or decarboxylated to acetone. Acetoacetate, β-hydroxybutyrate, and acetone are known collectively as *ketone bodies*. Their synthesis is inhibited by insulin, and normally they are produced only in small quantities. When insulin concentrations are low, as in fasting, diabetes, or with carbohydrate-free diets, their production increases and they are utilized in peripheral tissues as a source of acetyl-CoA. This is particularly important for the brain, which normally requires about 100 g glucose per day, but in prolonged fasting can replace more than one-half the glucose by ketone bodies.

Glucose is the only important nutrient which can be used for ATP formation without being oxidized. One mole of glucose, by glycolysis to pyruvate, yields 2 ATP and 4 H (Figure 7.1). Under hypoxic conditions, the 4 H are used to convert the 2 moles of pyruvate to lactate; otherwise the reaction would stop when all the NAD^+ was converted to NADH. Conversion of glucose to lactate then gives rise to only 2 ATP per glucose, one-nineteenth of the energy gained from complete oxidation of glucose. Nevertheless, certain tissues get most or all their energy from glycolysis, converting glucose to lactate, which then is reconverted to glucose in the liver and the kidney. These tissues include red and white blood cells, the lens of the eye, the kidney medulla, and very important in critically ill patients, wounds and regenerating tissues.

Although almost all the energy released by oxidation of nutrients is converted to the terminal ~P of ATP, there is not very much ATP in the cell. The whole body content of ATP is about 250 mmoles or 0.25 moles. This contains in the terminal ~P bond about 3 kcals (12 kJ). At rest, energy expenditure is about 1 kcal (4 kJ) per minute, so we have only a 3-minute supply. At maximal exertion, ordinary people can expend 10 to 15 kcal (42 to 63 kJ) per minute, and a trained athlete can expend 20 kcal (84 kJ) per minute. Thus the latter has only a 9-second supply. However, ATP concentrations change very little, even at maximal exercise, they will not decrease by more then 20%, and much less during ordinary activity. This means that the rate of ATP formation must always be almost exactly the same, within seconds, as the rate of ATP utilization. For many tissues, rates of utilization are quite constant and therefore the rate of production of ATP will be quite constant. However, in skeletal muscle the rate of ATP utilization for muscular work can increase 100-fold within 1 to 2 seconds and the rate of ATP production must also be able to increase 100-fold. The elegantly sensitive mechanisms which regulate the relations between ATP utilization and ATP production have been described in fascinating detail by Newsholme and Stark in their book *Regulation in Metabolism* (2).

Not only must the body produce ATP at the same rate it uses it, it must also select which fuels to use. Furthermore, for most tissues part or all of their fuel comes from the blood, in the form of fatty acids, glucose, amino acids, or ketone bodies; therefore the blood supply to tissues, particularly muscle, must be able to keep up with its demands. This means that adipose tissue, fat, and liver glycogen must be mobilized in response to changing activities of skeletal muscle or heart in order to maintain an adequate blood supply of nutrients. Some of these interrelations will be explored in the next sections.

COORDINATION OF ENERGY INTAKE WITH ENERGY CONSUMPTION

For most animals eating is episodic, occurring at certain times of day and not at others. Thus most humans eat three meals per day mostly during daylight hours, and go for long periods, 8-12 hours during the night, without eating. However, energy requirements remain quite constant for most organs, and if they change markedly, as for heart and skeletal muscle, they do so entirely unrelated to times of eating. Therefore, only some of the substrates secreted by the gut after a meal are immediately utilized by other tissues for energy production, the rest must be stored to be used later in the day, when the gut supply has stopped. In addition the proportions in the diet of the three major foodstuffs—proteins, carbohydrates and fat—can vary over a wide range and still remain adequate. For instance, a diet based almost entirely on unpolished rice contains about 85% of total energy as carbohydrate, 10% as protein, and 5% as fat; while a meat diet contains less than 5% as carbohydrate, about 40% as protein, and 60% as fat. Both of these diets are eaten in some parts of the globe and both are adequate. Thus the amounts of each foodstuff available, the amounts that need to be stored, and the amounts which may have to be converted to others will vary over a wide range, depending on the pattern of ingestion and the composition of the diet. This coordination of dietary intake with the energy needs of tissues and organs comprises a major aspect of metabolic regulation, and particularly involves insulin and glucagon, which might be termed the *dietary hormones*.

Protein

Minimum protein requirements, discussed in Chapter 3, are about 35 g per day. Daily protein intake however may be as high as 300 g or more. There are no storage proteins as such. Protein storage represents an increase in the amounts of functional proteins in the cell. The liver is the major organ of protein storage in terms of diurnal changes. It has first access to the gut output of amino acids carried in portal blood, and to a first approximation it absorbs the entire output except for the branched chain amino acids, leucine, isoleucine and valine (3). The liver's response to a meat meal given to dogs is shown in Figure 4.2. These animals were trained to eat all their requirements as a single meat meal given daily at noon (4). Urea synthesis was constant, at a rate of 25 mmole hr^{-1} kg^{-1}, during the postabsorptive period. With the meal it promptly increased five-fold for eight hours and then returned to postabsorptive values. Only part of the carbon skeletons of the amino acids, accounting for this rise in urea synthesis, were oxidized to CO_2; more than 50% were converted to glucose, accompanied by an increase in hepatic glucose output and presumably of glycogen storage in liver and muscle. Net protein synthesis was also abruptly induced by the meal and continued for ten hours when it returned to zero. This net synthesis is due mainly to an increase in unidirectional synthesis rather than a decrease in degradation. These two processes—protein synthesis and urea production in the liver—consumed the bulk of the ingested amino acids. The net positive 24-hour protein synthesis (Figure 4.2), is consistent with the role of the liver as an exporter of proteins. Most of the plasma proteins are synthesized in the liver, but a large part are degraded in peripheral tissues; thus, liver exports proteins to the periphery and receives back the amino acids from their degradation (3). Although the evidence is not conclusive, glucagon is probably the hormone most closely associated with the effects of a protein meal in the absence of carbohydrate (5). When smaller amounts of protein are fed together with carbohydrate, there is also an increase in net protein syn-

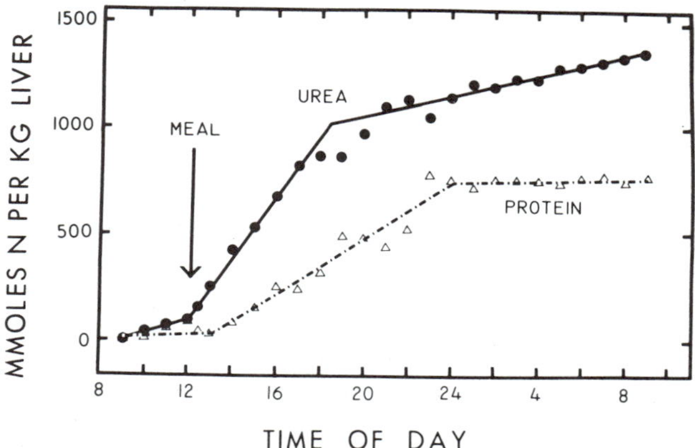

Figure 4.2. From Elwyn DH, Parikh HC, Shoemaker WC: Amino acid movements between gut, liver and periphery in unanesthetized dogs. *Am J Physiol* 215:1260-1275, 1968. The effect of a large meat meal eaten at 12:00 on urea and protein synthesis in dog liver, in vivo.

thesis (6). However this is due primarily to a decrease in unidirectional protein breakdown. The largest part of protein breakdown takes place in lysosomes (6) or in autophagic vacuoles, which appear to be related to lysosomes. Increased insulin due to eating carbohydrate decreases the number of both organelles, thus decreasing the rate of protein breakdown (6). Feeding carbohydrate also decreases gluconeogenesis and urea synthesis. Thus, ingestion of either carbohydrate or protein increases net protein synthesis in the liver, the first by decreasing degradation; the second by increasing synthesis. Carbohydrate decreases, while protein increases both gluconeogenesis and ureagenesis. The effects of carbohydrate are mainly mediated by insulin; those of protein mainly by glucagon. The effects of a mixed meal will depend on the relative proportions of carbohydrate and protein.

Normal adults, as discussed in Chapter 3, are in zero N balance. Therefore, despite diurnal deposition and loss of protein in the liver, all protein intake will be oxidized by the end of the day. Transient exceptions occur when abrupt changes in protein intake occur. By contrast, in adequately fed neonates, 80% to 90% of protein intake is used for growth and only a small fraction is oxidized (Chapter 3). Older children and malnourished adults lie between these extremes.

Carbohydrate

Carbohydrate is not generally considered to be a dietary essential since it can be synthesized from protein and to a lesser extent from fat (equations 3,4).

$$100\ g\ protein \rightleftarrows 55\ g\ carbohydrate \qquad (3)$$

$$100\ g\ fat \rightleftarrows 10 - 15\ g\ carbohydrate \qquad (4)$$

However, brain and some other tissues require glucose as the major source of energy. In prolonged fasting, more than 50% of the brain's glucose requirement may be replaced by ketone bodies derived from fat; but in the fed state, even on carbohydrate-free diets, the contribution of ketone bodies is very much smaller (7). The glucose requirements of tissues such as red and white blood cells, kidney medulla, and lens of the eye are small. Furthermore energy in these tissues is derived solely from glycolysis, with the resulting lactate reconverted to glucose in the liver. Therefore, these tissues have no net requirement for glucose. The brain and nervous tissue derive energy from the complete oxidation of glucose. In adult humans, energy expenditure of the brain accounts for 20% of whole body resting energy expenditure, while in children it can reach 40%-50% (8). This is much greater than the 2% to 3% required by most mammals or even the 8% required by other primates (Table 4.1). For the adult this comes to about 100 to 150 g of carbohydrate per day (9). This means that on a carbohydrate-free diet, roughly 150 to 200 g protein will be broken down to meet brain glucose requirements (Equations 3 and 4) (7). Put another way, if protein intake is less than 150 g per day, carbohydrate becomes an essential dietary ingredient to avoid negative N balance and loss of body cell mass. This is important for artificial nutrition, since protein is rarely given in excess of 150 g per day. There is evidence that severely stressed patients, with injury, sepsis or burns, may require higher amounts of glucose than normal subjects (10,11).

Table 4.1.
Rates of oxygen consumption in the brain compared to whole body (BMR) for various species of mammals.[a]

Species	Body Weight (kg)	Brain Weight (g)	Total O_2 Consumption (ml/min)	Brain O_2 Uptake Total[b] (ml/min)	Brain O_2 Uptake Percentage of BMR
Elephant	6650	5700	7800	200	2.5
Elephant	3752	4896	5960	171	2.9
Horse	600	670	1296	23	1.8
Horse	392	517	1000	18	1.8
Pig	125	120	400	4.2	1.0
Man	70	1400	250	49	19.6
Sheep	52	106	215	3.7	1.7
Chimpanzee	38	387	158	13.5	8.6
Dog	16.4	70	83.4	2.4	2.9
Monkey (ateles)	3.8	91	36.0	3.2	8.8
Rabbit	2.6	19	21.7	0.7	3.1
Guinea Pig	0.800	4.7	10.3	0.16	1.6
Rat	0.250	2.0	3.4	0.07	2.1
Mouse	0.027	0.37	0.75	0.013	1.7

[a]From Grande F: Energy expenditure of organs and tissues. In Kinney JM: *Assessment of Energy Metabolism in Health and Disease*, Columbus, Ross Laboratories, 1980, pp 88–92.
[b]Brain O_2 consumption = 3.5ml 100 g^{-1} $min^{-1}$for all the species.

Carbohydrate has more subtle effects than those on N balance, which may be largely unexplored. One such, is the effect on muscle concentrations of ATP, ADP, and creatine-P. Liaw et al. (12) maintained patients after total hip replacement on 90 g day^{-1} of glucose, 70 g day^{-1} of amino acids, or 90 g glucose + 70 g amino acids as sole nutrient support for four days. Muscle biopsies were taken prior to operation and on the fourth postoperative day. The patients given only amino acids had marked decreases in muscle ATP, ADP and creatine-P (Figure 4.3), while those receiving glucose, with or without amino acids, showed no changes. Normal subjects given the same diets had no decreases in high energy phosphates even without glucose. In another study, severely malnourished patients had marked decreases in muscle high energy phosphates even with 90 g of glucose. These were abolished with 600 g day^{-1} of glucose (13). Thus, although glucose is not required to maintain muscle high energy phosphates in normal subjects, 90 g day^{-1} is required after total hip replacement, and much more is required with severe stress. This property of glucose cannot be replaced by giving protein, so that in stressed patients carbohydrate becomes a dietary essential even in the presence of large quantities of protein.

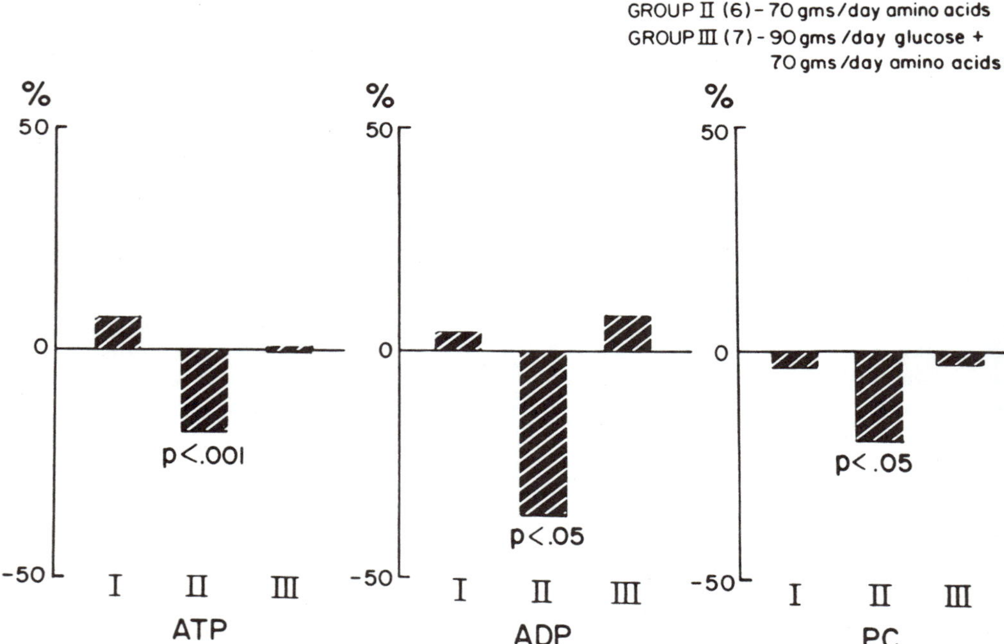

Figure 4.3. From Liaw KY, Askanazi J, Michelson CB et al.: Effects of postoperative nutrition on muscle high energy phosphates. *Ann Surg* 195:12-18,1982. With permission of the *Annals of Surgery*. Changes in muscle concentration of ATP, ADP and creatine-phosphate in patients 4 days after total hip replacement maintained with 90 g glucose day^{-1}, 70 g amino acids day^{-1}, or 90 g glucose + 70 g amino acids day^{-1} as sole sources of nutrients.

Ingested carbohydrate, after absorption by the gut, is in part oxidized and in part stored as glycogen for use in the postabsorptive period. If large amounts are ingested over long periods it may also be converted to fat (Figure 4.4), but this rarely occurs in normal subjects on normal oral diets, despite the wide range of possible diet compositions (14, 15).

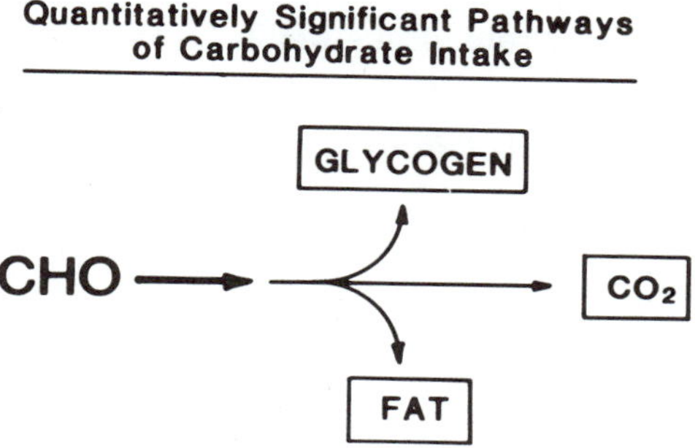

Figure 4.4. Major metabolic fates of carbohydrate.

Glycogen is stored in liver and in muscle. The amount of glycogen stored and the rate of glycogen storage is a complex function of the rate of carbohydrate intake over the past few days. Since meal-eating is episodic, glycogen will be stored during the absorptive period after a carbohydrate-containing meal, only to be utilized during the postabsorptive period. Despite diurnal variation, an individual who eats the same amount of a diet of constant overall composition, and who expends the same amount of energy each day, will have a constant mean daily store of glycogen. The amount is directly related to the daily carbohydrate intake. At carbohydrate intakes close to zero, both muscle and liver contain about 1% of wet weight as glycogen; at high intakes with diets not in excess of energy expenditure, glycogen content increases to about 2% in muscle and about 10% in liver (16, 17). In a 70 kg man, the maximum change in glycogen stores is about 430 g. With excessive amounts of carbohydrate intake, 1500 kcal (6276 kJ) per day in excess of the previous day's expenditure, glycogen stores can increase by 900 g (18). It takes three to four days to reach new steady-state levels of glycogen after a change in carbohydrate intake (19). This is illustrated in Figure 4.5 for ambulatory malnourished patients on continuous infusion of total parenteral nutrition, given either low (14 kcal [59 kJ] kg^{-1} day^{-1}) or high (32 kcal [134 kJ] kg^{-1} day^{-1}) intakes of carbohydrate. Initially, during the the high intake, there was extensive glycogen storage, 4 g kg^{-1} day^{-1} or 210 g day^{-1}per subject, which declined by day 5 to plateau values of about 1.4 g kg^{-1} day^{-1}. These constant values at rest indicate that mean daily glycogen stores are constant and that glycogen deposition at rest is equally balanced by glycogen utilization during physical acitivity in these ambulatory patients. The transient increase above plateau on days 1-4, represents net glycogen storage of about 300 g per subject. On the low intake, for those subjects previously on the high intake (Figure 4.5), there was a net loss of glycogen on day 1, with a gradual rise, by day 5, to plateau values of 1 g kg^{-1} day^{-1}. Even on a hypocaloric diet, with carbohydrate intake well below resting energy expendi-

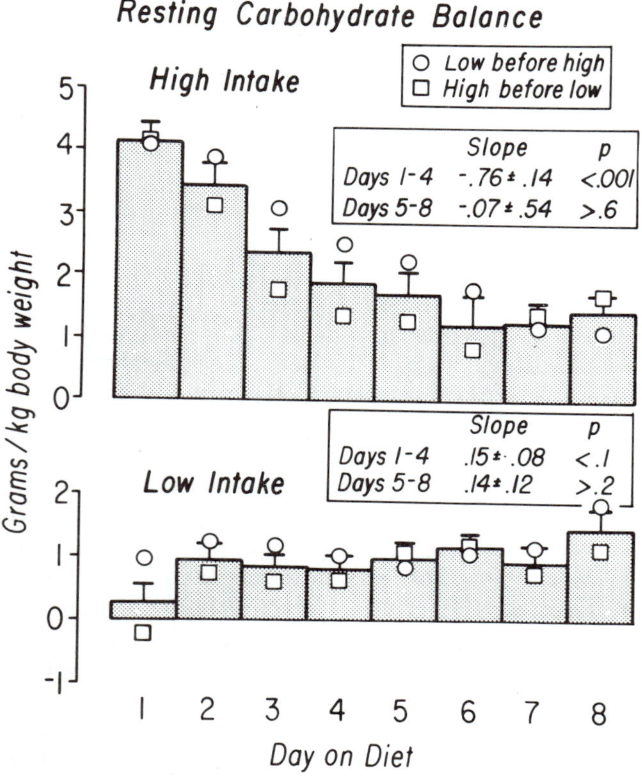

Figure 4.5. From Elwyn DH: The unique role of glucose in artificial nutrition: impact of injury and malnutrition. *Clin Nutr*, in press. With permission of *Clinical Nutrition.* Rates of glycogen deposition at rest (mean ± SE) in 11 malnourished patients for 8-day periods during administration of low or high glucose TPN. ○ low glucose diet given before high. □ high glucose diet given before low. Total energy and carbohydrate intake, respectively, were: 36.4 and 31.5 kcal (152 and 132 kJ) $kg^{-1}day^{-1}$ on the high diet, and 18.4 and 13.9 kcal (77 and 58 kJ) on the low diet.

ture, there was glycogen deposition at rest, with utilization of an equal amount of glycogen during physical activity. Approximately 200 g glycogen per subject was lost during the first 4 days for three subjects. The other patients on the low intake were previously given 5% dextrose and showed little change in rates of resting glycogen storage during the eight-day period.

The proportions of nonprotein energy derived from either fat or carbohydrate oxidation, represented by the nonprotein RQ, are controlled primarily by the overall rate of carbohydrate intake, since except transiently, all carbohydrate intake is oxidized, usually within 24 hours of administration. Changing rates of deposition or utilization of glycogen tend to buffer the impact of carbohydrate ingestion or of exercise on the nonprotein RQ. After a meal, the tendency to replace fat oxidation by carbohydrate oxidation, or to increase the nonprotein RQ, is buffered by increased rates of glycogen deposition. With physical activity or in the post absorptive period, the tendency to replace carbohydrate oxidation by fat oxidation, or to decrease the nonprotein RQ, is diminished or in the case of some exercise, may be completely overcome by utilization of glycogen stores.

For normal subjects on most diets, in which carbohydrate supplies 35%-70% of nonprotein energy intake, this buffering effect of carbohydrate means that the nonprotein RQ varies over only a limited range during the course of the day, either at rest or during moderate physical acitivity. The mean daily value of the nonprotein RQ will depend on intake, if carbohydrate is 35% and fat 65%, it will average about 0.80; if carbohydrate is 70% and fat 30%, the nonprotein RQ will average about 0.91. Daily excursions from this mean will seldom be greater than ± 0.05.

However, glycogen stores are limited. As they increase under any given set of circumstances, the rate of glycogen storage decreases, so that at any level of carbohydrate intake, there is a maximum level of glycogen stores. When this level is reached, all carbohydrate intake is utilized for other processes, either oxidation or lipogenesis (Figure 4.4). At very high rates of carbohydrate intake, as after a large meal, the nonprotein RQ may increase greatly and even exceed 1.0, indicating net lipogenesis is taking place (20,21). This is illustrated by a study of Acheson et al. (21), in which 500 g (2000 kcal, 8370 kJ) of carbohydrate was eaten by normal subjects, after an overnight fast, during a 5-hour period (Figure 4.6). For the previous six days, one group was maintained on a low-carbohydrate, high-fat regimen; a second group on a medium; and a third group on a high-carbohydrate diet. Postabsorptive nonprotein RQs, just before the meal, were about 0.92 on the high-, 0.82 on the medium- and 0.75 on the low-carbohydrate intake (Figure 4.6). At one hour after ingestion of the first 250 g of dextrin maltose, nonprotein RQs rose strongly, indicating replacement of fat oxidation by glucose oxidation, and for some hours were above 1.0 for the subjects who had been on the medium- and high-carbohydrate intakes. Thus in these two groups, there was no net fat oxidation but rather a small amount of lipogenesis for a substantial period of time. By 15 hours, RQs had returned to or below initial values. The fates of the 2000 kcal (8370 kJ), for the first 14 hours after ingestion, are shown in Table 4.2. Glycogen storage accounted for 50% to 65% of the amount ingested, depending on previous diet. Neverthless glucose oxidation completely or almost completely suppressed fat oxidation in all three groups. The extent of lipogenesis, however, was small, amounting to only 4% of the ingested meal even for the subjects who had previously been on a high-carbohydrate diet. A very similar pattern of response to a mixed meal of 900 kcal (3766 kJ) containing mostly carbohydrate and protein was reported by Bursztein et al. (20). Thus, even with carbohydrate meals much larger than are normally encountered, lipogenesis is minimal, supporting the view of Bjorntörp and Sjöström (14) that it is quantitatively unimportant in either normal or obese humans on oral diets.

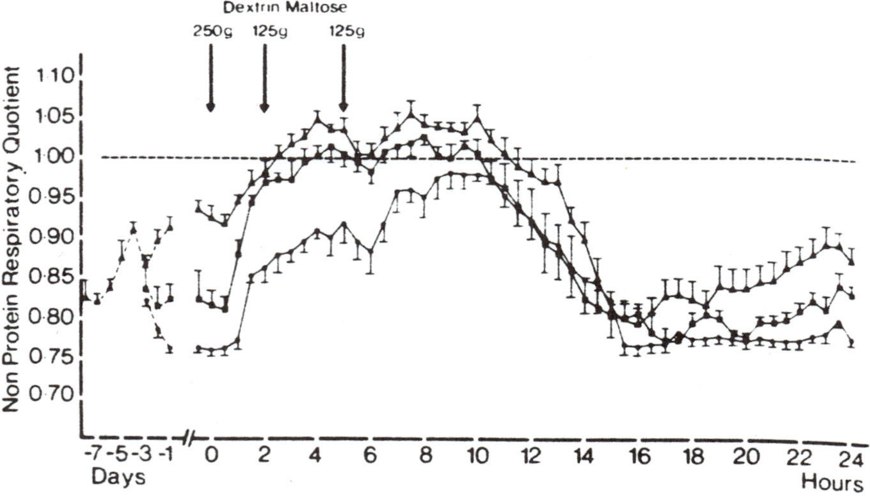

Figure 4.6. From Acheson KJ, Schutz Y, Bessard T et al.: Nutritional influences on lipogenesis and thermogenesis after a carbohydrate meal. *Am J Physiol* 246:E62-E70, 1984. With permission of the *American Journal of Physiology.* Changes in fasting nonprotein RQ each morning while subjects were on adaptive diets (· high fat, • medium carbohydrate, ▲ high carbohydrate) and before, during, and after ingestion of 500 g (2000 kcal, 8368 kJ) dextrin maltose.

Table 4.2.
Metabolic fate of 8368 kJ (2000 kcal) of dextrin maltose during 14 hours after ingestion in 3 groups of normal subjects maintained for 6 days previously on low, medium, or high fat diets. Mean ± SEM.

Previous diet		Stored as Glycogen	Oxidized	Converted to Fat
	kJ	5406±100	2933±84	29±21
Low CHO	kcal	1292±24	701±20	7±5
	kJ	4310±151	3925±184	134±25
Medium CHO	kcal	1030±36	938±44	32±6
	kJ	4058±84	3958±121	351±38
High CHO	kcal	970±20	946±29	84±9

[a]Data adapted from Acheson et al (21).

Nevertheless, it is very common to give patients who require parenteral nutrition energy intakes of 3000 kcal (12,550 kJ) per day or more, with most of it derived from carbohydrate and protein. Since energy expenditure of most patients averages under 2000 kcal (8370 kJ) per day, this means that for many patients there will be extensive lipogenesis from carbohydrate and protein, often in excess of 100 g fat per day (22). These high rates of fat synthesis with excess carbohydrate in parenteral nutrition are associated with: *(a)* development of fatty liver (23) and of hepatic dysfunction, as shown by increased blood levels of bilirubin and hepatic enzymes (24,25); *(b)* markedly increased thermogenesis, since the thermic effect of glucose is about 30%, given in excess, compared to 10% when given below energy requirements (15,18); and *(c)* marked increases in sympathetic activity as evidenced by urinary norepinephrine excretion (26). Intuitively these complications seem undesirable; however, there is no strong evidence that they contribute significantly to morbidity or mortality.

An important aspect of high-carbohydrate intakes is their effect on CO_2 production. The RQ of carbohydrate is 1.0, while that of fat is about 0.7; therefore as the amount of carbohydrate in the diet increases, CO_2 production and thereby the RQ increases, as illustrated in Figure 4.7. It is possible for a small patient to double his or her CO_2 production, going from 5% dextrose to 3000 kcal (12,550 kJ) per day of glucose-based TPN. For normal subjects, such an increase in CO_2 production, with its associated increase in minute ventilation, has no noticeable effect on breathing. It is roughly equivalent to the change in going from lying down to walking slowly (Table 2.9). For patients with poor pulmonary function the difference can be important (27). This is illustrated, in Figure 4.8, for a severely malnourished patient referred for parenteral nutrition. When given 5% dextrose, he was ambulatory with no breathing discomfort. When given glucose-based total parenteral nutrition, he became dyspneic and had to stay in bed. His minute ventilation at rest was 10.8 liters min^{-1}. When one-half the glucose was replaced by fat emulsion, his resting minute ventilation fell to 6.4 liters min^{-1} and he could again walk around without breathing discomfort.

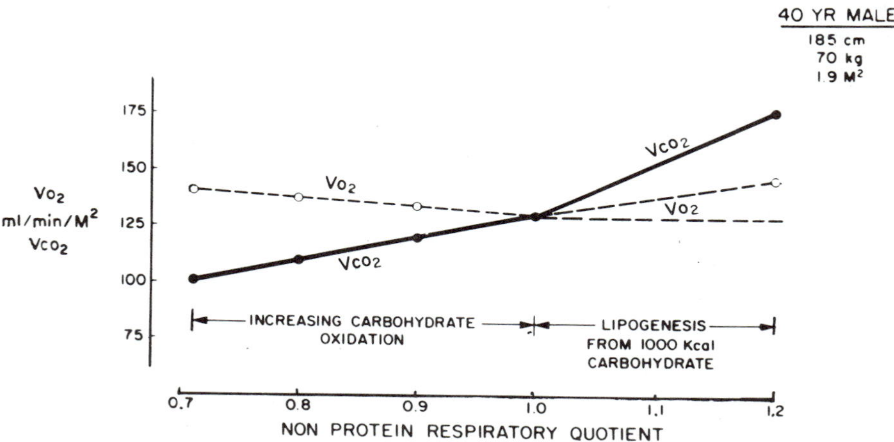

Figure 4.7. From Elwyn DH, Askanazi J, Kinney JM, Gump FE: Kinetics of energy substrates. *Acta Chir Scand* (Suppl) 507:209-219, 1981. With permission of *Acta Chirurgica Scandinavica.* Effects of increasing carbohydrate intake on CO_2 production, O_2 consumption, and RQ in normal subjects. Data derived from the literature.

Too high a carbohydrate intake can seriously interfere with weaning patients off of mechanical ventilation (27).

Fat

Dietary fat is less important than carbohydrate in influencing fuel utilization. Nevertheless, it can affect rates of carbohydrate and fat oxidation even though the effects may be transitory. This is illustrated for malnourished patients maintained on parenteral nutrition with all nonprotein energy supplied as glucose, or with one third of the glucose replaced by fat (28). The lipid was infused only during the hours of 09:00 to 17:00. During this period, fat oxidation was higher and carbohydrate

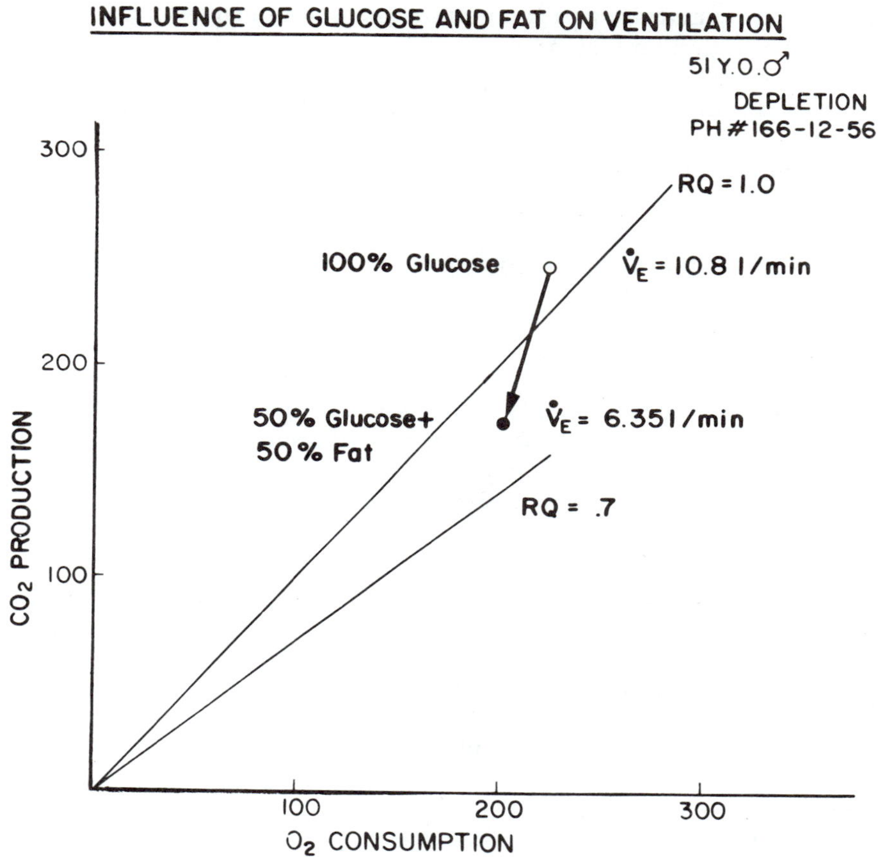

Figure 4.8. From Elwyn DH: Nutritional requirements of adult surgical patients. *Crit Care Med* 8:9-22, 1980. With permission of *Critical Care Medicine.* Effects of high and low carbohydrate intake on RQ and minute ventilation in a severely malnourished patient.

oxidation lower than during the other 16 hours when no lipid was infused (Figure 4.9). Thus lipid infusion caused an increase in rate of fat oxidation together with increases in rates of glycogen storage and decreases in carbohydrate oxidation. Presumably the major mediator of this effect was the increase in plasma-free fatty acid concentration. If this rate of lipid infusion had been continued indefinitely, instead of 8 hours only, we would expect this effect to disappear, since as glycogen increased, the rate of glycogen deposition would decrease until it returned to the rate occurring prior to lipid infusion. As a consequence, rates of carbohydrate and lipid oxidation would also return to their rates prior to lipid infusion.

The metabolic and hormonal mechanisms by which diet and exercise regulate the amounts of fat and carbohydrate oxidized, converted to ketone bodies or lactate, or stored, have been termed the *glucose fatty acid cycle* (29), which has been described in great detail by Newsholme and Start (2). The major effector, in relation to diet, is the rate of carbohydrate intake mediated by insulin. Increased insulin increases the rate of disposal of glucose: as glycogen, in liver or muscle; by glycolysis and oxidation; and rarely by conversion to fat. At the same time it decreases lipolysis and increases fatty acid esterification in adipose tissue, thus decreasing release of fatty acids and plasma fatty acid concentrations. Since fatty acid oxidation in all tissues, very low density lipoprotein synthesis in liver, and ketone body production in liver are all dependent on plasma fatty acid concentrations, all of these processes decrease. In addition insulin acts directly to suppress ketogenesis. Oral intake of fat, increases concentrations of chylomicrons which are acted on by lipoprotein lipase causing increased plasma FFA concentrations (infused lipid particles, after acquiring endogenous lipoproteins, are also hydrolyzed by lipoprotein lipase). These increased fatty acid concentrations act to increase fatty acid oxidation and to inhibit glycolysis and pyruvate oxidation due to increased acetyl-CoA and citrate concentrations (Figure 4.1), and thereby divert glucose-1-phosphate to glycogen synthesis. Exercise triggers release of epinephrine, which increases glycolysis and lipolysis, thereby increasing the availability of both fatty acids and glucose for muscle use.

In addition to their function as a major energy source, fats are required in mammalian diets as a source of essential fatty acids. These comprise two groups of polyunsaturated fatty acids, represented by linoleic and linolenic acids, which can be modified but not synthesized de novo by animal tissues. They constitute essential components of all cell membranes, and are precursors to several groups of hormone-like substances, the prostaglandins, thromboxanes, and leukotrienes, which are collectively referred to as eicosanoids. Linoleic acid is acted on by liver enzymes to form arachidonic acid. This is accomplished by introducing two double bonds in the omega-12 and omega-15 positions, and adding two carbons at the carboxyl end of the molecule (Figure 4.10). Arachidonic acid is the major polyunsaturated fatty acid of cell membranes, and the precursor of one group of prostaglandins, as well as serving a number of other key metabolic roles. Linolenic acid is acted on, in an exactly parallel manner to linoleic acid, to give 5,8,11,14,17-eicosapentaenoic acid (Figure 4.10), which is not quantitatively as important as arachidonic acid, but which also serves as a membrane constitu-

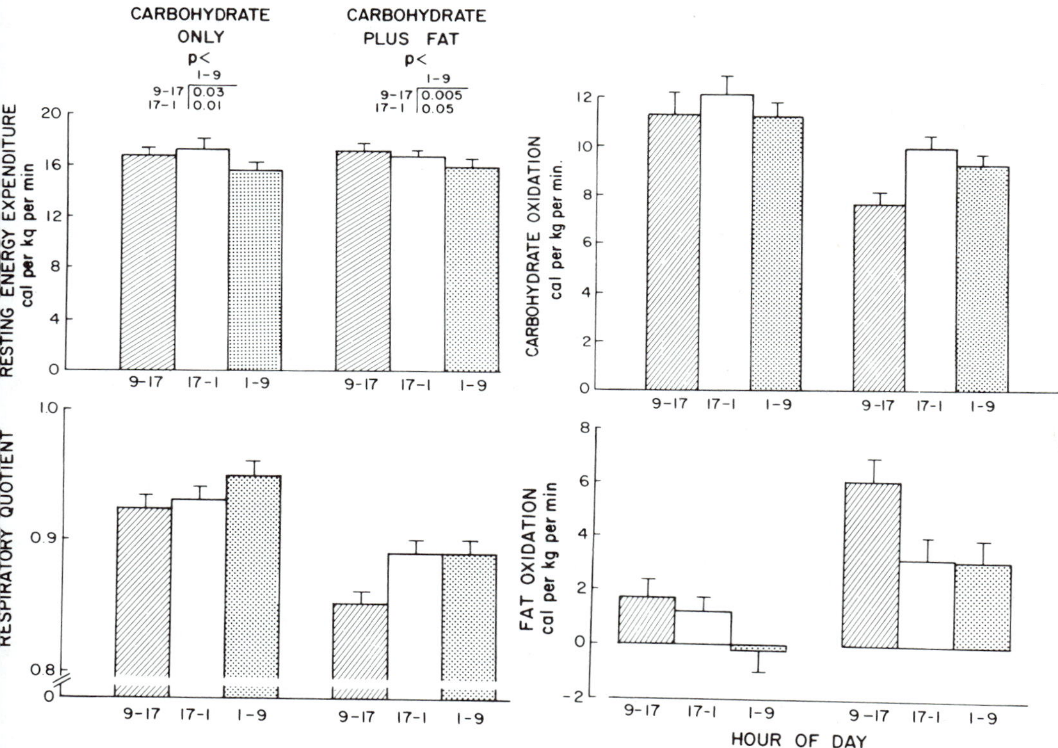

Figure 4.9. From Elwyn DH, Kinney JM, Gump FE et al.: Some metabolic effects of fat infusion in depleted patients. *Metabolism* 29:125-132, 1980. With permission of *Metabolism*. Rates of fat and carbohydrate oxidation and resting energy expenditure and RQ in malnourished patients given total parenteral nutrition with all nonprotein energy as glucose, or with 1/3 of the glucose replaced by lipid emulsion, which was infused only between the hours of 09.00 and 17.00.

ent and as a precursor of another group of prostaglandins. It also acts to inhibit prostaglandin synthesis from arachidonic acid (30). The essentiality of these fatty acids lies in the double bonds at position 12 in both linoleic and linolenic acid, and at position 15 in linolenic acid. These double bonds cannot be introduced by animal enzymes. Whereas chain lengthening, and introduction of double bonds between positions 10 and the carboxyl group of the 18 carbon fatty acid can be accomplished by animal enzymes. Thus oleic acid is readily synthesized by animal tissues and is a normal constituent of all fats and of cell membranes. In essential fatty acid deficiency, oleic acid substitutes for linoleic acid as a substrate for chain lengthening and introduction of more double bonds to give abnormally high concentrations of 5,8,11-eicosatrienoic acid (Figure 4.10). This is an inadequate substitute for arachidonic acid. In adults on oral diets it is almost impossible to demonstrate essential fatty acid deficiency, since adipose tissue triglycerides contain at least a year's supply of linoleic and linolenic acids which are released from adipose tissue in adequate amounts during postabsorptive periods. Adult essential fatty acid deficiency was first clearly demonstrated in patients given glucose-based, total parenteral nutrition (no fat) infused continuously over each 24-hour period. Continuous infusion of glucose, at rates close to or greater than energy requirements, almost completely inhibits release of fatty acids from adipose tissue. In healthy subjects this can produce essential fatty acid deficiency in less than two weeks (Figure 4.11), as evidenced by a decrease in linoleic acid content of plasma cholesterol esters to one-fourth normal concentrations and a more than 10-fold increase in 5, 8,11-eicosatrienoic acid (31).

There are three sets of nomenclature for the metabolically important unsaturated fatty acids. The standard, or *Geneva*, nomenclature is shown on the right side of Figure 4.10. The numbering starts at the carboxyl group. This has the disadvantage that the numbers associated with the double bonds change as the fatty acid chain is lengthened. Thus the double bond at position 9 in oleic, linoleic, or linolenic, shifts to position 11 as two carbons are added at the carboxyl end (Figure 4.10). To avoid this, the omega (ω) system of numbering from the other end has been adopted, as shown on the left side of Figure 4.10. In this system the numbers of the double bonds remain the same as the carbon chain is lengthened to 20 or even 22 or 24 atoms. In this system, all the derivatives of linoleic acid can be referred to collectively as omega-6 fatty acids, while those of linolenic acid are the omega-3 fatty acids. Since, from a dietary point of view, the omega-6, and omega-3 double bonds are the only essential features of these fatty acids, other members of either group of fatty acids can meet dietary requirements, and linoleic and li-

Omega -9-octadecenoic acid (18:1 ω9) **Oleic acid** *9 - Octadecenoic acid (18:1 Δ9)*

18 17 16 15 14 13 12 11 10 9 8 7 6 5 4 3 2 1

$CH_3-CH_2-CH_2-CH_2-CH_2-CH_2-CH_2-CH_2-\mathbf{CH{=}CH}-CH_2-CH_2-CH_2-CH_2-CH_2-CH_2-CH_2-COOH$

Omega -1 2 3 4 5 6 7 8 9 10 11 12 13 14 15 16 17 18

Omega -9-eicosatrienoic acid(20:3 ω9) *5,8,11 - Eicosatrienoic acid (20:3 Δ5,8,11)*

20 19 18 17 16 15 14 13 12 11 10 9 8 7 6 5 4 3 2 1

$CH_3-CH_2-CH_2-CH_2-CH_2-CH_2-CH_2-CH_2-\mathbf{CH{=}CH}-CH_2-\mathbf{CH{=}CH}-CH_2-\mathbf{CH{=}CH}-CH_2-CH_2-CH_2-COOH$

Omega -1 2 3 4 5 6 7 8 9 10 11 12 13 14 15 16 17 18 19 20

Omega -6-octadecadienoic acid(18:2 ω6) **Linoleic acid** *9,12 - Octadecadienoic acid (18: 2 Δ9, 12)*

$CH_3-CH_2-CH_2-CH_2-CH_2-\mathbf{CH{=}CH}-CH_2-\mathbf{CH{=}CH}-CH_2-CH_2-CH_2-CH_2-CH_2-CH_2-CH_2-COOH$

Omega -6-eicosatetraenoic acid (20:4 ω6) ***Arachidonic acid*** *5,8,11,14-Eicosatetraenoic acid (20:4 Δ5,8,11,14)*

$CH_3-CH_2-CH_2-CH_2-CH_2-\mathbf{CH{=}CH}-CH_2-\mathbf{CH{=}CH}-CH_2-\mathbf{CH{=}CH}-CH_2-\mathbf{CH{=}CH}-CH_2-CH_2-CH_2-COOH$

Omega -3-octadecatrienoic acid(18:3 ω3) ***Linolenic acid*** *9,12,15 -Octadecatrienoic acid (18:3 Δ9,12,15)*

$CH_3-CH_2-\mathbf{CH{=}CH}-CH_2-\mathbf{CH{=}CH}-CH_2-\mathbf{CH{=}CH}-CH_2-CH_2-CH_2-CH_2-CH_2-CH_2-CH_2-COOH$

Omega -3-eicosapentaenoic acid(20:5 ω3) *5,8,11,14,17-Eicosapentaenoic acid (20:5 Δ5,8,11,14,17)*

$CH_3-CH_2-\mathbf{CH{=}CH}-CH_2-\mathbf{CH{=}CH}-CH_2-\mathbf{CH{=}CH}-CH_2-\mathbf{CH{=}CH}-CH_2-\mathbf{CH{=}CH}-CH_2-CH_2-CH_2-COOH$

Figure 4.10. Structures, nomenclature, and numbering systems for oleic, linoleic, and linolenic acids and their 20 carbon derivatives. Numbering systems shown for oleic acid and 5,8,11-eicosatrienoic acid apply equally to the other 18 and 20 carbon acids.

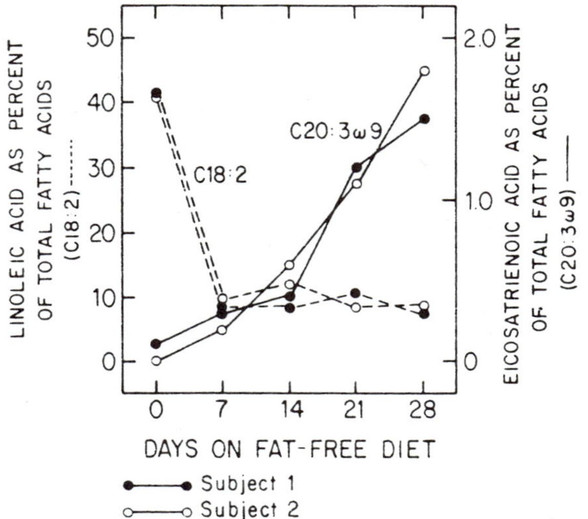

Figure 4.11. From Wene JP, Conner WE, Den Besten L: The development of essential fatty acid deficiency in healthy men fed fat free diets intravenously and orally. *J Clin Invest* 56: 127-137, 1975. With permission of the *Journal of Clinical Investigation.* Changes in linoleic and eicosatrienoic acid as percentage of total fatty acid composition of plasma cholesterol esters in two subjects given glucose based total parenteral nutrition continuously for two weeks.

nolenic acids are not required per se. Since the double bonds in all these fatty acids are always spaced at intervals of 3 carbon atoms, it is necessary to specify only the first double bond position. Thus 20:4 omega-6, specifies that the double bonds are at omega-6,9,12, and 15. In this system omega is often replaced by the symbol n. The third system of nomenclature involves the trivial names of each fatty acid. It is used frequently for the common fatty acids, but rarely for the others.

The requirement for the omega-6 fatty acids is about 10 g day^{-1} or 4% of energy intake. This is most easily met by vegetable oils such as corn, soy or safflower oils which contain 50% or more of their fatty acids as linoleic acid. Linolenic acid occurs to a much smaller extent in vegetable oils, there is none in safflower oil, but other members of the omega-3 series occur in many fish oils. Exact requirements for the omega-3 series have not been determined, but their physiological and nutritional effects are currently under active investigation. One of the most important nutritional aspects of the omega-6 and omega-3 series of fatty acids is their role in reducing the development of atherosclerosis.

Recently, use of polyunsaturated fats in parenteral and enteral feeding has disclosed some very important pharmacological effects. These effects are postulated to be mediated by prostaglandin E_2 (PGE_2), a derivative of arachidonic acid, and of other eicosanoids. Askanazi and colleagues (32–34) administered lipid containing total parenteral nutrition to cystic fibrosis patients. They found marked improvement within about six months with respect to thinning of secretions, lung function, exercise tolerance, body weight, and decreased hospitalization. By six months to a year, these changes became dramatic. Subjects previously confined to bed, breathing 40% O_2, were able to live an active physical life and work for a living. These results were achieved by administration of about 100 g lipid per day, as a slow infusion over 12 hours, with appropriate amounts of other nutrients. If the lipid was infused too rapidly or in excessive amounts, chest secretions became thicker and lung function poorer. The authors postulate that the improvements were due primarily to PGE_2, which is known to cause pulmonary vasodilatation and depresses inflammation and immunity, but that at high rates of lipid infusion increased rates of synthesis of other eicosanoids, such as prostaglandin F_2, and some of the thromboxanes and leukotrienes predominate, which cause pulmonary vasoconstriction and increase immunity and inflammation.

In other experiments, Alexander and coworkers (35-38) investigated the effects of enteral nutrition on gut mucosa, metabolism, immunity and morbidity in guinea pigs given 30% third-degree burns. They found that when adequate enteral feeding was given immediately after the burns, rather than parenteral nutrition or delayed enteral feeding, there was greatly improved maintenance of mucosal morphology, improved N content in muscle and other organs at autopsy, a much reduced hypermetabolic and hypercatabolic response to the burn injury, and reduced morbidity in general. Optimal effects were achieved when lipid comprised 5% to 15% of total energy intake. When lipid was supplied at 30% or 50% as safflower oil, there were marked decreases in immune responses, and reduced nitrogen retention. When supplied as fish oil, there was a reduction of similar magnitude in N retention, but no decrease in immune responses. These authors postulate that the immunosuppressive effects were due to excess production of PGE_2, which would be high with safflower oil, which contains over 70% of linoleic acid and negligible amounts of omega-3 fatty acids. By contrast fish oil contains mainly omega-3 fatty acids, which not only produce no PGE_2 but inhibit PGE_2 synthesis from endogenous arachidonic acid. A personal communication from Dr. J. W. Alexander indicates that similar results to the guinea pig studies have been obtained with humans.

These two exciting sets of studies on the pharmacological effects of lipids represent only the beginnings of a new field of investigation. At present it seems highly likely that these effects are mediated by prostaglandins, thromboxanes, and leukotrienes, some of which are inflammatory, immunostimulatory, and vasoconstrictive, while others are antiinflammatory, immunosuppressive, and vasodilatory. The amounts and proportions of these hormone-like substances can be strongly influenced by the composition and amount of administered lipids. Decisions as to how much and which type of lipid to give, will therefore depend not only on its use for energy purposes, but also on the possible pharmacological effects both beneficial and harmful. As indicated by the examples cited, these findings open up the possibility for the future of using disease-specific lipid regimens for therapeutic purposes in many illnesses.

Metabolic Effects of Fasting

In fasting the body derives its energy only from its own stores of fat and glycogen and from functional intracellular proteins. During the first few days, marked metabolic changes occur which serve to conserve energy and particularly protein; subsequent adaptations proceed at a slower rate.

The classical study of fasting was performed by Benedict (39). He advertised for a subject, and accepted Mr. A. Levanzin of Malta. Levanzin was a strong advocate of fasting as a therapeutic measure, and claimed that his daughter was cured of smallpox through fasting for 17 days. His fascinating autobiographical notes are included in Benedict 's report. He fasted for 31 days, which he spent continuously in an indirect calorimetry chamber. Continuous measurements were made of O_2 consumption and CO_2 production. Daily measurements were made of N balance and urinary constituents. Daily weight loss was rapid at first (Figure 4.12), in large part due to an initial water loss, and continued at a decreasing rate throughout the 31 days. Nitrogen losses were also rapid at first, reaching a maximum of 12 g per day on day 4 and decreasing to a constant value of 7 g per day by day 20. This is still higher than rates of N excretion measured in obese patients or other normal subjects as discussed below. Weight decreased by 23% in 31 days and BCM, estimated from N losses by 24%. (For comparison to partial starvation see Figure 3.6.) Total energy expenditure, which includes physical activity, decreased by 30%, from 1770 kcal (7406 kJ) day^{-1} to a plateau of 1250 kcal (5230 kJ) day^{-1} by day 18. Available glycogen stores were almost completely gone by day 6. Excretion of betahydroxybutyrate increased sharply until day 4 and then

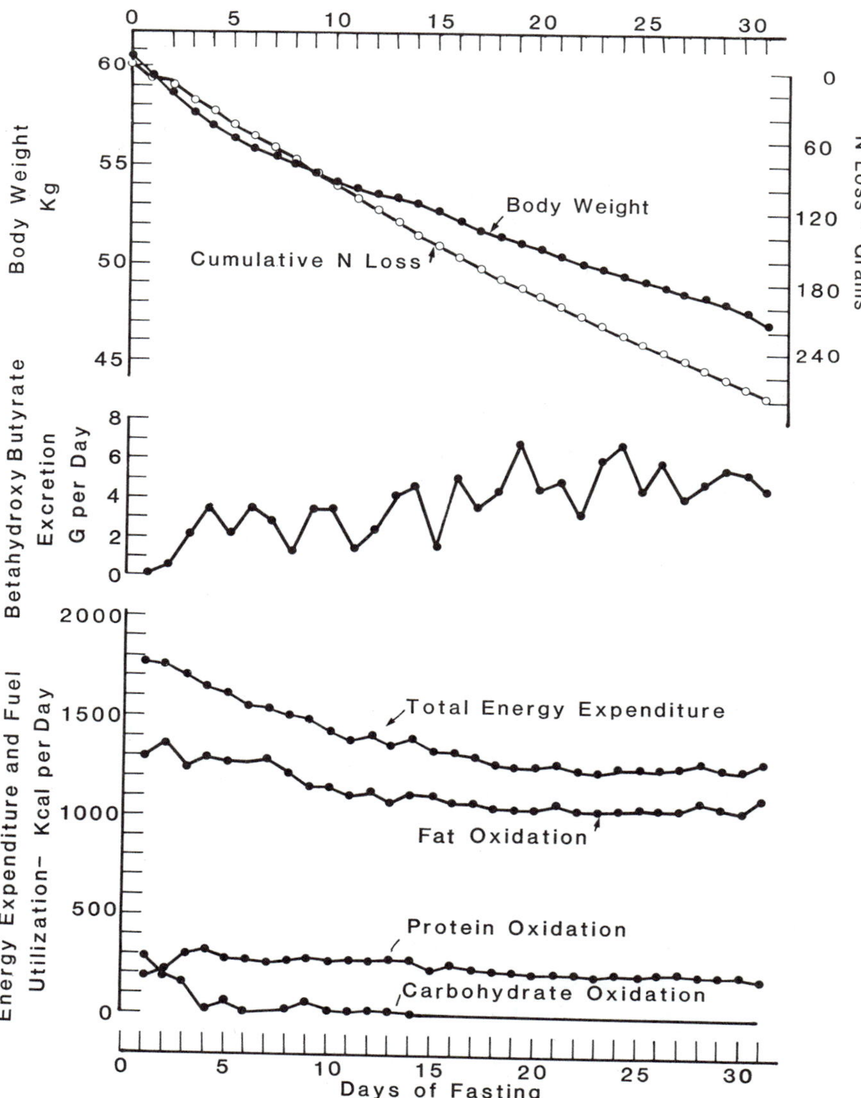

Figure 4.12. Data adapted from Benedict (39). Loss of body weight and N, and daily values of total energy expenditure, fat, protein, and carbohydrate oxidation, and beta-hydroxybutyrate excretion in a man fasted for 31 days.

more slowly to a plateau averaging 5 g day^{-1} by day 16. Blood constituents were not measured in this study, but are shown for a later study of obese patients in Figure 4.13. This shows the dramatic rise in blood ketone bodies and in plasma fatty acids, and the decrease in plasma glucose and insulin characteristic of prolonged fasting (40).

The metabolic mechanisms by which N is conserved in fasting have been extensively studied by Cahill, Owen and colleagues (9, 40-45). Approximate rates of metabolic processes somewhat modified from those of Cahill (41), are shown for a 24-hour fast (Figure 4.14) and a five- to six-weeks fast (Figure 4.15).

After 24 hours of fasting, both liver and muscle retain some available glycogen, the actual amount dependent on previous diet intake. In this scheme, liver glycogen is shown to supply 30 g day^{-1} to blood glucose, while muscles are shown to oxidize another 30 g (Figure 4.14). Brain glucose requirements of 94 g are much greater than can be supplied by liver glycogen, and the rest is obtained from gluconeogenesis in liver, using amino acids, primarily from breakdown of muscle protein, and glycerol derived from lipolysis of adipose tissue triglycerides. Lactate and pyruvate, produced by red and white cells and other glycolizing tissues such as the kidney medulla and lens of the eye, are also substrates for glucose production in the liver; however, an exactly equal amount of glucose is reconverted to lactate and pyruvate in these tissues, thereby constituting a metabolic cycle in which there is no net gain or destruction of glucose. The brain also obtains a small amount of energy from oxidation of ketone bodies, even at this early stage of fasting. It was formerly thought that the brain had to adapt to oxidation of ketone bodies, but it is now clear that the proportions of glucose and ketone bodies utilized by the brain depend on their relative concentrations in blood (40). In the fed state, concentrations of ketone bodies are 1/500 those of glucose and they are used to a negligible extent. After one day's fast the ratio increases to 1/10 (Figure 4.13) and they provide about 10% of brain requirements (Figure 4.14). By 5 to 6 weeks, ketone body concentrations are higher than those of glucose, and they provide more than one-half of brain requirements (Figure 4.15).

By the third day of fasting, both ketogenesis and gluconeogenesis are proceeding at nearly maximal rates because blood levels of glucose and particularly of insulin have declined markedly from the fed state, releasing the inhibition of these processes, and concentrations of glucagon, which stimulate gluconeogenesis, have increased (46). However, muscle and heart also utilize ketone bodies at this stage, and the increase in blood ketone bodies is intermediate between the fed and prolonged fasting states (Figure 4.13). As fasting continues for several

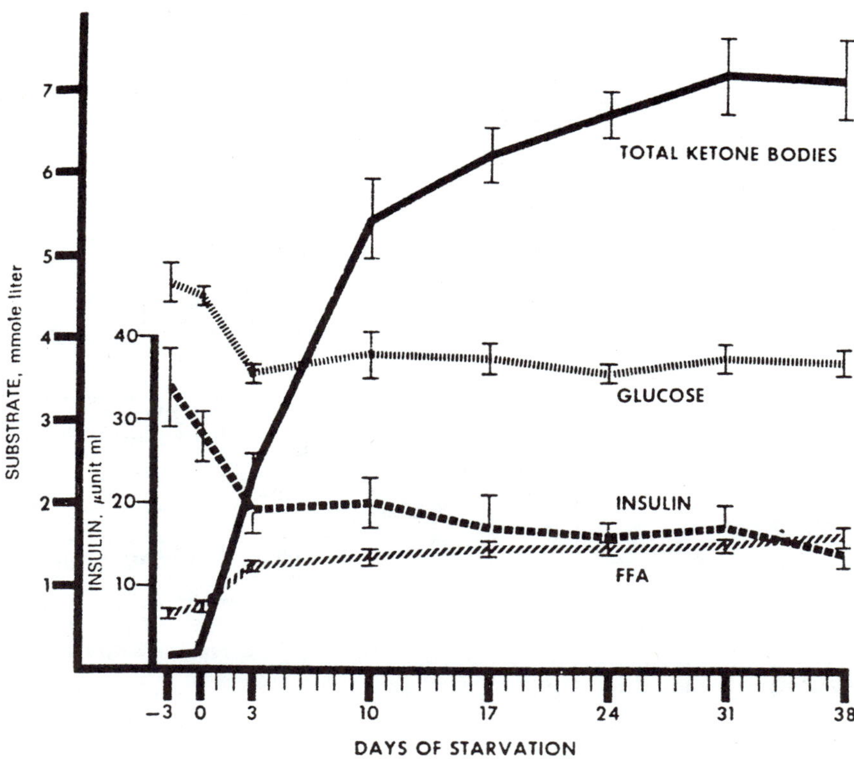

Figure 4.13 From Owen OE, Reichard GA Jr: Ketone body metabolism in normal, obese and diabetic subjects. *Israel J Med Sci* 11: 560-570, 1975. With permission of the *Israel Journal of Medical Sciences.* Concentrations of blood glucose and ketone bodies, plasma-free fatty acids, and serum insulin in 37 obese patients during prolonged starvation.

more days, ketone body oxidation in heart and skeletal muscle decreases. This causes a further increase in ketone body concentrations, to 5-10 mmolar, and subsequently the brain obtains more than 50% of its energy requirements from ketones (Figure 4.15). When ketone body concentrations reach these high levels, substantial amounts are excreted in the urine (Figure 4.15) and fasting of more than 3 or 4 days is associated with metabolic acidosis.

The weights and intracellular N contents of all organs and tissues decrease more or less in parallel during fasting or starvation (47), except for the brain and nervous tissue which show negligible changes. However, muscle comprises about 72% of body cell mass; therefore, it is the major contributor to the 75 g protein (12 g N) loss, shown in Figure 4.14.

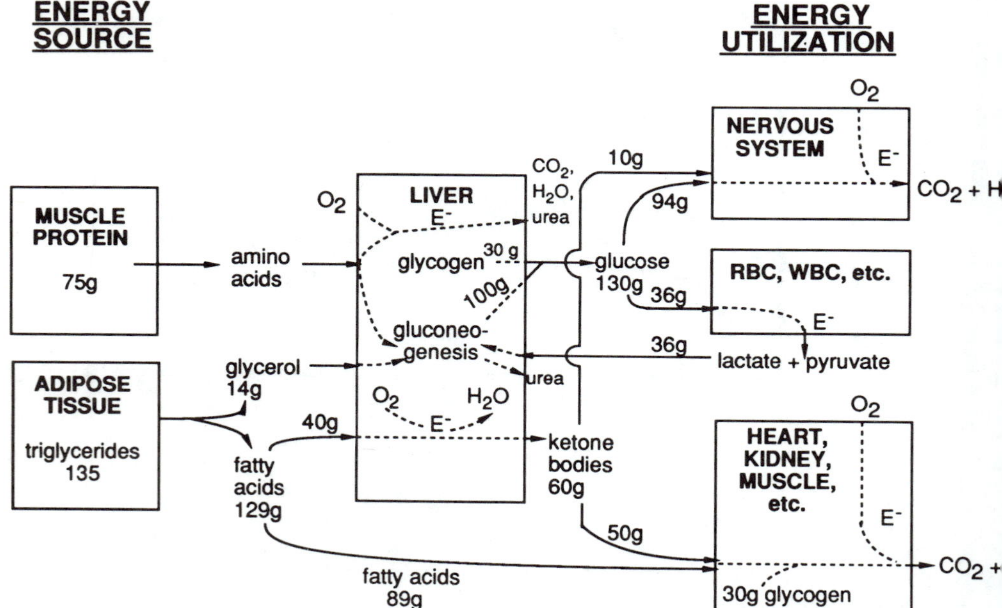

Figure 4.14. Modified from Cahill GF Jr: Starvation in man. *New Eng J Med*, 282:668-675, 1970. Metabolic rates in g day^{-1} after a brief fast of 24 hours. Energy expenditure = 1800 kcal (7531 kJ) day^{-1}, RQ =0.76.

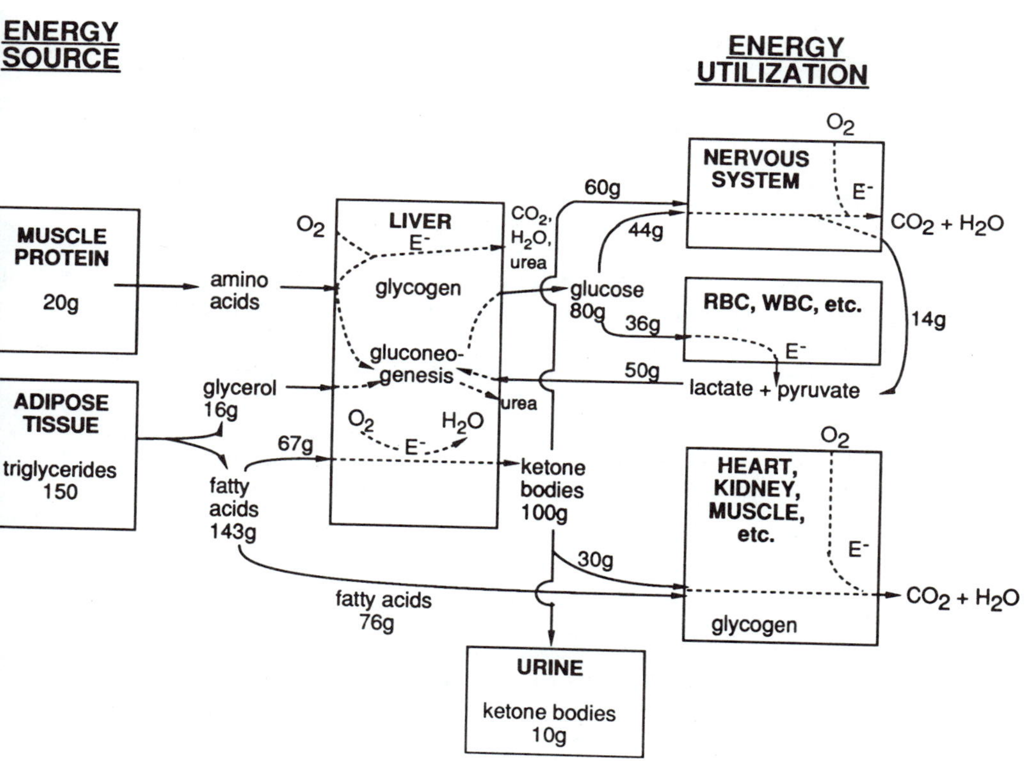

Figure 4.15. Modified from Cahill GF Jr: Starvation in man. *N Engl J Med*, 282:668-675, 1970. Metabolic rates in g day^{-1} after a prolonged fast of 5-6 weeks. Energy expenditure = 1450 kcal (6067 kJ) day^{-1}, RQ = 0.73.

Only about 60% of protein can be converted to glucose; the rest is oxidized, mainly in the liver. This, together with the energy derived from ketogenesis, just meets liver requirements during fasting.

After 24 hours, oxidation of protein and glycogen account for about 570 kcal (2385 kJ) day^{-1}; the remaining energy ,for a total of 1800 kcal (7531 kJ) day^{-1}, is supplied by 135 g of triglycerides from adipose tissue, which on hydrolysis, with addition of water, produces 14 g of glycerol and 129 g of fatty acids (Figure 4.14). The calculated RQ of 0.76 indicates the predominant role of fat as an energy source under these conditions.

After 4 or 5 days of fasting, available glycogen stores have been completely depleted (48) and glucose and insulin concentrations are at minimum levels. Subsequently, further adaptations take place at a slower pace. With decreases in heart and muscle oxidation, blood concentrations of ketone bodies reach maximal levels only after 3 to 4 weeks. Energy expenditure declines. Rates of muscle protein breakdown and of gluconeogenesis decrease. An increasing portion of gluconeogenesis takes place in the kidney, associated with increased excretion of ammonia in response to the metabolic acidosis caused by excretion of the ketone bodies—betahydroxybutyrate, and acetoacetate.

With time these processes develop into the picture shown in Figure 4.15. Energy expenditure has declined by about 20%, from 1800 to 1450 kcal (7531 to 6067 kJ) day^{-1}. There is no further contribution from glycogen; 20 g protein (3.2 g N) supplies only 85 kcal (356 kJ); and the remainder comes from 150 g of fat, which gives rise to 16 g of glycerol and 143 g of fatty acids. The calculated RQ of 0.73 reflects the increased role of fat. More than one-half of the brain's energy now comes from ketone bodies. Except for the glycolyzing tissues, and protein oxidation in the liver, all other organs obtain all of their energy requirements from fatty acids.

The adaptations to fasting, in which the brain minimizes glucose oxidation, replacing it with ketone body oxidation, permit a reduction in protein loss from 75 g, initially, to 20 g day^{-1} after several weeks. This is reflected in a decrease in urea excretion nearly to zero (Figure 4.16). Twenty g of protein correspond to 90 g of body cell mass. Since almost all the muscle mass, approximately 28 kg, can be lost before death ensues, it should be theoretically possible to fast for about 200 days if loss of muscle were the limiting factor. However, as discussed in Chapter 2, fat stores are more limiting and fasts of 60 days usually end in death.

Hormonal Mediators of Fasting

The initial reduction in insulin is probably the most important endocrine change mediating the effect of early fasting. However, insulin concentration remains very constant after the third day (Figure 4.13).

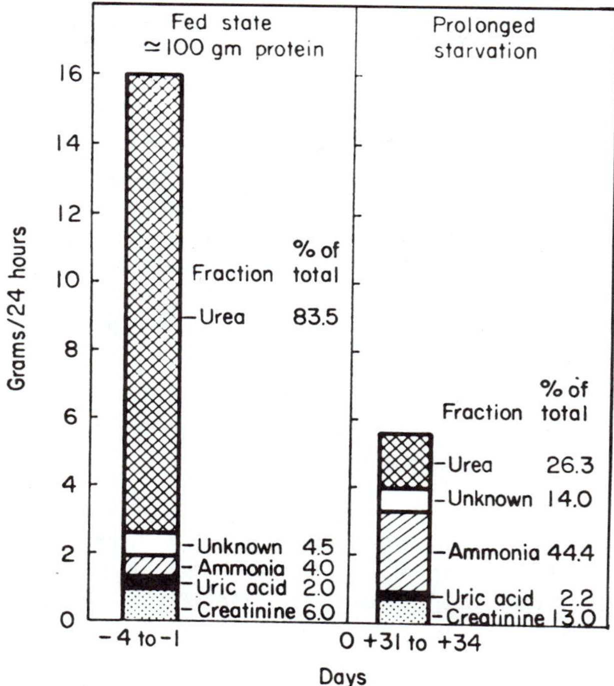

Figure 4.16. Adapted from Cahill (41). Components of urinary N excretion after a 24-hour or 5- to 6-week fast.

Glucagon concentrations increase steadily during fasting, at least up to six or seven days (46), which may account for some of the slower changes. Glucocorticoid concentrations rise during fasting (41).

Concentrations of T_3 decrease and of T_3r increase (49,50) during fasting, and concentrations of growth hormone show erratic changes (41). What specific roles these changes play in the metabolic adaptation to fasting is not clear.

Sympathetic activity decreases in fasting as a result of decreased carbohydrate intake (50-52) and is unlikely to account for the major metabolic changes such as increased lipolysis, gluconeogenesis, and ketogenesis . In some instances increased concentrations of both epinephrine and norepinephrine have been reported. These seem to be of adrenal origin and to be associated with hypoglycemia and perhaps exercise (48,53).

Effects of Carbohydrate Intake on Fasting Metabolism

The metabolic rates seen in uncomplicated fasting are very sensitive to small amounts of carbohydrate. Gamble (54) showed, with healthy young men, that 100 g glucose per day would reduce N excretion to one-half of fasting rates (Figure 7.2). Even in prolonged fasting, when N excretion was already low (7 g per day) infusion of 100 g of dextrose per day reduced it to less than 3 g day^{-1} (48). This daily amount of dextrose is also sufficient to completely suppress gluconeogenesis in normal subjects (55) and both gluconeogenesis and ketogenesis in malnourished patients (56). This 100 g of glucose just meets brain requirements. Thus it seems likely that the metabolic changes which take place in fasting are primarily a mechanism to supply adequate energy to the brain. We may surmise that this is a very human characteristic, shared in part perhaps with our primate relations, since the brain requirements for glucose in other mammals account for only 3% or less of energy expenditure, which can be met entirely from the glycerol released from fat oxidation (Table 4.1).

HYPERMETABOLIC, HYPERCATABOLIC STRESSED STATES

Mechanical injury, burns, and sepsis share a number of pathological conditions, which include marked alterations in metabolism and response to nutrients.

Cuthbertson defined two phases in the response to injury, the *ebb* or *shock* phase followed by the *flow phase* (57). The flow phase has been further divided into a *catabolic* and an *anabolic* phase (58). Stoner (59) distinguished two flow phases: the *flow phase proper* in which oxidation is adequate leading to recovery, and a *necrobiosis phase* leading to death. The duration of these phases depends on both the type and severity of the insult. The ebb phase may last a few hours after uncomplicated surgery, but two to three days after severe accidental injury, burns or sepsis.

The ebb or shock phase is characterized by loss of intravascular fluids to interstitial fluid, transcellular spaces, or by hemorrhage. Blood pressure and blood flow fall, and there is greatly increased sympathetic activity, although energy expenditure falls (60). There is marked initial hyperglycemia derived mainly from glycogen stores. Subsequent development of hypoglycemia with exhaustion of glycogen has a poor prognosis. Reduced energy expenditure is accompanied by lowered body temperature and seems to be related to changes in thermoregulation in the hypothalamus (60).

The catabolic flow phase may last from a few days to several weeks or longer with severe burns or sepsis. This is the hypermetabolic, hypercatabolic stress state which is generally associated with trauma.

Energy expenditure is increased (Figure 7.3) by about 10% postoperatively, from 10% to 30% with accidental injury, 30% to 50% with sepsis, and up to 100% with severe burns (61). Starvation reduces energy expenditure up to 40%. Since injured or septic patients are often starved to some extent, their change in energy expenditure will be the algebraic sum of the two effects. Indeed, energy expenditure of patients under intensive care can range from about 40% below to 60% above normal values (62). Measurements of 100% increases after severe burns were made before the awareness that high ambient temperature and minimization of evaporative loss were important therapeutic procedures. With modern treatment, it is only rarely that increases would be expected to be greater than 50% to 60%. The increased energy expenditure, or hypermetabolism, of injured and septic patients is associated with increased body temperature. This increase in temperature in the flow phase, like the decrease in the ebb phase, is related to thermoregulation in the hypothalamus which results in a change in the thermoneutral temperature range, that is, the range of temperature in which the nude subject feels most comfortable and expends the minimum energy at rest (63). In the flow phase the thermoneutral zone is increased several degrees above normal values of 27° to 29° C (64,65).

Protein Metabolism

The injured, septic, or burned patient is hypercatabolic as well as hypermetabolic. As in fasting normal subjects the bulk of N loss comes from skeletal muscle. Since N losses are markedly affected by diet, quantitative comparison to normals can be made only at constant diet intake. This has been discussed in detail in Chapter 3, which presents rates of N loss in various pathological states during 5% dextrose administration (Figure 3.7) As with energy expenditure, the extent of the N loss is dependent on the severity of the stress. In fasting patients it can exceed 30 g N or 150 g protein per day.

Carbohydrate Metabolism

A characteristic feature of injury, sepsis, and burns is hyperglycemia. This may range from just above normal after elective surgery to as high as 800 mg dl^{-1} (45 mmolar) in severe cases. The hyperosmolarity of blood with these very high glucose concentrations can have severe clinical consequences. These high blood glucose concentrations have been termed the "diabetes of injury." However, unlike diabetes mellitus, they are associated with increased rather than decreased concentrations of insulin. Long and colleagues (66) demonstrated with tracer techniques that hyperglycemia was associated with increased production of glucose and that gluconeogenesis in septic patients was much higher than in normal subjects (55). This higher than normal rate of glucose production is associated with a decreased rate of oxidation of preformed glucose, whether in the form of glycogen or of administered carbohydrate, as measured by indirect calorimetry (15,66a). Glucose, fat, and protein oxidation in normal subjects and injured and septic patients at two different levels of glucose intake are shown in Figure 4.17. At each level of intake, glucose oxidation was lower in the patients than in the normal subjects, while fat and protein oxidations were higher. Thus in the hypermetabolic state, glucose production is higher but utilization of preformed glucose is lower than normal. If, however, one adds the amount of glucose produced by gluconeogenesis from noncarbohydrate precursors, which is oxidized, to the amount of preformed glucose oxidized, total glucose oxidation is greater than normal in stressed patients.

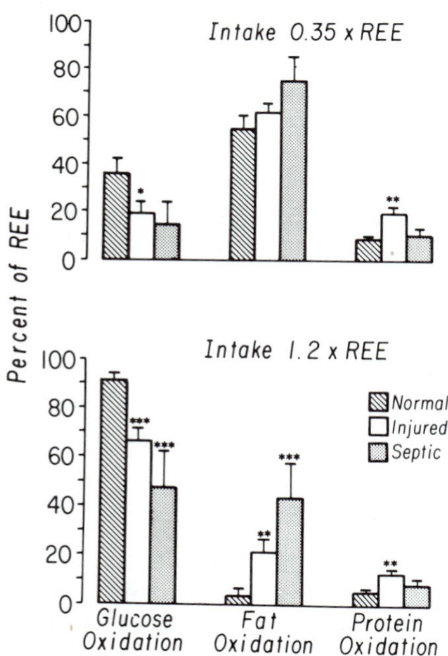

Figure 4.17. Reproduced from Elwyn DH: The unique role of glucose in artificial nutrition: Impact of injury and malnutrition. *Clin Nutr*, in Press. With permission of *Clinical Nutrition.* Glucose, fat and protein oxidation in 6 normal subjects, 6 injured patients and 3 septic patients at low (0.35 x resting energy expenditure) and high (1.2 x resting energy expenditure) glucose intake given intravenously, as sole source of calories, for 3 days. Differs from normal: * $P<0.05$, ** $P<0.01$, *** $P<0.005$.

Glucose turnover increases even more than glucose oxidation in trauma and sepsis (66,67), due to an increase in glycolysis, which is a requirement of the wound or septic region. In sepsis there is an increase in white blood cells at the site of infection which use glucose for glycolysis rather than oxidation. In injury or burn the healing tissue also uses glucose for glycolysis rather than oxidation. Wound requirements have been measured by Wilmore et al. (68) in severely burned patients in whom one leg was either severely burned (50%) or lightly burned (10%). Blood flow and O_2consumption were measured for the whole body and for a single leg. Glucose consumption and lactate production were also measured in the leg (Table 4.3). There were no significant differences in whole body percentage of burn, blood flow, or O_2 consumption between the patients with the large or the small leg burns, leg blood flow; glucose consumption, and lactate production were much higher with the large than the small leg burn, but there was little difference in O_2 consumption. Almost all the glucose consumed was recovered as lactate. Thus the major difference between the legs with large and small burns was due to a difference in the amount of glucose used for glycolysis, not for oxidation. This difference, of 0.30 mg glucose min^{-1} per 100 ml leg, may be attributed to the burn, amounting to 40% of the leg area (50% minus 10%). Extrapolated to the whole body, the amount of glucose glycolized by the burn wound in a patient with a 40% burn is about 200-300 g per day. The energy derived from glycolysis of glucose is about one-twentieth of that obtained from oxidation or 0.2 kcal (0.8 kJ) g^{-1}. Thus although the glucose requirements of the wound are very large, the energy requirements of the wound itself are modest, about 60 kcal (251 kJ) day^{-1}, much less than the increase in energy expenditure in the body generally, due to the presence of the wound, which is closer to 500-1000 kcal (2100-4200 kJ) day^{-1}. Wolfe et al. (69) found glycolytic gluconeogenic cycling of glucose, measured isotopically, in severely burned patients to be about 170 g day^{-1} for a 70-kg man. If we consider that most of this is required for the wound, it is in reasonable agreement with the 200-300 g day^{-1} derived from Wilmore's data (Table 4.3), especially considering the difference in techniques and problems in extrapolating from the leg to the whole body.

At any given level of carbohydrate intake, glycogen storage is increased and glycogenolysis is decreased in stressed patients compared to normal (15).

Fat Metabolism

Fat oxidation tends to be higher in hypermetabolic patients than in normal subjects (Figure 4.17) or than in malnourished patients (70).

Table 4.3.
Effects of leg burn size on leg blood flow and glucose metabolism in severely burned patients.

	Size of Leg Burn		
	Small (10%)	Large (50%)	P<
Total Body			
% Burn	41	42	NS
Cardiac index (liter m^{-2} min^{-1})	7.8	7.5	NS
O_2 consumption (ml m^{-2} min^{-1})	204	241	NS
Leg			
Blood flow (ml min^{-1}/100 ml leg)	4.2	8.0	0.001
O_2 consumption (ml min^{-1}/100 ml leg)	0.19	0.24	NS
Glucose consumption (mg min^{-1}/100 ml leg)	0.04	0.34	0.01
Lactate production (mg min^{-1}/100 ml leg)	0.06	0.30	0.05

[a]Reproduced from Wilmore DW, Aulick LH, Mason AD Jr et al.: The influence of the burn wound on local and systemic responses to injury. *Ann Surg* 186:444-458, 1977. With permission of the *Annals of Surgery*.

Carpentier et al. found that lipolysis of triglycerides in adipose tissue increases to a much greater extent than fat oxidation (70). The excess fatty acids must be reesterified, constituting what has been termed a *substrate cycle* (71). In malnourished patients, this substrate cycle accounted for 100 g fat day^{-1} per subject and was independent of the dietary intake or rate of oxidation of fat (72). With injury or sepsis this increased to about 200 g fat per day (70). Wolfe et al. (69) found values of about 100 g fat per day in normal subjects, which rose to about 450 g in severely burned patients (74% of surface area). This increase in fat mobilization is accompanied by marked increases in plasma concentrations of glycerol but not of fatty acids. Thus there is a dissociation of the normal relations between fatty acid turnover and concentration (72). These increases in fat mobilization and glycerol concentration and maintainence of normal concentrations of fatty acids occur despite the increases in insulin concentrations associated with trauma.

Although fat metabolism and oxidation are increased with stress, ketogenesis is decreased compared to normal fasted subjects (73). The blood concentration of betahydroxybutyrate has been used to distinguish severe injury, less than 200 μmole $liter^{-1}$, from mild or moderate injury, greater than 200 (73).

These metabolic changes with trauma are summarized for a typical severely hypermetabolic, hypercatabolic patient in Figure 4.18. For comparison with normal patients (Figures 4.14 and 4.15) this hypothetical patient is shown as fasting. However, for ethical reasons, severely stressed patients are rarely fasted for 24 hours or more for study purposes. Therefore the actual figures shown are extrapolated from studies of patients receiving some nutrients, mostly 5% dextrose, and include a fair amount of guess-work. Also the metabolic rate will vary with the severity of the stress, being much greater after a 75%, third-degree burn than after an abdominal operation. Nevertheless, Figure 4.18 serves to summarize the typical metabolic changes which accompany severe injury under fasting conditions.

A major difference from normal patients is the threefold increase in glucose production mainly used for glycolysis in the wound. However, glycogenolysis is suppressed and all the glucose comes from gluconeogenesis. Since ketogenesis is partly inhibited by high glucose and insulin concentrations, all the brain requirements are met by glucose, and in addition, under these conditions, other tissues oxidize some glucose. This increased glucose oxidation is derived almost entirely from degradation of muscle protein, which proceeds at 2.5 times the rate in normal subjects. The RQ is reduced from 0.76 in fasting normals (Figure 4.14) to 0.74, reflecting the lack of glycogen utilization.

Hormonal Changes in Trauma and Sepsis

The metabolic pattern in the stressed patient does not undergo the same adaptation with time as is seen in the normal fasting patient. This is because the normal regulatory mechanisms which are very sensitive to insulin concentration and glucose intake are overwhelmed by increases in counterregulatory hormones. There are many hormone changes which accompany injury, burns, or sepsis, and this subject has been reviewed in detail elsewhere (74,75). For many of these, the connections to the changes in metabolism are obscure. The best understood and most important changes are the increases in epinephrine and norepinephrine, cortisol, and glucagon. Increases in norepinephrine mainly reflect increases in sympathetic activity. They occur immediately after the insult, are very high in the ebb phase, and continue at high but declining rates during the catabolic part of the flow phase. Increases in cortisol occur more gradually but are evident throughout the flow phase. Hormone concentrations in patients with severe burns, compared to normal subjects (69), are shown in Table 4.4.

Infusion of cortisol, glucagon, and epinephrine into normal subjects at rates which maintain blood concentrations in the range seen in stressed patients (Table 4.4) causes metabolic changes which mimic those seen in injury and sepsis (76,77). These include hypermetabolism, hypercatabolism, hyperglycemia, and hyperinsulinemia, together with

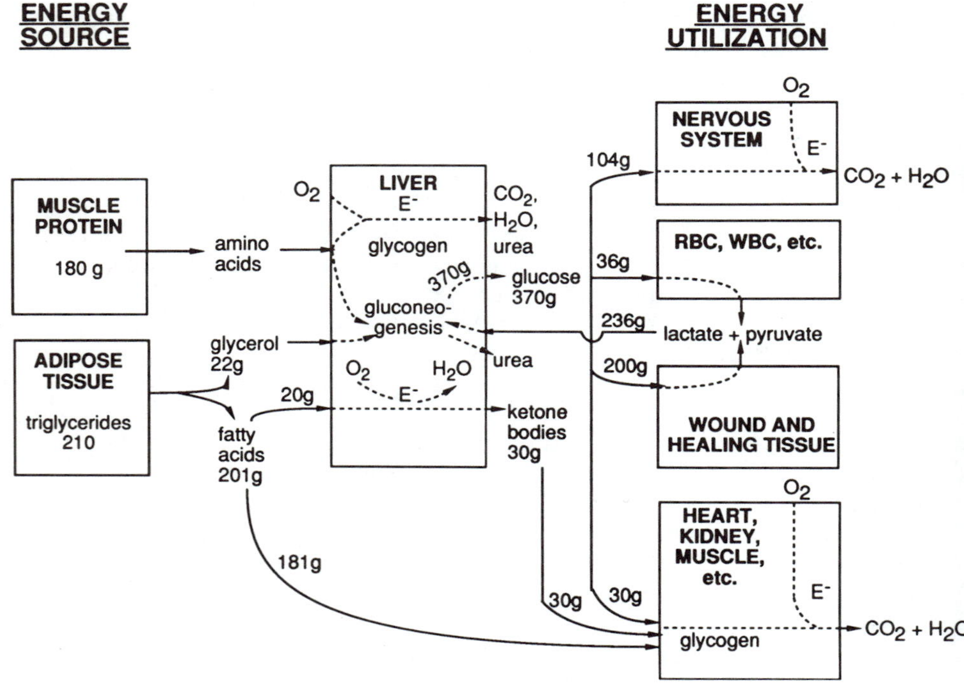

Figure 4.18. Metabolic rates in g day^{-1} after a brief fast in a hypothetical severely injured subject. Energy expenditure 2700 kcal (11,297 kJ) day^{-1}, RQ-0.74.

Table 4.4.
Hormone concentrations in normal volunteers and in patients with burns. Samples taken after a fast of 8 hours or more. Mean ± SEM. All values in patients are significantly different from normal ($P < 0.01$).[a]

Subjects	Insulin $\mu U\ ml^{-1}$	Glucagon $pg\ ml^{-1}$	Cortisol $ng\ dl^{-1}$	Epinephrine $pg\ ml^{-1}$	Norepinephrine $pg\ ml^{-1}$
Normal volunteers	11.3±0.9	143±28	8±1.8	35±5	184±34
Patients with burns	19.6±4.2	325±53	32±4.8	376±74	1,558±295

[a]Reproduced from Wolfe RR, Herndon DN, Jahoor F et al: Effect of severe burn injury on substrate cycling by glucose and fatty acids. *N Engl J Med* 317:403-408, 1987. With permission of the *New England Journal of Medicine.*

increased glucose and insulin resistance. The hyperglycemia results from both increased production and decreased clearance of glucose.

There are two main pathways by which the wound or septic insult causes this change in the neuroendocrine milieu. One of these involves stimulation of a variety of receptors, which send impulses via the afferent nervous system to be coordinated in the hypothalamus (74). Nerve endings, including pain receptors at the site of injury, are stimulated. Epidural analgesia prevents transmission of the stimuli and blocks the development of the stress response immediately after injury (78). Baroreceptors respond to the low volume and flow in the ebb phase and chemoreceptors respond to variations in O_2, CO_2, and pH. Fear, anxiety, temperature, and other physiological and environmental factors also have input into the metabolic response to injury. These various signals are coordinated or integrated in the hypothalamus (79) and appropriate efferent signals are transmitted through the sympathetic system and adrenal medulla, which respond rapidly, and the pituitary gland, which responds more slowly.

The other pathway, mediating the effects of injury or sepsis on metabolism, involves secretion of a number of polypeptide hormones or groups of hormones by white blood cells at the site of injury or infection. Some of these polypeptides have been isolated and characterized and there may be others. Endogenous pyrogen, leukocyte endogenous mediator, and lymphocyte-activating factor constitute either one or a family of polypeptides of 13-16,000 daltons, secreted by a wide variety of phagocytic cell types under appropriate stimulation (80).

One of these is the same as interleukin-1, a peptide of 17,000 daltons. Once released this peptide, or peptides, acts directly on the hypothalamus, augmenting and supplementing the effects of afferent nervous stimuli. In addition they influence the activity of many tissues, including lymphocytes, granulocytes, macrophages, bone marrow, the reticuloendothelial system, liver, muscle, and endocrine organs. Among their actions are to stimulate induction of fever, granulopoiesis, synthesis of acute phase proteins, hyperinsulinemia, and uptake of zinc and iron by the liver. Interleukin-1 acts directly on muscle to increase proteolysis and net breakdown of protein (81), providing an increased supply of amino acids for use by the liver and hematopoietic tissues. This action appears to be mediated by prostaglandin E_2 (81). A second peptide of about 4000 daltons has been isolated from plasma of septic patients. This also directly stimulates proteolysis in muscle and may be a degradation product of interleukin-1 (82). A third peptide, cachectin or tumor necrosis factor, is released by stimulated macrophages. It has many pathophysiological effects which overlap those of interleukin-1; it also stimulates release of interleukin-1, and appears to be the major factor mediating the lethal effects of endotoxin (83).

Although afferent neurogenic pathways and these various peptides can account for the ability of injury and sepsis to effect neuroendocrine and metabolic changes, the detailed mechanisms of their actions, the relative importance of each, and whether other factors play a role remain to be determined.

Why Does the Stress Response Occur?

It seems reasonable to assume that these metabolic changes, which are shared by humans with many other species, are adaptive, at least in the short term of days to weeks. The injured organism has increased nutrient requirements in order to cope with wound healing and infection, but particularly in the wild state, must obtain these nutrients from its own body stores. Some have suggested that the increased muscle protein breakdown is needed as an energy source per se. However, even in most severe stress, endogenous protein accounts for only 25% of total energy requirements (84). Furthermore mobilization of fat, which is the major endogenous source of fuel, is greatly increased with stress (70). It seems more likely that increased muscle proteolysis is needed to supply specific nutrients, glucose, and amino acids, which cannot be derived from fat.

An increased supply of amino acids is required by the liver and hematopoietic tissues for synthesis of acute phase proteins and for increased production of white blood cells. These are needed to control infection, to clear up necrotic tissues, and to take part in wound healing. In particular, an increased supply of glutamine may be important for white blood cells, the gut, the wound, and other rapidly dividing tissues since it plays a critical role in biosynthesis of nucleic acids and other cell constituents and is a major source of energy (85,86). The sharp decrease in muscle glutamine concentrations immediately following injury or other stress may reflect this requirement for glutamine of other tissues (87). Glutamine, administered intravenously, also serves to protect the structure and function of intestinal mucosa in the absence of oral or enteral intake. (88). In addition, in the absence of carbohydrate, amino acids are the main source of synthesis of the glucose needed for the brain and other glucose-requiring tissues and particularly for the wound itself.

Perhaps the most significant metabolic change due to injury is the occurrence of hyperglycemia in the absence of carbohydrate intake. In fasting normal subjects, blood glucose concentrations are decreased and extensive ketogenesis greatly reduces the amount of glucose required by the brain. Nitrogen excretion will drop below 5 g day^{-1} (80 mg kg^{-1} day^{-1}) in prolonged fasting (41).

Why does the stressed, fasted patient become hyperglycemic? It is not to meet brain requirements for glucose, which are readily met in the normal subject who is hypoglycemic. Rather it seems to be a requirement of the wound itself. As discussed above, the wound may require 200 g or more of glucose per day (Figure 4.18) which it needs for glycolysis rather than oxidation. We may calculate from Wilmore's study (Table 4.3) that the A-V difference in glucose concentration across the 50% burn leg was 4.3 mg dl^{-1} ($0.34 \times 100/8$). If we assume that the wound receives 10% of the leg blood supply and uses all the glucose, the calculated A-V difference across the wound itself is 43 mg dl^{-1}, more than one-half the arterial concentration in fasting normal subjects. This enormous extraction of glucose must take place even though the wound and regenerating tissues are poorly vascularized and would therefore require a high glucose concentration gradient. It thus seems very likely that hyperglycemia is an effective adaptive response to meet the glucose requirements of the wound or septic site. If this is true then in treatment of injured or septic patients, one should not make strong efforts to lower glucose concentrations of critically ill patients to normal values of 90-120 mg dl^{-1}.

While the requirements of the wound appear to be responsible for the hyperglycemia, they are not directly responsible for increased glucose consumption, since the wound converts glucose to lactate and pyruvate, which are used by the liver to resynthesize glucose. However, maintenance of hyperglycemia in a fasting subject is possible only by disruption of the normal regulation of carbohydrate and fat oxidation, the glucose fatty acid cycle (2, 29). Normally hyperglycemia, particularly when accompanied by hyperinsulinemia, would suppress fat mobilization and oxidation. In the fasting, hyperglycemic, hyperinsulinemic, stressed patient, fat mobilization is above normal, and roughly 75%-90 % of energy is supplied by oxidation of fat. Thus tissues such as skeletal muscle, heart, and liver utilize fatty acids preferentially, despite high glucose concentrations. These changes appear to be largely due to increases in sympathetic activity and of glucagon and cortisol (76, 77). The high concentrations of glucose and insulin also decrease ketogenesis as compared to normal fasting (73). With less ketones available, the brain requires much more glucose in the fasted stressed patients than in fasted controls. It is this high net requirement of the brain for glucose which is oxidized, much more than the wound requirement for glucose for glycolysis, which determines the amount of protein that must be broken down for gluconeogenic purposes in the stressed patient.

Thus the need of the wound for hyperglycemia is seen as a major etiological cause of the neuroendocrine changes in injury and sepsis. This disrupts the usual relations by which glucose intake or production and insulin concentration regulate fuel utilization. Brain requirement for glucose remains high and some glucose is oxidized by other tissues (Figure 4.18). This amount of glucose oxidized must be synthesized from muscle protein producing a hypercatabolic state.

The increased substrate cycles discussed above, lipolysis and triglyceride synthesis, and glycolysis and gluconeogenesis, which are energy-producing processes and an obligatory part of the changed neuro-endocrine and metabolic conditions, cause increases in energy expenditure (69). In addition, increase in protein turnover, another form of substrate cycling, occurs which also increases energy expenditure (89). These changes can account for much if not all of the increase in energy expenditure in injury and sepsis. We may speculate that the increase in core temperature and the thermoneutral zone, which accompany the increase in energy expenditure, provide, as does hyperglycemia, a more favorable environment for tissue regeneration and host defense.

Response to Nutrients

The changed neuroendocrine milieu in stressed patients changes the response to nutrients. Since fuel utilization patterns are now largely determined by the increased sympathetic activity and counterregulatory hormones, the ability of exogenous nutrients, particularly glucose, to change these patterns is attenuated.

In fasting normal subjects there is substantial incorporation of isotopically labeled alanine into blood glucose indicating extensive gluconeogenesis (Figure 4.19)(55). Administration of 3 liters of 5% dextrose per day completely suppresses it. In septic or injured patients receiving 3 liters of 5% dextrose, gluconeogenesis is twice as high as in fasting normal subjects, and is not completely suppressed until at least 600 g day^{-1} of glucose is given (Figure 4.19) (90). Injury or sepsis also attenuates the effect of administered glucose to decrease fat oxidation and increase glucose oxidation. Increasing glucose intake from 0.35 to 1.2 times resting energy expenditure (REE) for three days in normal subjects (Figure 4.17) increased glucose oxidation from 36% to 92% of REE; on average, for injured and septic patients, glucose oxidation increased from 16% to 57%. In normals, fat oxidation decreased from 55% to 5% of REE, in the patients from 68% to 34%. So that even with glucose intakes in excess of energy expenditure, the injured and septic patients derived one-third of their energy from endogenous fat. Askanazi et al. (91) compared fuel utilization and energy expenditure in malnourished and injured or septic patients maintained on 5% dex-

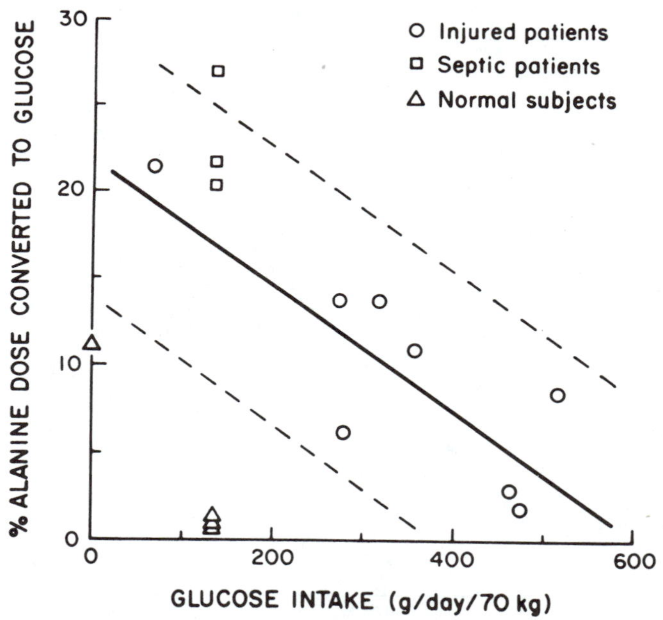

Figure 4.19. Data for injured patients and for the regression line and 95% confidence limits (*dotted lines*) from Elwyn DH et al. (90). Data for septic patients and normal subjects from Long et al. (55). Reproduced from Elwyn DH, Kinney JM, Jeevanandam M et al.: Influence of increasing carbohydrate intake on glucose kinetics in injured patients. *Ann Surg* 190:117-127, 1979. With permission of *Annals of Surgery.* Effect of glucose on gluconeogenesis measured by incorporation of isotopic alanine into blood glucose.

trose or glucose and amino acid based TPN given in excess of energy requirements (Figure 4.20). In the depleted patients, VCO_2 increased by 32%, VO_2 by only 3%. Thus RQ increased to 1.05 and there was substantial lipogenesis, producing 427 kcal (1787 kJ) day^{-1} of fat. The increase in REE was 9%, reflecting the diet-induced thermogenesis of the protein component of TPN. The septic/injured patients increased VCO_2 by 56%, more than for the depleted patients, but this was accompanied by a 29% increase in VO_2. The RQ increased only to 0.95 and there was continued fat oxidation of 474 kcal (1983 kJ) day^{-1}, although glucose intake was in excess of energy expenditure. Energy expenditure increased by 34%, far more than in the depleted patients or than would be expected in normal subjects. Thus in this study, also, injury or sepsis attenuated the usual effects of glucose intake to suppress fat oxidation and increase glucose oxidation. Accompanying this effect was an increase in diet-induced thermogenesis of glucose and amino acids above that of depleted patients and what would be expected in normal subjects (92).

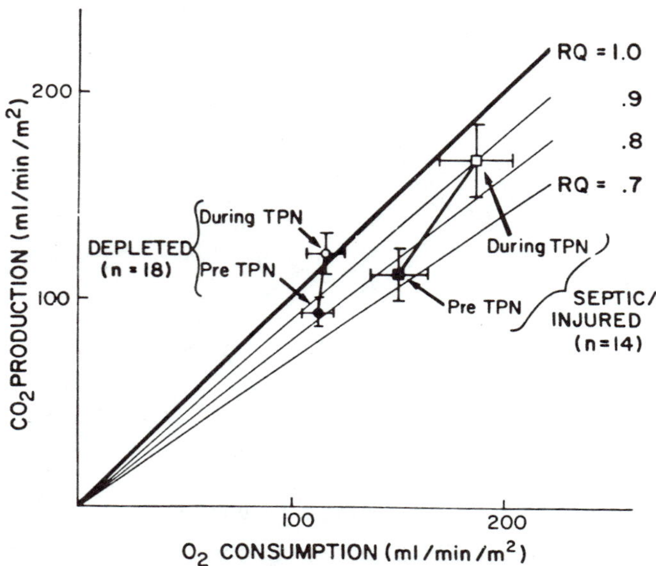

Figure 4.20. Reproduced from Askanazi J, Carpentier YA, Elwyn DH et al.: Influence of total parenteral nutrition on fuel utilization in injury and sepsis. *Ann Surg* 191:40-46, 1980. With permission of *Annals of Surgery*. Alterations in gas exchange in depleted or septic/injured patients when 5% dextrose infusions are replaced by glucose and amino acid based TPN.

All these effects of injury and sepsis, to attenuate the effects of glucose intake on gluconeogenesis, and on fat and glucose oxidation, and to increase the diet induced-thermogenesis of glucose and protein, occur despite that blood glucose and insulin concentrations are consistently higher, and increase more in response to glucose intake, than in normal subjects. A consequence of decreased glucose oxidation and increased fat oxidation in stressed patients, at any given level of glucose intake, is that glycogen storage is much greater than normal (15, 90) and can reach levels as high as 2000 g (93).

The effect of protein intake to improve N balance is also attenuated in injured, septic, or burned patients, as discussed in detail in Chapter 3. Normal subjects attain zero N balance at zero energy balance with an intake of 80 mg N kg^{-1} day^{-1}, whereas severely stressed patients (Figure 3.10) are in negative N balance of 3-4 g per day with N intakes of 200 to 300 mg kg^{-1} day^{-1} and energy intake in excess of expenditure (94).

The effects of nutrient administration on metabolic rates after four days of TPN are summarized in Figure 4.21 for the hypothetical severely injured patient shown fasting in Figure 4.18. Resting energy expenditure has increased to 3250 kcal (13,600 kJ) day^{-1} due to diet-induced thermogenesis, which is greater than in normal subjects (15, 91). Nutrient intake, as total parenteral nutrition, has been set at 3900 kcal (16,320 kJ) day^{-1}, 1.2 times energy expenditure in this bedridden patient. Nonprotein energy intake is given as equicaloric amounts of lipid emulsion and glucose. Protein intake is 210 g day^{-1} (33.6 g N day^{-1}, or 420 mg N kg^{-1} day^{-1}, if we assume a body weight of 80 kg), giving a calorie to N ratio of 116:1. This amount of protein is higher than would be given in most institutions (or than the authors would recommend [see Chapter 7]) and is greater than the amount of muscle protein broken down when the patient was fasting [Figure 4.18]. Nevertheless, and even though energy intake is in excess of expenditure, this amount of protein does not completely suppress catabolism of endogenous protein, and an additional 20 g of muscle protein are degraded, leaving the patient in a negative N balance of 3.2 g day^{-1}. Although the 400 g of glucose infused is more than is required by the brain for oxidation, a high rate of gluconeogenesis, 250 g day^{-1}, persists. This is largely because of the enormous supply of lactate and pyruvate produced by the wound and other glycolyzing tissues. Although we postulate that some of the lactate and pyruvate is oxidized by other tissues, most goes back to the liver to be reconverted to glucose. An additional 60 g of glucose is synthesized from glycerol released by hydrolysis of administered lipid and from protein. Since glucose intake is well in excess of brain requirements, substantial amounts are oxidized

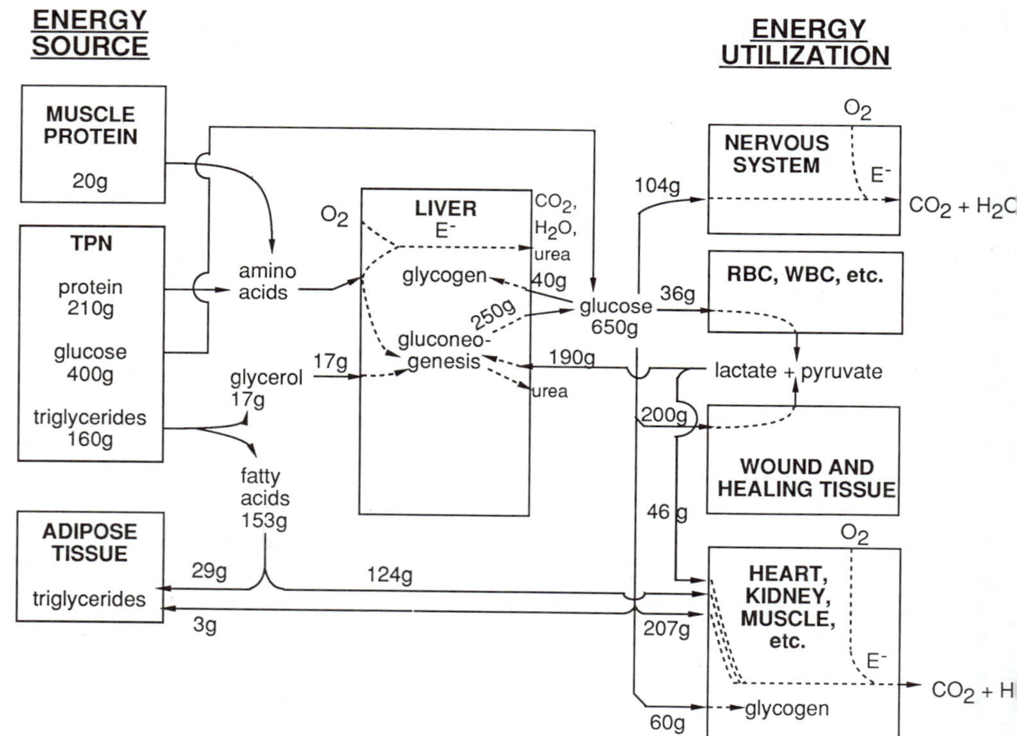

Figure 4.21. Metabolic rates in g day^{-1} in the severely injured patient of Figure 4.18 when given total parenteral nutrition at 1.2 times energy expenditure. Energy expenditure = 3250 kcal (13,598 kJ) day^{-1}, RQ = .82.

by other tissues. Nevertheless, substantial amounts are stored as glycogen in muscle and liver, much more than would be expected in normal subjects after four days on this diet. Because of the high rate of glycogen storage, storage of fat in adipose tissue is minimal. The RQ of 0.82 reflects the high rates of fat and protein oxidation, despite the large glucose intake.

REFERENCES

1. Lehninger AL: *Biochemistry, the Molecular Basis of Cell Structure and Function*, ed 2, New York, Worth, 1975.
2. Newsholme EA, Start C: *Regulation in Metabolism*, London, Wiley, 1973.
3. Elwyn DH: The role of the liver in regulation of amino acid and protein metabolism. In Munro HN (ed): *Mammalian Protein Metabolism*, New York, Academic Press, 1970, Vol. 4, pp 523–527.
4. Elwyn DH, Parikh HC, Shoemaker WC: Amino acid movements between gut, liver and periphery in unanesthetized dogs. *Am J Physiol* 215:1260-1275, 1968.
5. Bartlett EJ, Gusberg R, Ferrannini E et al.: Amino acid and glucose metabolism in the postabsorptive state and following amino acid ingestion in the dog. *Metabolism* 35:709-717, 1986.
6. Khairallah EA: In vivo determination of rates of protein degradation in livers of meal-fed rats: implications of amino acid compartmentation. In: Segal HL, Doyle DJ (eds): *Protein Turnover and Lysosome Function*, New York, Academic Press, 1978, pp 89–104.
7. Silwer H: Studien uber die N-Auscheidung im Harn bei einshrunkung des Kohlehydrates der Nahrung ohne wesentliche Veranderung des Energiengehaltes derselben. Acta Med Scand 79 (Suppl): 1-273, 1937.
8. Grande F: Energy expenditure of organs and tissues. In Kinney JM (ed): *Assessment of Energy Metabolism in Health and Disease*, Columbus, Ross Laboratories, 1980, pp 88–92.
9. Cahill GF Jr, Owen OE: Some observations on carbohydrate metabolism in man. In Dickens F, Randle PJ, Whelan J (eds): *Carbohydrate Metabolism and its Disorders*, New York, Academic Press, 1968, pp 497–522.
10. Wolfson AMJ, Heatly RV, Allison SP: Insulin to inhibit protein catabolism after injury. *New Engl J Med* 300:14-17, 1979.
11. Long JM, Wilmore DW, Mason AD Jr, Pruitt BA Jr: Effect of carbohydrate and fat intake on nitrogen excretion during total intravenous feeding. *Ann Surg* 185:417-422, 1977.
12. Liaw KY, Askanazi J, Michelsen CB et al.: Effect of postoperative nutrition on muscle high energy phosphates. *Ann Surg* 195:12-18, 1982.
13. Fürst P: Nutritional induced changes in muscle biochemistry in various catabolic states. *Boll Soc Ital Biol Sper* 59 (Suppl D):31-47, 1983.
14. Bjorntörp P, Sjöström L: Carbohydrate storage in man: Speculations and some quantitative considerations. *Metabolism* 27 (Suppl 2): 1853-1865, 1978.
15. Elwyn DH: The unique role of glucose in artificial nutrition: impact of injury and malnutrition. *Clin Nutr.*, 7:195-202, 1988.
16. Hultman E, Bergström J, Roch-Norlund AE: Glycogen storage in human skeletal muscle. In: Pernow B, Saltin B (eds): *Muscle Metabolism During Exercise*, New York, Plenum Press, 1971, pp 273–278.

17. Hultman E, Nilsson LH: Liver glycogen in man. Effect of different diets and muscular exercise. In: Pernow B, Saltin B (eds): *Muscle Metabolism During Exercise*, New York, Plenum Press, 1971, pp 143–151.
18. Schutz Y, Acheson JK, Jéquier E: Twenty-four hour energy expenditure and thermogenesis: response to progressive carbohydrate feeding in man. *Intl J Obesity* 9 (Suppl 2):111-114, 1985.
19. Chikenji T, Elwyn DH, Gil KM et al.: Effects of increasing glucose intake on nitrogen balance and energy expenditure in malnourished adult patients receiving parenteral nutrition. *Clin Sci* 72:489-501, 1985.
20. Bursztein S, Glaser P, Trichet B et al.: Utilization of protein carbohydrate and fat in fasting and postabsorptive subjects. *Am J Clin Nutr* 33:998-1001, 1980.
21. Acheson KJ, Schutz Y, Bessard T et al.: Nutritional influences on lipogenesis and thermogenesis after a carbohydrate meal. *Am J Physiol* 246: E62-E70, 1984.
22. Chascione C, Elwyn DH, Davila M et al.: Effect of carbohydrate intake on de novo lipogenesis in human adipose tissue. *Am J Physiol* 253:E664-E669, 1987.
23. Burke JF, Wolfe RR, Mullany CJ et al.: Glucose requirements following burn injury. *Ann Surg* 190:274-285, 1979.
24. Sheldon G, Baker C: Complications of nutritional support. *Crit Care Med* 8:35-37, 1980.
25. Lowery SF, Brennan MF: Abnormal liver function during parenteral nutrition: Relation to infusion excess. *J Surg Res* 26:300-307, 1979.
26. Nordenström J, Jeevanandam M, Elwyn DH et al.: Increasing glucose intake during total parenteral nutrition increases norepinephrine excretion in trauma and sepsis. *Clin Physiol* 1:525-534, 1981.
27. Askanazi J, Weissman C, Rosenbaum SH et al.: Nutrition and the respiratory system. *Crit Care Med.* 10:163-172, 1982.
28. Elwyn DH, Kinney JM, Gump FE et al.: Some metabolic effects of fat infusion in depleted patients. *Metabolism* 29: 125-132, 1980.
29. Randle PJ, Garland PB, Hales CN, Newsholme EA: The glucose and fatty acid cycle: Its role in insulin sensitivity and the metabolic disturbances of diabetes mellitus. *Lancet* i:785-789, 1963.
30. Culp BR, Titus BJ, Lands WEM: Inhibition of prostaglandin biosynthesis by eicosapentaenoic acid. *Prostagl Med* 5:269-278, 1979.
31. Wene JD, Connor WE, DenBesten L: The development of essential fatty acid deficiency in healthy men fed fat free diets intravenously and orally. *J Clin Invest* 56:127-134,1975.
32. Skeie B, Askanazi J, Rothkopf MM et al.: The beneficial effects of fat on ventilation and pulmonary function. *Nutrition* 3:149-154, 1987.
33. Askanazi J, Rothkopf MM, Rosenbaum SH, Ross E: Treatment of cystic fibrosis with long term home total parenteral nutrition. *Nutrition* 3:277-279, 1987.
34. Skeie B, Askanazi J, Rothkopf MM et al.: Improved tolerance with long-term parenteral nutrition in cystic fibrosis. *Crit Care Med* 15: 960-962, 1987.
35. Mochizuki H, Trocki O, Dominioni L et al.: Optimal lipid content for enteral diets following thermal injury. *JPEN* 8: 638-646, 1984.
36. Mochizuki H, Trocki O, Dominioni L et al.: Mechanism of prevention of postburn hypermetabolism and catabolism by early enteral feeding. *Ann Surg* 200:297-310, 1984.
37. Trocki O, Heyd TJ, Waymack JP, Alexander JW: Effects of fish oil on postburn metabolism and immunity. *JPEN* 11:521-528, 1987
38. Dominioni L, Trocki O, Mochizuki H et al: Prevention of severe postburn

hypermetabolism and catabolism by means of immediate intragastric feeding. *J Burn Care Rehab* 5:106-112, 1984

39. Benedict FG: *A study of prolonged fasting* . Washington D.C, Carnegie Institute Publ No. 203, 1915.
40. Owen OE, Reichard GA Jr: Ketone body metabolism in normal, obese and diabetic subjects. *Israel J Med Sci* 11:560-570, 1975
41. Cahill GF Jr: Starvation in man. *New Engl J Med* 282:668-675, 1970.
42. Cahill GF Jr , Herrera MG, Morgan AP et al.: Hormone-fuel interrelationships during fasting. *J Clin Invest* 45:1751-1768, 1966.
43. Owen OE, Felig P, Morgan AP et al.: Liver and kidney metabolism during prolonged starvation. *J Clin Invest* 48:574-583, 1969.
44. Owen OE, Morgan AP, Kemp HG et al.: Brain metabolism during fasting. *J Clin Invest* 46:1589-1595, 1967.
45. Felig P, Owen OE, Wahren J, Cahill GF Jr: Amino acid metabolism in prolonged starvation. *J Clin Invest* 48: 584-594, 1969.
46. Lawrence AM: Radioimmuno assayable glucagon in man: Effects of starvation, hypoglycemia and glucose administration. *Proc Nat Acad Sci* 55:316-320, 1966.
47. Grant JP: Clinical impact of protein malnutrition on organ mass and function. In Blackburn GL, Grant JP, Young VR (eds): *Amino acids: Metabolism and Medical Application.* Littleton MA, Wright PSG, 1983, pp 347–358.
48. Elwyn DH, Kinney JM, Gump FE et al.: Metabolic and endocrine effects of fasting followed by infusion of five percent glucose. *Surgery* 90:810-816, 1981.
49. Burman KD, Dimond RC ,Harvey GS et al.: Glucose modulation of alterations in serum iodothyronine concentration induced by fasting. *Metabolism* 28:291-299, 1979.
50. Palmblad J, Levi L, Burger H et al.: Effects of total energy withdrawal (fasting) on the level of growth hormone, thyrotropin, cortisol, adrenalin, noradrenaline, T^4, T^3, and RT^3 in healthy males. *Acta Med Scand* 201:15-22, 1977.
51. Jung RI, Shetty PS, Barrand M et al.: Role of catecholamines in hypotensive response to dieting. *Br Med J* 1:12-13, 1979.
52. Landsberg L, Young JB: Fasting, feeding and regulation of the sympathetic nervous system. *N Engl J Med* 298:1295-1301, 1978.
53. Pequignot JM, Peyrin L, Peres G: Catechol-fuel interrelationships during exercise in fasting men. *J Appl Physiol* 48:109-113,1980.
54. Gamble JL: Physiological information gained from studies on the life raft ration. *Harvey Lect* 42:247-273, 1947.
55. Long CL, Kinney JM, Geiger JM: Nonsuppressibility of gluconeogenesis by glucose in septic patients. *Metabolism* 25:193-201, 1976.
56. Gil KM, Gump FE, Starker PM et al.: Splanchnic substrate balance in malnourished patients during parenteral nutrition. *Am J Physiol* 248:E409-E419, 1985.
57. Cuthbertson DP: Post-shock metabolic response. *Lancet* i:433-437, 1942.
58. Moore FD: Bodily changes in surgical convalescence. I. The normal sequence—Observations and interpretations. *Ann Surg* 137:289-315, 1953.
59. Stoner HB, Heath DF: The effect of trauma on carbohydrate metabolism. *Br J Anesthes* 45:244-251, 1973.
60. Stoner HB: The acute effects of trauma on heat production. In Porter R and Knight J (eds): *Energy Metabolism in Trauma*, London, Churchill, 1970, pp 1–22.
61. Kinney JM, Duke JH Jr, Long CL, Gump F: Tissue fuel and weight loss after injury. *J Clin Path* 23 (Suppl 4):65-72, 1970.

62. Weissman C, Kemper M, Askanazi J et al.: Resting metabolic rate of the critically ill patient: Measured versus predicted. *Anesthesiology* 64:673-679, 1986.
63. Elwyn DH, Kinney JM, Askanzi J: Energy expenditure in surgical patients. *Surg Clin N Am* 61:545-556, 1981.
64. Tilstone WJ, Cuthbertson DP: The protein component of the disturbance of energy metabolism in trauma. In Porter R and Knight J (eds): *Energy Metabolism in Trauma* , London, Churchill, 1970, pp 43–58, 1970.
65. Aulick LH: Studies in heat transport and heat loss in thermally injured patients. In Kinney JM (ed): *Assessment of Energy Metabolism in Health and Disease*, Columbus, Ross Laboratories, 1980, pp 141–144.
66a. Jeevanandam M, Grote-Holman AE, Chikenji T et al.: Effects of glucose on fuel utilization and glycerol turnover in normal, injured and septic man. *Crit Car Med* 1989, in press.
66. Long CL, Spencer JL, Kinney JM and Geiger JW: Carbohydrate metabolism in man: Effect of elective operations and major injury. *J Appl Physiol* 31:110-116, 1971.
67. Wolfe RR, Durhot MJ, Allsop JR, Burke JF: Glucose metabolism in severely burned patients. *Metabolism* 28:1031-1039, 1979.
68. Wilmore DW, Aulick LH, Mason AD Jr et al: The influence of the burn wound on local and systemic responses to injury. *Ann Surg* 186:444-458, 1977.
69. Wolfe RR, Herndon DN, Jahoor F et al.: Effect of severe burn injury on substrate cycling by glucose and fatty acids. *N Engl J Med* 317:403-408, 1987.
70. Carpentier YA, Askanazi J, Elwyn DH: Effects of hypercaloric glucose infusion on lipid metabolism in injury and sepsis. *J Trauma* 19:649-654, 1979.
71. Newsholm EA, Gevers W: Control of glycolysis and gluconeogenesis in liver and kidney cortex. *Vitam Horm* 25:1-87, 1967.
72. Carpentier YA, Askanazi J, Elwyn DH et al.: The effect of carbohydrate intake on the lipolytic rate in depleted patients. *Metabolism* 29:974-979, 1980.
73. Smith R, Fuller DJ, Wedge JH et al.: Initial effect of injury on ketone bodies and other blood metabolites. *Lancet* i:1-3, 1975.
74. Suchner U, Rothkopf MM: Metabolic effects of the neuroendocrine stress response. *Clin Anesthesiol*, 6:1-22, 1988.
75. Kinney JM, Felig P: The metabolic response to injury and infection. In De Groot LJ (ed): *Endocrinology*, New York, Grune and Stratton, 1979, Vol 3, pp 1963–1985.
76. Shamoon HR, Hendler R, Sherwin RS: Synergistic interaction among antiinsulin hormones in the pathogenesis of stress hyperglycemia in humans. *J Clin Endocrinol Metab* 52:1235-1241, 1981.
77. Bessy PQ, Watters JM, Aoki TT, Wilmore DW: Combined hormonal infusion simulates the metabolic response to injury. *Ann Surg* 200: 264-281, 1984.
78. Kehlet H, Moller IW: The effects of regional anaesthesia on the endocrine-metabolic response to surgery and infection. In Oyama T (ed): *Endocrinology and the Anaesthetist: Monographs in Anaesthesiology.* Amsterdam, Elsevier, 1983, pp 23–35.
79. Stoner HB: Hypothalamic involvement in the response to injury. In Richards JR, Kinney JM (ed): *Nutritional Aspects of Care in the Critically Ill*, Edinburgh, Churchill Livingston, 1977, pp 257–271.
80. Powanda MC, Beisel WR: Hypothesis: Leukocyte endogenous mediator/endogenous pyrogen/lymphocyte-activating factor modulates the development of nonspecific and specific immunity and affects nutritional status. *Am J Clin Nutr* 35:762-768, 1982.
81. Barracos V, Rodemann HP, Dinarello CA, Goldberg AL: Stimulation of muscle pro-

tein degradation and prostaglandin E_2 release by leukocytic pyrogen (interleukin-1). *New Engl J Med* 308:553-558, 1983.
82. Clowes GH, George BC, Villee CA Jr, Saravis CA: Muscle proteolysis induced by circulating peptide in patients with sepsis or trauma. *N Engl J Med* 308:545-552, 1983.
83. Beutler B, Milsark IW, Cerami AC: Passive immunization against cachectin/tumor necrosis factor protects mice from lethal effect of endotoxin. *Science* 229:869-871, 1985.
84. Kinney JM: The tissue composition of surgical weight loss. In Johnson IDA (ed): *Advances in Parenteral Nutrition*, Lancaster, MTP Press, 1977, pp 511–519.
85. Ardawi MSM, Newsholme EA: Metabolism in lymphocytes and its importance in the immune response. *Essays in Biochem* 21:1-44, 1985
86. Newsholme EA, Crabtree B, Ardawi MSM: Glutamine metabolism in lymphocytes: Its biochemical, physiological, and clinical importance. *Q J Exp Physiol* 70:473-489, 1985.
87. Askanazi J, Elwyn DH, Kinney JM et al.: Muscle and plasma amino acids following injury: Influence of intercurrent infection. *Ann Surg* 192:78-85, 1980.
88. Grant JP, Snyder PJ: Use of L-glutamine in total parenteral nutrition. *J Surg Res* 44:506-513, 1988
89. Kinney JM, Elwyn DH: Protein metabolism in injury. *Ann Rev Nutr* 3:433-466, 1983.
90. Elwyn DH, Kinney JM, Jeevanandam M et al.: Influence of increasing carbohydrate intake on glucose kinetics in injured patients. *Ann Surg* 190: 117-127, 1979.
91. Askanazi J, Carpentier YA, Elwyn DH et al.: Influence of total parenteral nutrition on fuel utilization in injury and sepsis. *Ann Surg* 191:40-46, 1980.
92. Jéquier E: Influence of nutrient administration on energy expenditure in man. *Clin Nutr* 5:181-186, 1986.
93. Askanazi J, Elwyn DH, Silverberg PA et al.: Respiratory distress secondary to a high carbohydrate load: A case report. *Surgery* 87:596-598, 1980.
94. Larssen J, Martenssen J, Vinnars F: Nitrogen requirements in hypermetabolic patients. *Clin Nutr* (Special Suppl) 4: O.4, 1984.

CHAPTER

5

Methods of Measurement and Interpretation of Indirect Calorimetry

> *When you can measure what you are speaking about and express it in numbers, you know something about it, but when you cannot express it in numbers, your knowledge is of a meager and unsatisfactory kind.*
>
> Lord Kelvin

Calculation of energy expenditure and fuel utilization is based on solving the equations described in Chapter 2, and requires:

1. Measurement of the three variables-VO_2, VCO_2, and NM.
2. Use of a series of constants representing: the amount of calories produced by the metabolism of 1 g of carbohydrate,1 g of protein, and 1 g of fat; the quantities of oxygen necessary to metabolize 1 g of carbohydrate, 1 g of protein, and 1 g of fat; and the quantities of carbon dioxide produced by the metabolism of 1 g of carbohydrate,1 g of protein, and 1 g of fat.

In this chapter we shall discuss the methods of measurement and the errors involved in each of these measurements and try to understand the meaning of their variation in various cirumstances.

OXYGEN CONSUMPTION AND CARBON DIOXIDE PRODUCTION

Although what characterizes indirect calorimetry is that it is a non invasive technique and that all measurements are performed on urine, and inspired and expired gases, it would be incomplete not to remind the reader that once oxygen is taken up by the lungs it will be carried by the blood to the mitochondria of each single cell. Only in the cell and mainly in the mitochondria is O_2 actually consumed. In the same way, carbon dioxide is produced at the cellular level and must come all the way to the lungs to be exhaled.

For purposes of indirect calorimetry we need to know the volume of O_2 consumed and CO_2 produced by the cell. What we measure is the volume of gases (VO_2 and VCO_2) exchanged by the lungs, which is not always the same thing. The ratio of CO_2 to O_2 exchanged at the lungs, or the *respiratory exchange ratio*, is traditionally represented by R. The ratio of CO_2 produced and O_2 consumed at the cellular level is traditionally represented by RQ, or the respiratory quotient. The RQ will be equal to R only when no changes are occurring in body O_2 and, more important, CO_2 stores.

Some Theoretical Considerations in the Measurement of Respiratory Gas Exchange

Let us assume that a man breathes with a frequency (F) of about 20 times per minute, and that each time he will inhale and exhale a tidal volume (VT) of about 500 ml of air. In this situation the minute volume (V) will be:

$$V = VT \times F = 500 \times 20 = 10{,}000\ ml\ min^{-1}$$

During inspiration, the concentration of both inspiratory gases, O_2 and CO_2 (FIO_2 and $FICO_2$), remain constant. During expiration the concentration of CO_2 increases, from close to 0% to a maximum value around 6%, and the concentration of O_2 decreases, from approximatively 21% to a minimum value around 16%. In Figure 5.1 the variation of the concentrations in oxygen (FO_2) and in carbon dioxide (FCO_2) are represented, during the inspiratory phase *a* and the expiratory phase *b*. The extreme values of O_2 and of CO_2, at the end of the expiratory phase, represent the concentrations of O_2 and CO_2 in alveolar air; this is why they are called alveolar concentrations of O_2 and of CO_2 and are designated as FAO_2 and $FACO_2$.

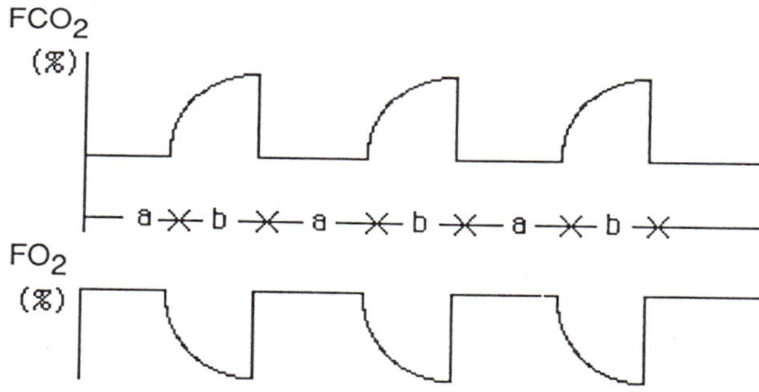

Figure 5.1. Variation of the concentrations of oxygen (FO_2) and of carbon dioxide (FCO_2) during the inspiratory (*a*) and the expiratory phase (*b*) of a normal respiratory cycle.

When the expired air is mixed in a Douglas bag or other mixing chamber, the concentration of expired gases becomes homogeneous, representing the mean value of the variations represented in Figure 5.1. Homogenization of expired gases is necessary to obtain on-line measurements of VO_2 and VCO_2. In 1934, Margaria built a mixing bottle for obtaining homogenous gases (1). Even earlier, Bock, in 1929 designed a mixing chamber for metabolic measurements (2). Figure 5.2 shows how expired gases become progressively more homogeneous in a system with two mixing chambers for measuring on line-gas exchange (3).

There are methods for obtaining breath-by-breath values for O_2 and CO_2 exchange. These are difficult to achieve and are not important for evaluating rates of tissue O_2 consumption and CO_2 production. The more usual approach is to average values for expired O_2 (FEO_2) and CO_2 ($FECO_2$). Multiplying these by the respiratory volume gives values for VO_2 and VCO_2.

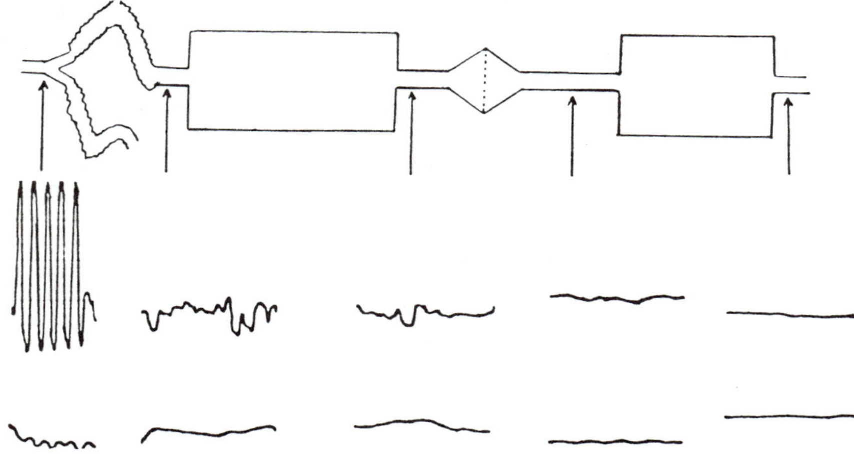

Figure 5.2. Adapted from Glaser and Bursztein (3). Degree of mixing of CO_2 (upper) and O_2 (lower) at various stages along a mixing apparatus.

The only situation where the inspiratory minute volume (VI), will be equal to the expiratory volume (VE) is if VO_2 is equal to VCO_2, or when R equals 1. Therefore, for calculation of VO_2 and VCO_2, it is necessary to use the different values of VI and VE, instead of V. In Figure 5.3 a schema of a simple open circuit for metabolic measurements is represented. With this scheme, VO_2 and VCO_2 can be calculated by the following procedures. As an example we may assume that VI = VE = 10,000 ml; that FIO_2 and $FICO_2$ are, respectively, 21% (0.21) and 0% (the concentration of CO_2 equals 0.03% in inspired air which is close enough to zero to be neglected)[a]; and that the values of FEO_2 and of $FECO_2$ as measured by O_2 and CO_2 analyzers are, respectively, 18% (0.18) and 3% (0.03). Then:

$$\begin{aligned} VO_2\,(ml\ min^{-1}) &= VI \times FIO_2 - VE \times FEO_2 \qquad (1) \\ &= 10{,}000 \times 0.21 - 10{,}000 \times 0.18 \\ &= 300\ ml\ min^{-1} \end{aligned}$$

[a] For very accurate work the exact values of CO_2 and O_2 in inspired air may need to be used. These are usually taken to be 0.03% (0.0003) for CO_2 and 20.93% for O_2. With many people in a room the value for O_2 will decrease and that for CO_2 will increase, therefore for accurate work inspired air should be obtained outside the building or from an intake duct providing fresh air to the room. Alternatively, the actual values for FIO_2 and $FICO_2$ may be measured, in addition to values for FEO_2 and $FECO_2$.

and

$$VCO_2\ (ml\ min^{-1}) = VE \times FECO_2 - VI \times FICO_2 \qquad (2)$$

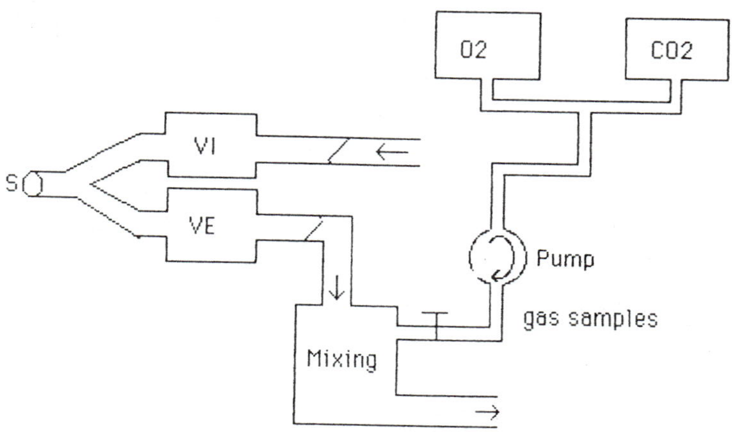

Figure 5.3. Representation of a simple system for metabolic measurements. The patient is connected to the system at S by a mouthpiece, a naso- or oro-tracheal tube, or a tracheotomy cannula. At each inspiration, the one-way valve VI opens, while the one-way valve VE closes and before reaching the patient, the inspired volume (VI) is measured by a flowmeter, which integrates the amount of air that will be inhaled by the patient. When the patient exhales the air, the valve VE opens while the valve VI closes and the expired volume of air (VE), after being measured by an identical flowmeter, is collected in a mixing chamber or a Douglas bag. From this mixing chamber, or this bag, samples of mixed expired air can be analyzed, off line or on line, by an oxygen analyzer and a carbon dioxide analyzer to give FEO_2 and $FECO_2$.

Since in room air $FICO_2$ is considered to be equal to zero, the second term of equation 2 is deleted and the equation becomes

$$\begin{aligned} VCO_2 &= VE \times FECO_2 \\ &= 10{,}000 \times 0.03 \\ &= 300\ ml\ min^{-1} \end{aligned} \qquad (3)$$

In practice, measurements should be made during at least 20 to 30 minutes and the total volume should then be divided by the time of measurement in order to express the values per minute. This is because FEO_2, $FECO_2$, respiratory rate, and respiratory volume may vary from minute to minute, and sampling over a longer period of time will improve accuracy . By definition the respiratory exchange ratio is equal to VCO_2/VO_2:

$$R = VCO_2/VO_2 = 300/300 = 1$$

In this example we assumed that VI was equal to VE and therefore VO_2 was equal to VCO_2 and R equaled 1. In most cases R will not be equal to 1, and VE will not equal VI. In order to calculate VO_2 and VCO_2 as shown in equations 1 and 3 we need to determine values for VI, VE, FIO_2, FEO_2, and $FECO_2$. However, we need not make separate measurements for VI and VE as shown in Figure 5.3, since they are interrelated and measurement of only one will suffice. Since nitrogen is not metabolized in the body (see discussion in Chapter 3), the amount of N_2 exhaled is equal to the amount inhaled. If FIN_2 is the concentration of inspired nitrogen and FEN_2 the concentration of expired nitrogen, we may write:

$$VI \times FIN_2 = VE \times FEN_2 \tag{4}$$

From equation 4, VI and VE can be derived:

$$VI = VE \times \frac{FEN_2}{FIN_2} \quad (5) \quad VE = VI \times \frac{FIN_2}{FEN_2} \quad (6)$$

Nitrogen analyzers are not commonly used in the clinical setting but it is not necessary to measure N_2 since it can be determined by difference. By definition, inspiratory air and expiratory air are composed of all the gases that are contained in air. If we assume dry air (without water vapor) and, as we did before, neglect $FICO_2$, this may be expressed by the following equations.[b] For inspiratory gas:

$$FIO_2 + FIN_2 = 1\ (100\%)\ or\ FIN_2 = 1 - FIO_2 \tag{7}$$

For expiratory gas:

$$FEO_2 + FECO_2 + FEN_2 = 1\ (100\%)\ or\ FEN_2 = 1 - FEO_2 - FECO_2 \tag{8}$$

By replacing FIN_2 and FEN_2 in equations 5 and 6 by their values in equations 7 and 8, VI and VE can be obtained from the measurement of one volume instead of two, and from the measurement of the concentra-

---

[b] These equations appear to neglect the trace amounts of gases such as argon and helium in the air. However, these gases, like N_2, are not metabolized, and therefore FIN_2 and FEN_2 actually represent the sum of all gases other than O_2, CO_2 and H_2O in air and no error is introduced by neglecting to mention these trace gases.

tions of O_2 in inspired gas and of O_2 and CO_2 in expired gas. Then equations 5 and 6 become

$$VI = VE \times \frac{1 - FEO_2 - FECO_2}{1 - FIO_2} \tag{9}$$

and

$$VE = VI \times \frac{1 - FIO_2}{1 - FEO_2 - FECO_2} \tag{10}$$

If we use the values from our previous example of $FIO_2 = 0.21$, $FEO_2 = 0.18$, and $FECO_2 = 0.03$, and substitute in equations 9 and 10, the values of the fractions equal 1 and so VI = VE:

$$\frac{1 - FIO_2}{1 - FEO_2 - FECO_2} \text{ or } \frac{1 - 0.21}{1 - 0.18 - 0.03} = \frac{0.79}{0.79} = 1$$

$$\frac{1 - FEO2 - FECO2}{1 - FIO_2} \text{ or } \frac{1 - 0.18 - 0.03}{1 - 0.21} = \frac{0.79}{0.79} = 1$$

If we assume the following values—$FIO_2 = 0.21$, $FEO_2 = 0.18$, $FECO_2 = 0.025$, and VE = 10,000—the calculation of VI will give

$$VI = 10{,}000 \times \frac{1 - 0.18 - 0.025}{1 - 0.21} = 10{,}000 \times \frac{0.795}{0.79} = 10{,}063\ ml\ min^{-1}$$

From equations 1 and 3, $VO_2 = 313$ ml min^{-1}, $VCO_2 = 250$ ml min^{-1}, and R = 0.80. Since the difference between VI and VE is small, one might consider neglecting it for clinical purposes and use only the measured value, in this example VE, for both VI and VE. If we do this, the values of VO_2 and VCO_2 calculated from equations 1 and 3 become 300 and 250, respectively, and R becomes 0.83. Thus with a difference of only 0.6% between VI and VE we have a 4% error in VO_2 and an error of 0.03 in R. For R values further removed from 1 and for increases in the ratio of VO_2/VI the errors will even be larger. Since all that is saved in this simplification is one or two steps in a calculation, in practice the exact calculation should always be used.

Normally R is less than 1, which means that VO_2 is greater then VCO_2 and VI is greater than VE. One may wonder why this situation will not inflate the subject with air. This does not occur because the higher amount of oxygen inhaled than carbon dioxide exhaled is utilized in the formation of metabolic water, which is eliminated in the urine or by evaporation, and of urea, uric acid, and other oxygen-containing compounds excreted in the urine.

If for any reason there is an increase in the energy needs, because of exercise or because of acute disease associated with hypermetabolism, the only way to meet this increased energy expenditure is to burn more substrate, which requires higher oxygen consumption and carbon dioxide production. The normal adaptation of the body to high oxygen demands is to increase minute ventilation. In equations 1 and 3, FIO_2 is always constant, and there are only two possible ways of increasing VO_2 and VCO_2: *(a)* by decreasing FEO_2 and increasing $FECO_2$, which is economical for the body since it requires no change in the work of breathing, but occurs to only a small extent; and *(b)* by increasing VI and VE, which is the main mechanism, and which increases the work of breathing. The work of breathing requires about 3% to 5% of the total VO_2 at rest in normal subjects, and increases exponentially when minute ventilation is increased. All types of respiratory impairments increase the work of breathing during both rest and exercise. This work of breathing is not easy to evaluate. Nevertheless differences of about 24% in VO_2 between ventilated and nonventilated patients demonstrate the approximate magnitude of respiratory work in acutely ill patients, much greater than is seen in normal subjects (4).

The R value can be obtained from the concentrations of gases without the necessity of measuring volume. This might be useful when apparatus for volume measurement is not available, since it gives some, if limited, information as to a patient's metabolic status. An equation for R can be developed, first by combining equations 1 and 3 to give equation 11:

$$R = \frac{VCO_2}{VO_2} = \frac{VE \times FECO2}{VI \times FIO_2 - VE \times FEO_2} \tag{11}$$

Then if we replace VI by its value as calculated in equation 9, we get equation 12,

$$R = \frac{VE \times FECO_2}{\dfrac{(VE \times (1 - FEO_2 - FECO_2) \times FIO_2)}{1 - FIO_2} - VE \times FEO_2} \tag{12}$$

which can be rearranged into equation 13:

$$R = \frac{FECO_2\,(1 - FIO_2)}{FIO_2\,(1 - FECO_2) - FEO_2} \tag{13}$$

In this way we can calculate R solely from values of O_2 and CO_2 concentrations in inspired and expired air.

Techniques for Measuring Gas Exchange

The simplest system for measuring gas exchange is probably the spirometer attached to a kymograph as shown in Figure 5.4. This consists of a bell containing pure O_2 placed in a water seal. The subject breathes in pure O_2, and the expired gas containing O_2 and CO_2 is passed through an absorbant to remove CO_2 before the O_2 is returned to the bell. The top of the bell is attached to a pen or stylus, which traces a line on a revolving drum (kymograph). As the patient breathes in, the bell goes down and the pen goes up, thus the upstroke on the pen is equal to VI. As the patient breathes out, the bell goes up, and the pen goes down. The downstroke represents only the O_2 exhaled since the CO_2 is absorbed. The mean value for VO_2 is obtained by dividing the change in volume by the change in time on the kymograph record. The value for VCO_2 can only be obtained by measuring the weight of CO_2 added to the absorbent.

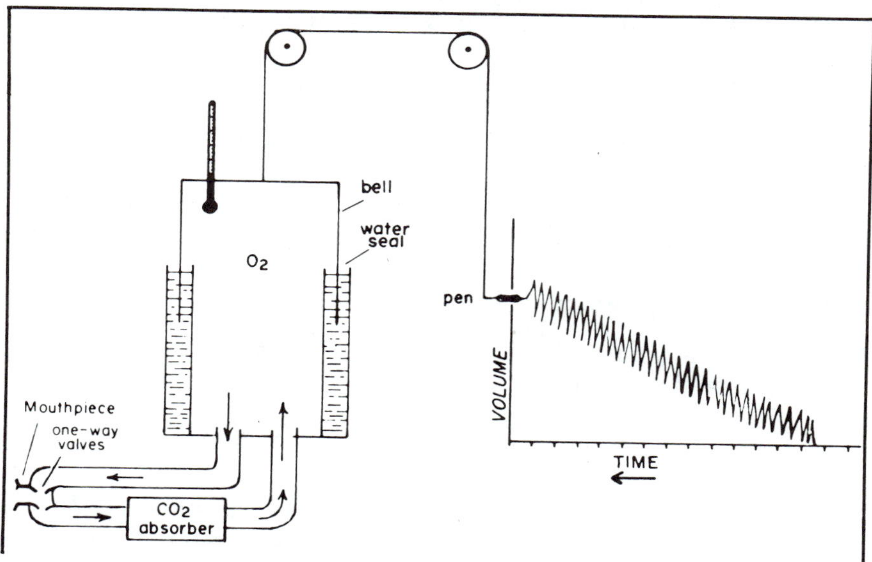

Figure 5.4. Closed circuit spirometer.

An important aspect of measuring gas exchange is that all determinations are performed at room temperature, which is usually around 20° C, whereas body temperature is usually 37° C. A correction of volumes is necessary and special formulas are used to correct the measured volumes from ambient to body temperature. Values of V, VI, and

VE are measured, usually at room temperature, at the ambient barometric pressure, and are saturated with water vapor (ATPS); however, they should be expressed at body temperature, at the ambient barometric pressure, and are saturated with water vapor (BTPS). VO_2 and VCO_2, which are usually calculated from VI and VE measured under ATPS conditions, are by convention expressed at standard conditions, namely 0° C for temperature, 760 mm Hg for barometric pressure, and as dry gases (STPD). To convert volumes measured at ATPS to BTPS conditions, these volumes have to be multiplied by the factor K1:

$$K1 = \frac{273 + 37°\,C}{273 + T°A} \times \frac{BP - PA\,H_2O}{BP - PH_2O\ at\ 37°\,C} \tag{14}$$

where:

- $K1$ = conversion factor of ATPS into BTPS
- 273 = the absolute temperature (in degrees Kelvin) at 0° C
- BP = barometric pressure (although many factors alter barometric pressure, the main factor is altitude and Table 5.1 gives the relation among altitude, temperature, and barometric pressure),
- $T°A$ = the ambient temperature at which the measurement was performed
- PAH_2O = the pressure of water vapor at the ambient temperature (Table 5.2 gives water vapor pressures for temperatures varying from 20° to 37° C)
- PH_2O = the pressure of water vapor

To convert VO_2 and VCO_2, measured at ATPS to STPD conditions, these measured values have to be multiplied by the factor K2:

$$K2 = \frac{273}{273 + T°A} \times \frac{BP - PAH_2O}{760} \tag{15}$$

where all factors are as defined for K1, 760 being the standard BP.

Figure 5.3 represents the classical schema of any open system for the measurement of respiratory volumes and O_2 and CO_2 concentrations. In Figures 5.5 to 5.7, we show possible variations of this system that can be adapted to the needs of any starting "metabolician" who is eager to perform indirect calorimetry measurements before he has the financial possibilities to acquire one of the sophisticated, specially designed instruments described in Chapter 6. In the system represented in Figure 5.5, the inspired volume (VI) is measured and the expired volume (VE) has to be calculated. Temperature is measured in order to correct

Table 5.1.
Relationship between altitude, barometric pressure and temperature.[a]

Altitude		Pressures		Temperature
Feet	Meters	Barometric	O_2	°C
0	0	760.0	159.1	+15.0
2000	610	706.6	147.9	+11.0
4000	1219	656.3	137.4	+7.1
6000	1829	609.0	127.5	+3.1
8000	2438	564.4	118.1	−0.8
10000	3048	522.6	109.4	−4.8
12000	3658	483.3	101.2	−8.8
14000	4267	446.4	93.4	−12.7
16000	4877	411.8	86.2	−16.7
18000	5486	379.4	79.4	−20.7
20000	6096	349.1	73.1	−24.6
22000	6706	320.8	67.1	−28.6
24000	7315	294.4	61.6	−32.5
26000	7925	269.8	56.5	−36.5
28000	8534	246.9	51.7	−40.5
30000	9144	225.6	47.2	−44.6
32000	9754	205.8	43.1	−48.4
34000	10363	187.4	39.2	−52.4
36000	10973	170.4	35.7	−55.0
38000	11582	154.9	32.4	−55.0
40000	12192	140.7	29.4	−55.0
42000	12802	127.9	26.8	−55.0
44000	13411	116.3	24.3	−55.0
46000	14021	105.7	22.1	−55.0
48000	14630	96.1	20.1	−55.0
50000	15240	87.3	18.3	−55.0
52000	15850	79.3	16.6	−55.0
54000	16459	72.1	15.1	−55.0
56000	17069	65.6	13.7	−55.0
58000	17678	54.2	12.5	−55.0
60000	18288	54.2	11.3	−55.0

[a]Adapted from Consolazio et al. (5).

VO_2 and VCO_2 to STPD conditions. The mixing chamber can be a Douglas bag or any mixing container with a 100- to 150-cm long outlet tube to avoid contamination of the expired gases of the container by ambient air. There is some controversy about the reliability of CO_2 measurements coming from rubber or plastic bags. Many investigators claim that measurements of CO_2 have to be performed within minutes because of the high diffusibility of this gas. Table 5.3 shows the variation

Table 5.2.
Pressure of water vapor (mmHg) at various temperatures.[a]

°C	PH_2O	°C	PH_2O	°C	PH_2O	°C	PH_2O
10	9.2	20	17.5	30	31.8	40	55.3
11	9.8	21	18.6	31	33.7	41	58.3
12	10.5	22	19.8	32	35.7	42	61.5
13	11.2	23	21.1	33	37.7	43	64.8
14	11.9	24	22.4	34	39.9	44	68.3
15	12.8	25	23.8	35	42.2	45	71.9
16	13.6	26	25.2	36	44.5	46	75.6
17	14.5	27	26.8	37	47.1	47	79.6
18	15.5	28	28.3	38	49.7	48	83.7
19	16.5	29	30.0	39	52.4	49	88.0

[a]Adapted from Consolazio et al. (5).

of CO_2 concentration with time in different types of containers. It appears that with small rubber bags the CO_2 concentration is stable for at least one hour, and that with most of the common equipment it is stable for 3 hours or more. From the sampling outlet, 50 ml of expired gas can be collected with a syringe, which is oiled to prevent gas leaks, and off-line measurements can be performed, even with a blood gas machine that is properly calibrated. The results obtained as partial pressure in expired gas of O_2 (PEO_2) and of CO_2 ($PECO_2$) can then be converted to fractional concentrations of the two gases (FEO_2, $FECO_2$) by the following formulas:

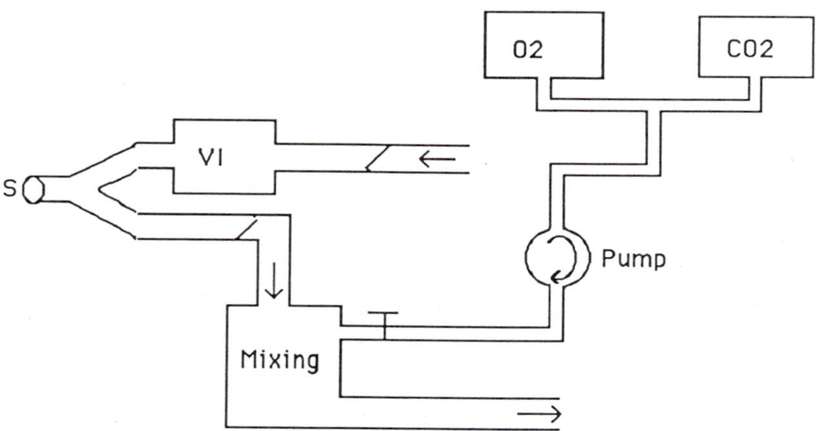

Figure 5.5. VO_2-VCO_2 measuring system with the volume measured at the inspiratory line.

Table 5.3.
The storage and diffusion of carbon dioxide.[a]

Time (Hours)	Oiled Syringes	Douglas Bags (200 liter)		Small Rubber Bags	Tissot Gasometer
		Rubber	Plastic		
0	4.32	4.34	4.29	4.32	4.32
1	4.32	4.33	4.33	4.23	4.35
2	4.29	4.29	4.31	4.20	4.32
3	4.32	4.13	4.30	—	4.29

[a]Reproduced from Consolazio CF, Johnson RE and Pecora LJ: *Physiologic Measurements of Metabolic Functions in Man.* New York, McGraw-Hill, 1963, p 22. With permission of McGraw-Hill.

$$FEO_2 = \frac{PEO_2}{BP - PH_2O} \quad (16) \qquad FECO_2 = \frac{PECO_2}{BP - PH_2O} \quad (17)$$

where:

PEO_2 = partial pressure of O_2 as measured from the sample
$PECO_2$ = partial pressure of CO_2 as measured from the sample
BP = barometric pressure
PH_2O = pressure of water vapor

Let us assume that the measurements gave a PEO_2 of 128 mm Hg and a $PECO_2$ of 18 mm Hg, and a VI of 10,000 ml min^{-1}, that BP is 758, and that the pressure measurements were made at 37°C so that PH_2O was 47. From equations 16 and 17, $FEO_2 = 0.180$ and $FECO_2 = 0.0253$. From equation 10, VE = 9933, and from equations 1 and 3, $VO_2 = 312$ and $VCO_2 = 251$ ml min^{-1}.

Figure 5.6 shows exactly the same system, but with the device for measuring volume on the expiratory line. In this case VI will have to be calculated from VE, FIO_2, FEO_2, and $FECO_2$. Another system with two mixing bottles and a calibration system previously described by the authors is presented in Figure 5.7 (6).

Volume Measurements

Several different instruments are available for measuring respiratory volumes, but most of them give results with errors of 5% to 10%. Such errors are acceptable for evaluating respiratory function in ventilated or spontaneously breathing patients or even to evaluate the efficacy of physiotherapy, but when the measured value has to be used for VO_2 and VCO_2 calculations, a greater precision is required.

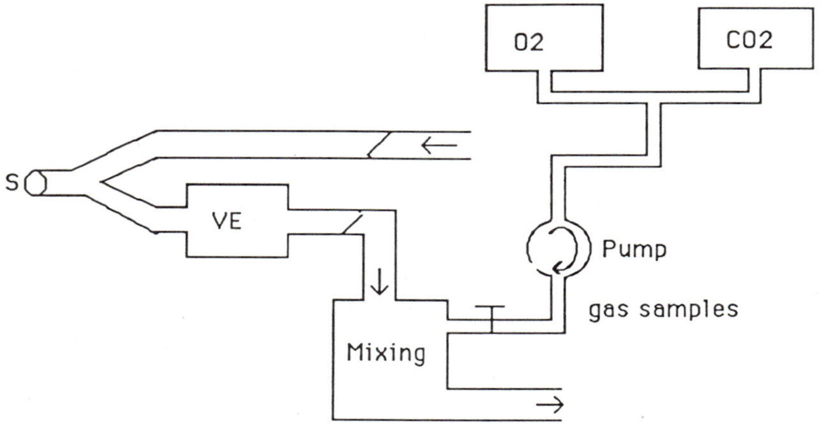

Figure 5.6. VO_2 -VCO_2 measuring system, with the volume measured at the expiratory line.

Pneumotachograph

Among the most precise tools for measuring respiratory volumes, when correctly calibrated, is the pneumotachograph (Figures 5.8 and 5.9). It is based on the property that the drop in pressure, as a fluid flows through a screen, is proportional to the flow. This mechanical measurement is converted to an electronic signal by a pressure transducer, amplified, and then integrated over a defined period of time to give the respiratory volume for this period of time. In most instances this screen is built of metal and is heated to 37 ° C, avoiding, according to the manufacturers, the problem of correcting the measured volumes from ATPS to BTPS conditions.

Exhaled gases are saturated with water vapor; if the pneumotachograph is placed close to the patient's mouth the screen may often be partially occluded with sputum or other secretions, altering the properties of the system. To avoid this, many investigators will place the apparatus at a distance from the patient. In this situation, since temperature is decreasing along the tube there will be condensation of water on the walls of the tube, but the expired gases will remain saturated as long as the temperature continues to decrease. If, at the level of the pneumotachograph, the temperature is again raised to 37° C the expired gases will no longer be saturated, introducing an error. This inconvenience is avoided by placing the captor of the pneumotachograph at the inspiratory line (VI in Figure 5.5). Finally, some systems are built with the pneumotachograph placed between the subject and the Y piece; in this

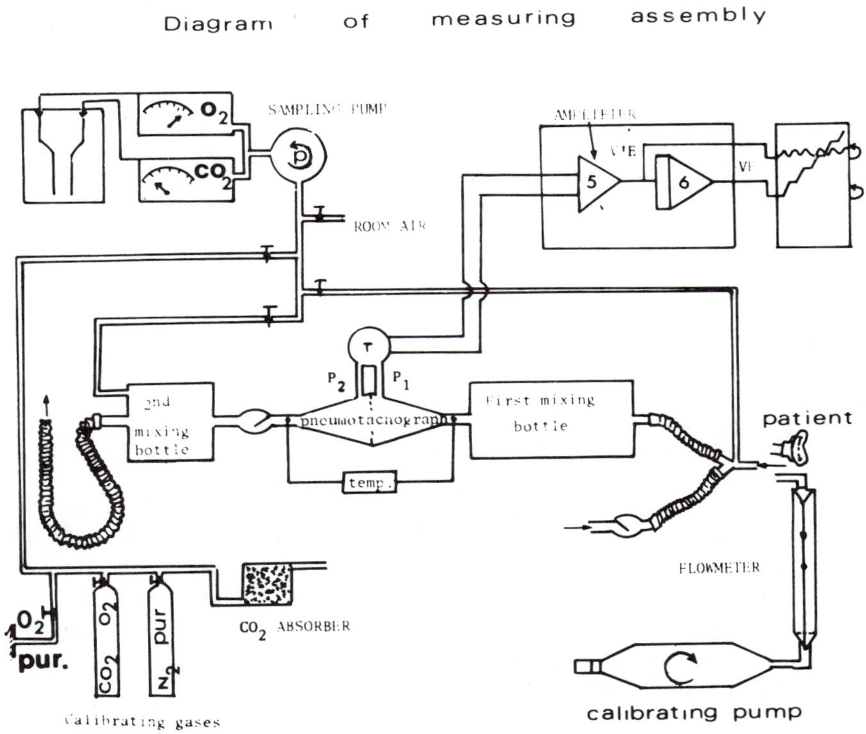

Figure 5.7. System for measuring VO_2 and VCO_2.

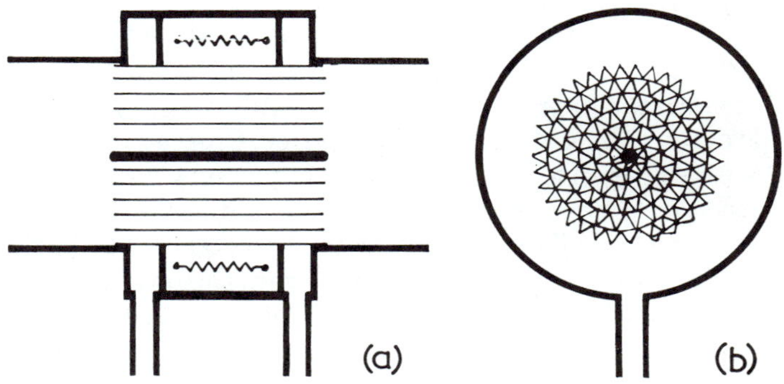

Figure 5.8. Schematic representation of the Fleisch pneumotachograph airflow resistance: *a*, longitudinal section; *b*, transverse section through the pressure-sensing connection.

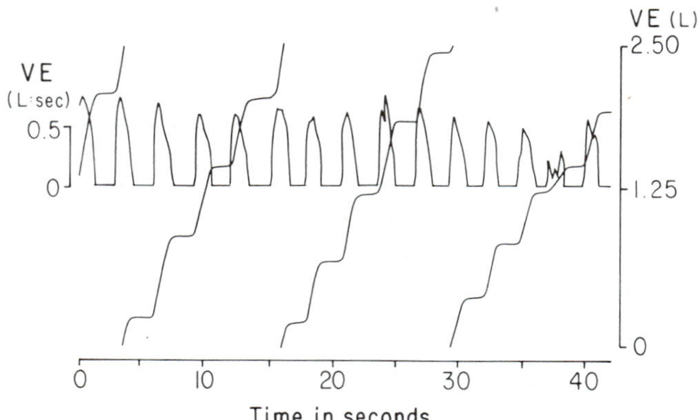

Figure 5.9. Pneumotachograph recording of expiratory flow rate and expiratory volume (integration of flow rate over time).

case both inspiratory and expiratory volumes can be recorded separately by appropriate electronic devices and both can be displayed. The calibration of the pneumotachograph can be performed with different known flows, and the simplest tool to obtain precise flows is the rotameter from Fischer and Porter. This provides a constant exact flow through the pneumotachograph, permitting an accurate calibration.

Airflow varies continuously throughout the respiratory cycle (Figure 5.9), reaching a maximum value in the middle of each inspiration or expiration and a minimum value of zero at the start and end of each inspiration and expiration. Since the calibration is performed with a flow rather close to the maximum value (60 to 80 liters min^{-1}), there may be some lack of precision at low flow values.

Tissot Gasometer

This apparatus, represented in Figure 5.10, is mentioned more for historical reasons than for practical purposes. Created in 1904, by Tissot, it was a very precise tool for measuring expiratory gases when carefully calibrated (7). Used in exercise tests, the subject breathes through a two-way valve and all expired gases are collected in a cylinder of either 100- or 250-liter capacity, that is sealed from the outside by using a water seal contained in a second cylinder. Total exhaled gas can be determined over a known period of time by noting the level of the internal cylinder, which is accurately counterpoised so as not to impede respiration. In this method the subject is connected to the gasometer by a mouthpiece, his nose being occluded with an uncomfortable noseclip. The temperature in the cylinder is measured in order to correct volumes to body or to standard conditions. From the cylinder, gas samples can be collected for measuring FEO_2 and $FECO_2$. Although it seems a museum item, the Tissot gasometer can still be found in many respiratory laboratories and is still used for volume measurements. The main source of inaccuracies, as in most of the following methods, is related to leaks that may occur at the level of the mouthpiece, the noseclip or the mask (more convenient than a mouthpiece and a noseclip). Leaks also may occur in all tube connections and in the valves. The precise reading of the cylinder level is also a source of error since a rise in the Tissot bell of 1 cm corresponds to an increase of 1 liter of gas in the bell.

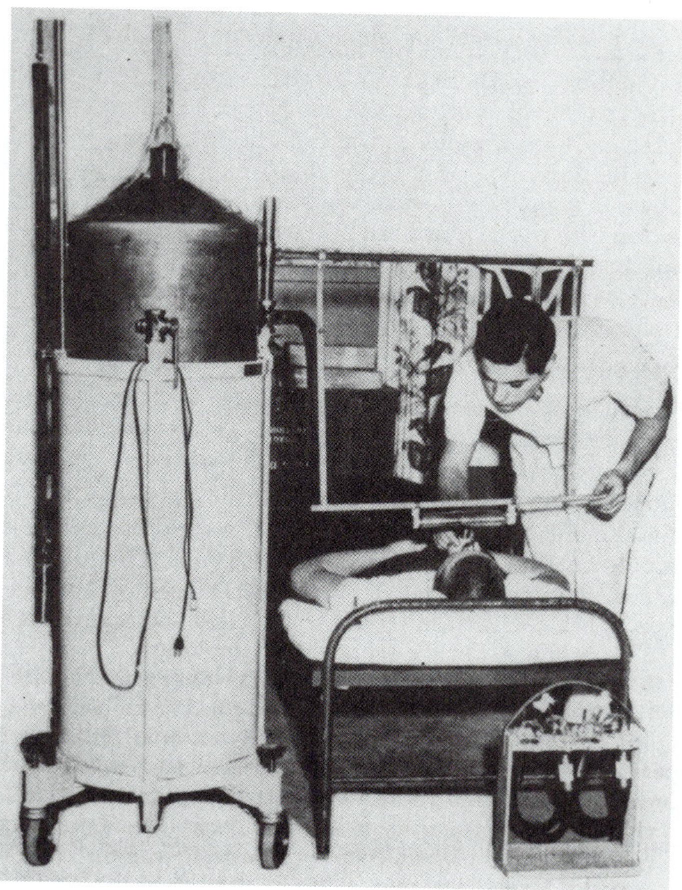

Figure 5.10. The Tissot gasometer.

Closed Circuit Spirometer

Both Benedict in 1918 and Krogh in 1923 performed important parts of their metabolic investigations using closed circuit spirometers of the type that we have already discussed (Figure 5.4) (8,9). For metabolic measurements, the bell of a volume of about 8 liters is usually filled with pure oxygen and the subject rebreathes the same gas, while the CO_2 from the expired gas is absorbed by soda lime. The subject is connected with a mouthpiece and a noseclip or with a face mask and breathes for 6 to 10 minutes into the system. At the end of the test, the slope of the line read on the kymograph gives the amount of oxygen consumed (Figure 5.4). Widely used in functional pulmonary laboratories and by clinicians, this method, improved by the apparatus built by Collins, is now considered as less accurate than open circuit methods, giving results that are between 5% and 12% lower than those obtained with the open circuit methods(10). Most of the errors which occur with the closed circuit systems, besides those related to leaks, are due to the calibration of the spirometer or to inaccuracies in the kymograph. If the soda lime is not replaced frequently enough, there may be incomplete absorption of CO_2. Leaks of the mouthpiece, the noseclip, or the mask affect the closed circuit system similarly to other methods, but when leaks occur in the inspiratory line, the effects are much larger since the subject will inspire a lower oxygen concentration than the 100% contained in the spirometer.

Wright Spirometer

The Wright spirometer represented in Figure 5.11, is a light and small instrument easy to use at the bedside of patients and is based on the principle of a rotor that turns at a speed proportional to the flow of air passing through the instrument (Figure 5.12). This nice but very fragile instrument, widely used for clinical measurements, is not precise enough to be used for metabolic computations. The same applies to tools of a similar type built by Bennett and Drager.

Douglas Bags

Many investigators collect all expired air in Douglas bags of 60-, 120- or even 200-liter capacity. The total volume of the bag is then measured by emptying it through an appropriate volume meter. It is important that the temperature of the volume meter be precisely determined so that the volume measured can be corrected to ATPS or BTPS conditions.

VO_2 Measured from Blood Flow and Arterio-Venous O_2 Concentration Difference

An alternative to measuring VO_2 from the difference in amounts of O_2 in, and volumes of, inspired and expired air, is to measure the difference

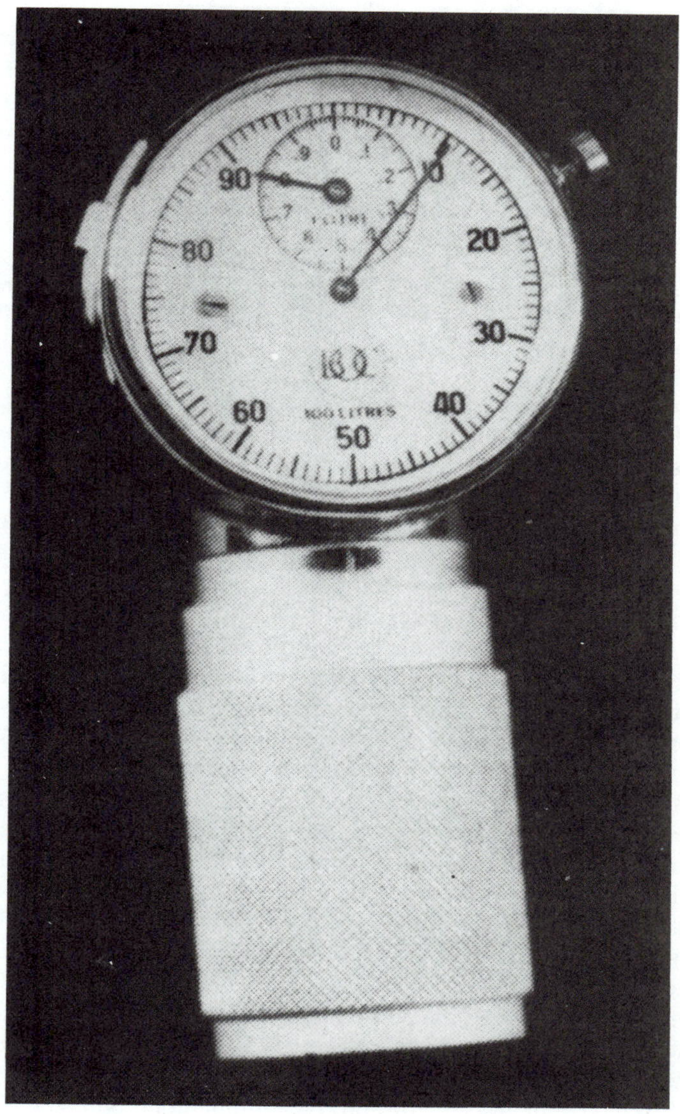

Figure 5.11. The Wright spirometer.

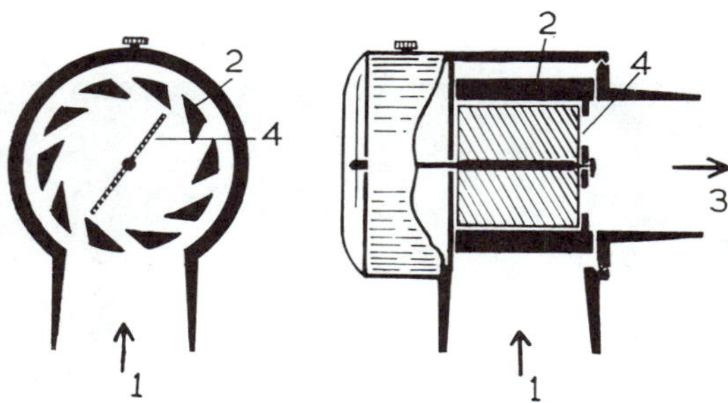

Figure 5.12. Diagram of the Wright spirometer: *1*, gas inlet. *2*, stator ring with 10 tangential slots. *3*, gas outlet. *4*, two-bladed rotor running on jeweled bearings.

in O_2 content of arterial and mixed venous blood (a-v DO_2) and multiply it by blood flow or cardiac output (CO). This method is much more invasive then measurements of inspired and expired air since it requires samples of arterial blood and of mixed venous blood obtained from the right heart or pulmonary artery. This method is never used when the sole object in obtaining such blood samples is to measure VO_2, since it would constitute an unreasonable risk compared to measurements of gas exchange. However, for those critically ill patients who have Swan-Ganz and arterial catheters in place for hemodynamic monitoring, as a necessary part of patient care, drawing additional small blood samples for measurement of VO_2 represents a very minor additional risk and is often more appropriate then measuring gas exchange. Cardiac output, in such patients, is generally considered a necessary part of patient care.

Equipment for measuring the O_2 and CO_2 contents of blood by manometric techniques has been available since the beginning of the century (11), has been modified for use with small samples (12), and is relatively inexpensive to acquire. However, the methodology is tedious, requires technicians who are highly trained in use of the instrumentation, and must be performed within an hour of sampling, since even in oiled syringes the blood samples deteriorate.

A more practical procedure, which uses equipment readily available to the intensive care unit, is to measure the O_2 pressure of arterial (PaO_2) and of mixed venous (PvO_2) blood, the percentage of saturation of hemoglobin (Hb) in arterial and mixed venous blood, and the Hb content. PaO_2 and PvO_2 can be measured in any blood gas analyzer. The percentage of saturation of Hb can be measured by a Cooximeter or other instrument which measures the proportions of reduced and oxidized Hb by spectral analysis. If such an instrument is not available the percentage of saturation can be calculated from PaO_2 and PvO_2 and the O_2 dissociation curve for Hb. The O_2 dissociation curve can be quite abnormal in acutely ill patients, introducing an additional source of error. However, since the errors will be in the same direction for both arterial and venous blood, they tend to cancel out each other.

Oxygen is carried in blood in two forms: in combination with hemoglobin (HbO_2) and simply as dissolved O_2. The amount of O_2 dissolved in blood is dependent on the pressure (PO_2) and the temperature. By definition the solubility factor of a gas in a fluid is the volume dissolved in 1 ml of fluid at 1 atmosphere (760 mm Hg) pressure. The experimentally established solubility for O_2 in blood (or water) at 37 ° C is 0.0228. For most purposes we express the amount of O_2 in blood as ml O_2 per 100 ml blood, and pressure in mm Hg. In those units the solubility factor becomes $(0.0228 / 760) \times 100$ or 0.00301 ml of O_2 per 100 ml of blood per 1 mm Hg. If the PaO_2 of arterial blood is 90, the amount of dissolved O_2 will be $90 \times 0.003 = 0.27$ ml O_2 per 100 ml. If the PvO_2 of mixed venous blood is 45 mm Hg, then the amount of dissolved O_2 will be $45 \times 0.003 = 0.135$ ml O_2 per 100 ml blood.

One g of hemoglobin, fully saturated, combines[c] with 1.38 ml of O_2. If we assume that there is 15 g Hb per 100 ml blood and that Hb in arterial blood is 100% saturated, then the amount of O_2 combined with Hb in 100 ml of arterial blood will be

$$(1.38\ ml\ O2\ /g\ Hb) \times (15\ g\ Hb\ /100\ ml) \times (100\%\ /100\%) = 20.7\ ml\ O_2\ per\ 100\ ml\ arterial\ blood.$$

If the percentage of saturation of venous blood (Satv %) is 72, the amount of O_2 combined with Hb will be

$$(1.38 \times 15) \times (72 / 100) = 14.9\ ml\ O_2\ per\ 100ml\ venous\ blood.$$

The general equation for calculating the amount of O_2 combined with Hb is

$$1.38 \times Hb\ (g) \times Sat\ (\%) / 100\ . \qquad (18)$$

The total concentration of oxygen in arterial and in venous blood may be expressed by the following formulas:

$$CaO_2 = 1.38 \times Hb(g) \times Sata(\%)/100 + 0.003 \times PaO_2. \qquad (19)$$

[c] Because of uncertainties in determining the molecular weight of Hb other values for its O_2 combining ability have been reported, ranging from 1.34 to 1.39. Nowadays the generally accepted value is 1.38, but for practical purposes these differences are not important.

and

$$CvO_2 = 1.38 \times Hb(g) \times Satv(\%)/100 + 0.003 \times PvO_2. \quad (20)$$

The only factors different in these two equations are the Sat and the PO_2, so that the difference in oxygen between arterial and venous blood can be expressed by the equation

$$a\text{-}vDO_2 = 1.38 \times Hb \times (Sat\ a - Sat\ v)/100 + 0.003 \times (PaO_2 - PvO_2). \quad (21)$$

By replacing with the numerical values, as in the above example, the CaO_2 is 20.7 ml O_2 per 100 ml arterial blood and CvO_2 is 14.9 ml O_2 per 100 ml venous blood. The difference, a-vDO_2, of 5.8 ml of O_2 per 100 ml of blood, indicates that each 100 ml of arterial blood will on average release 5.8 ml of oxygen while passing through the various tissues of the body, since the CvO_2 will of course be obtained from mixed venous blood (drawn from the pulmonary artery or from the right heart). The total oxygen extracted from arterial blood, corresponding to the VO_2, can then be expressed by the formula:

$$VO_2\ (ml\ min^{-1}) = CO\ (ml\ min^{-1}) \times [a\text{-}vDO_2]\ (ml\ per\ 100\ ml)/100. \quad (22)$$

Assuming a cardiac output (CO) of 5000 ml min^{-1}, we have

$$290\ ml\ min^{-1} = 5000\ ml\ min^{-1} \times 5.8\ ml\ per\ 100\ ml/100.$$

In principle, VCO_2 can be measured by the same type of procedures as shown in equation 23

$$VCO_2 = CO \times [v\text{-}aDCO_2]. \quad (23)$$

In practice, and for good reasons, VCO_2 is rarely measured in this manner. As discussed in Chapter 2, if we make reasonable assumptions for RQ and N excretion, energy expenditure can be accurately calculated from accurate measurements of VO_2. In the procedures we have just described, the accuracy of VO_2 depends on the accuracy of measurements of cardiac output and of arterial and venous O_2 content. An error of 2% in CO will give an error of 2% in VO_2. Errors of 2% in O_2 content are magnified because we are looking at the a-v difference. In the example cited above, where CaO_2 was 20.7 and CvO_2 was 14.9 ml per 100 ml, an error of 2% in each determination translates into an error of 8% for the difference of 5.8 ml per 100 ml. Critically ill patients usually have much lower hematocrits and CaO_2 and CvO_2 are more likely to be in the range of 14 and 8 ml per 100 ml blood, respectively. In this case errors of 2% in each determination translate into an error of only 5% in the difference of 6 ml per 100 ml. Such errors are acceptable, particularly since they can be reduced by multiple sampling, which is quite feasible. Furthermore values for CaO_2 and CvO_2 are readily available in the ICU, even if a Cooximeter is lacking, since most automatic blood gas analyzers calculate and display CaO_2 and CvO_2 as a part of routine blood analysis. Thus, with a few sequential blood samples it is possible to obtain VO_2, and thus resting energy expenditure, with an accuracy of better then 5%, a very useful value for the care of the ICU patient.

It is much more difficult to obtain accurate values for blood content of CO_2. It is present in a variety of interconvertible forms: *(a)* as carbamino derivatives of Hb and of plasma proteins; *(b)* as dissolved molecular CO_2; *(c)* as carbonic acid, H_2CO_3, which is the monohydrate of CO_2; and (*d*) as bicarbonate, HCO_3^-, derived by dissociation of H_2CO_3. Therefore, calculation of total CO_2 content from measurement of PCO_2 by the blood gas machine is less accurate than for O_2. More important, concentrations of CO_2 in blood are much higher then for O_2. Typical values for $CaCO_2$ and $CvCO_2$ are 50 and 55 ml per 100 ml, respectively. This means that a 2% error in each determination translates into a 30% error in the difference of 5 ml per 100 ml. Since measurement of VCO_2 is not required for energy expenditure, the only reason for measuring it would be to estimate rate of fat and carbohydrate oxidation. However, the inherent inaccuracy of the method makes it useless for this purpose as well.

Thus while measurement of VO_2 and energy expenditure from blood gases and cardiac output is accurate and useful in the care of the critically ill patient, measurement of VCO_2 by this procedure is too inaccurate to serve any useful function.

Theoretically, similar results should be obtained when VO_2 is measured from respiratory gases as when it is measured from CO and a-vDO_2. One small difference is that the latter method does not measure O_2 consumption by the lung parenchyma, since this tissue does not derive its O_2 from arterial blood. Liggett et al. measured REE both by gas exchange and from cardiac output and blood gas measurements, and found the mean values for 19 critically ill patients to differ by only 1.5% (13). The average difference between the two methods without regard to sign was 10%. This indicates that use of blood gas measurements for critically ill patients, instead of measuring respiratory gases, is adequate for estimating energy expenditure. If the authors had included the contribution of dissolved O_2 and taken three blood samples instead of one, the agreement might have been closer.

Homogenization of Expired Gases

To multiply two variables, VE and FEO_2 or VE and $FECO_2$, the signals can be synchronized and VO_2 and VCO_2 can then be calculated breath by breath (14). Another possibility is to transform the variable gas concentration into a constant by using a mixing system. Figure 5.2 shows how in a model of two mixing bottles an acceptable mixing of FEO_2 and of $FECO_2$ is obtained. This system was previously described (4) and is composed of two mixing bottles of 1550 and 800 ml placed on either side of the pneumotachograph and the expiratory valve (Figure 5.7). In order to obtain a stable value of FEO_2 and of $FECO_2$ the sampling has to be performed beyond the second mixing bottle. The time necessary to reach stable gas concentrations for 10 normal subjects at rest was 92.5 seconds for FEO_2 and 83.4 sec for $FECO_2$. Although this stabilization time may seem long, it is suitable for studying metabolic variations in patients.

Gas Concentration Measurements

Mass Spectrometer

All respiratory gases can be measured by a mass spectrometer (15). Gases are aspirated into a chamber by a vacuum pump, where they are ionized with an electron beam. The ionized molecules are accelerated by a potential difference before passing through a magnetic field that separates them as a function of their mass and electrical charge. This allows detection of the different constituents of the gas mixture, each one of the different gases producing a signal proportional to its concentration in the mixture. This expensive tool is very accurate and gives simultaneously a precise reading of O_2, CO_2, N_2, and other gases if desired. The sampling rate is not more then 20 to 30 ml per minute and the response time is no longer than about 200 milliseconds. The main problems with the mass spectrometer occur with the vacuum pump and capillary sampling tubes, which clog easily.

Some gases, like CO_2 and N_2O which have the same molecular weight can only be separated by special devices. A very important feature of the mass spectrometer is that it provides instantaneous values for CO_2 and O_2, but at a high cost. Since prolonged measurements of VO_2 and VCO_2 are required for indirect calorimetry, expensive instantaneous values are of little use and the mass spectrometer is not the method of choice.

Oxygen Concentration Measurements in Respiratory Gases

The volume of oxygen consumed can be evaluated by the amount of oxygen that has been removed from a spirometer, as we have shown for the closed circuit system. For many years in the first half of this century this was the most common technique used for the evaluation of "basal metabolic rate" from oxygen consumption. This method is easy and inexpensive to perform, since it does not use gas analyzers or sophisticated volume measurement devices. However, the likelihood of leaks in the inspiratory or the expiratory lines, the use of 100% FIO_2, and the limitation to 10-15 minutes of measurement makes the use of this method not reliable enough for metabolic evaluations.

Micro-Scholander

This chemical technique permits the determination of CO_2, O_2, and N_2 in a gas sample of 0.5 ml with an accuracy of 0.015 volume percent. It can handle samples containing between 0% and 99% of absorbable gases. The sample is introduced into a reaction chamber, connected to a micrometer burette and is balanced by means of an indicator drop in a capillary against a compensatory chamber. The volume of the air bubble is measured initially and after sequential mixing with CO_2 and O_2 absorbing fluids. The total amount of liquid in the system remains constant. Mercury is introduced in the reaction chamber to maintain the balance of the gas against the compensating chamber during the absorption of the gas, and the volume can be read on the micrometer divisions of the burette. This method is mainly used for measuring the concentration of calibrating gases. Since it is an off-line technique and time consuming it is not used for practical clinical metabolic evaluations, although some investgators have used this technique for research purposes (16).

Polarographic Oxygen Analyzer

This analyzer measures the partial pressure of O_2. It consists of platinum and silver electrodes placed in a potassium chloride electrolyte solution. The constant voltage applied between the two electrodes is modified by the partial pressure of O_2 and the current generated is measured. This Clark-type O_2 electrode, used also for blood PO_2 analysis, has a rapid response time, but loses accuracy after a relatively short time. The electrode is also sensitive to temperature and to barometric pressure variations (17).

Fuel Cell Oxygen Analyzer

Built with a lead cathode and a gold anode in a bath of potassium hydroxide, this PO_2 fuel cell analyzer generates its own voltage. Thus, acting like a battery, it does not need any external power supply. This type of fuel cell has a limited lifetime. New types of fuel cells for PO_2 analysis operated at high temperatures have recently been developed and their application for metabolic use is under investigation (18).

High Temperature Oxygen Analyzer

At a temperature of 900 ° C, in the presence of platinum, oxygen is ionized. A zirconium oxide ceramic tube is coated, on both the inside and outside, with thin layers of platinum. It is permeable to the ionized oxygen, which generates a potential between the two platinum surfaces as a function of the oxygen concentration. This method has a very short response time but requires a high temperature sensor.

Paramagnetic Oxygen Analyzer

Oxygen and, to a smaller degree, nitrous monoxide have paramagnetic properties. They have the ability to modify a magnetic field which is proportional to the partial pressure of the gas. It has been shown by Ellis and Nunn (19) to be a very reliable and accurate tool. It has a slow response time, up to 60 seconds, and is sensitive to flow and to water content of gas. However, ensuring that the gases are dry and the flow constant is quite feasible. Since a fast reaction time is not important for indirect calorimetry, this method is highly suitable for metabolic evaluation (19). Recently a fast response paramagnetic oxygen analyzer was developed which represents a serious improvement for this type of analyzer.

Carbon Dioxide by Weighing

The volume of carbon dioxide produced can be calculated from the weight of gas absorbed by soda lime. This method has been generally used with closed circuit instruments.

Infrared CO_2 Analyzer

The most common analyzer used today for on-line end-tidal or mixed expired CO_2 analysis is the infrared absorption analyzer. Carbon dioxide, as well as several other gases, absorb specific wavelengths of infrared rays. When a beam of infrared light passes through a sample of a gas containing CO_2, a certain amount of the beam is absorbed, and this absorption is compared to a reference sample with a known concentration of CO_2. One of the problems of these analyzers is that the output signal is not linearily related to the CO_2 concentration and that a linearization system has to be built into the apparatus. The absorption CO_2 analyzers are very stable and reliable, if careful calibrations are performed (5).

INTERPRETATION OF RESULTS AND DESIGN OF MEASUREMENTS

The design of indirect calorimetry measurements, which includes the purchase of equipment, the frequency and duration of measurements, and what parameters should be measured, is inextricably related to the particular goals to be obtained, and how the results of measurements are interpreted with particular reference to their accuracy and reliability. We may generalize the goals of indirect calorimetry into two main categories; research and patient care. The major use of indirect calorimetry over the 100 years of its existence has been for research in a wide variety of aspects of energy metabolism, research which is mainly responsible for our present understanding of energy metabolism and exercise physiology. There remains much more to learn about energy metabolism, and we can expect indirect calorimetry to be a major research tool in the years to come. However, each individual research project has its own unique goals and it is the responsibility of each investigator to determine whether and how the tools available can be used appropriately, or if, perhaps, new tools must be invented. Indirect calorimetry has also been used in the diagnosis and treatment of individual patients. For many years measurement of basal metabolic rate was used in the diagnosis of hyper- and hypothyroidism, and every hospital had instruments for routine measurements of VO_2. Since World War II measurement of circulating thyroid hormones has replaced measurements of BMR and these instruments have been abandoned. In the past 10 years, more sophisticated instruments have become commercially available (see Chapter 6), which are suitable for measuring VO_2 and VCO_2 in critically ill patients as well as in normal subjects. These are increasingly used to measure energy expenditure as a guide to energy intake for patients who require parenteral or non-oral enteral diets. While the ensuing discussion will deal with some questions relating to design of experimental research, it will be mainly directed to questions relating to nutritional therapy of the critically ill patient.

It should be kept in mind that any discussion of this type is dependent on the tools presently available, and with technological changes it will become outdated. For instance we will conclude that measurement of energy expenditure is very useful for care of critically ill patients and that measurement of N excretion is of less value. Ten years ago such a statement would have been impossible, since equipment for measuring energy expenditure was not available to the ICU. With the recent introduction of chemiluminescent techniques (Chapter 3) for detection of total N in urine, N excretion measurements may become more useful in the future.

Energy Expenditure

Energy expenditure is the single most useful measurement of indirect calorimetry for care of the patient on parenteral or enteral diets.

With present equipment, 24-hour resting energy expenditure can be measured with an accuracy approaching 5% or less, which is more then adequate to serve as a basis for nutritional requirements of the critically ill or malnourished patient. By comparison estimates of energy expenditure from formulas such as the Harris- Benedict equations modified for stress and malnutrition will differ from measured values by about 18% on the average (Chapter 7) and often by as much as 50%. This is due to the very wide dispersal of energy expenditures in critically ill patients (20) as illustrated in Figure 7.3 and Table 7.3.

For very precise measurements of energy expenditure we must measure VO_2, VCO_2, and urinary N. However, estimating N excretion, instead of measuring it leads to errors of no more than 1% or 2 %. Equations which neglect N excretion, suitable for critically ill patients, are given and discussed in Chapter 2 (equations 34 and 35). Thus for care of critically ill patients it is not necessary to measure N excretion in order to accurately calculate energy expenditure. As also discussed in Chapter 2 (see equations 36–38) quite accurate values for energy expenditure may be obtained only from VO_2, neglecting both CO_2 and N measurements. Indeed, many studies of exercise physiology, and of subjects studied in normal settings rather than in the laboratory or hospital, make use of instruments such as the Kofrany-Michaelis meter or the Pauling oxygen meter without measuring VCO_2 or urinary N (Chapter 1). In principle there is no need to measure VCO_2 to estimate energy expenditure in critically ill patients. Indeed if VO_2 is calculated from measurements of blood gases and cardiac output, it is a waste of time to attempt also a measurement of VCO_2. If, however, VO_2 is calculated from respiratory gases, then VCO_2 should also be measured, since equipment available to the ICU measures VCO_2 simultaneously with, and as accurately as it measures, VO_2. Accurate measurements of VCO_2 will provide more accurate estimates of energy expenditure than assumptions as to probable RQ. Energy expenditure does not remain constant during the day, even in bedridden patients. Furthermore, the process of fitting a patient with mask, noseclip or mouthpiece will often cause both hyperventilation and increase in energy expenditure. In ambulatory subjects we also have the problem of estimating activity energy expenditure (AEE).

For measurements of resting energy expenditure (REE), we must consider both the duration of each measurement and the number of measurements per day required to achieve any desired accuracy for 24-hour estimates of REE. Van Lanschot and coworkers (21) performed an ingenious experiment with patients on respirators. They measured REE, using gas exchange, continuously for 24-hour periods and then examined the number of periods per day required to estimate 24-hour REE with any particular degree of accuracy. They found that two 15-minute measurements at an approximately 12-hour interval, gave a 24-hour estimate within 4%. To improve this to less than 2% required four 60-minute periods more or less evenly dispersed throughout the day. For patient nutritional care, estimates within 4% are more than adequate, particularly since substantial improvement in accuracy requires 240 min instead of 30 min of measurement time. Measurement periods as short as 15 minutes are suitable for patients on respirators, since the apparatus is attached to the respirator system, and not to the patient, and therefore will have no effect on ventilatory rate or energy expenditure. A different problem with ventilated patients is that they are often given enriched O_2 mixtures with FIO_2 ranging from 40% to 100%. With many systems the accuracy of VO_2 measurements decreases with increasing FIO_2(22).

The situation is quite different for patients who are not on ventilators. Putting on a mask or a noseclip and mouthpiece may cause both an increase in energy expenditure and hyperventilation, which can take many minutes to subside. Indeed since some discomfort is associated with the apparatus, periods of measurement are limited to 10 to 15 minutes and respiratory gas exchange may never revert to resting values during that period. Thus this apparatus is difficult to use with such patients. More suitable is the use of either a *closed* or *open canopy system*. A closed system designed by Kinney and colleagues (23,24) is shown in Figure 5.13. The patient lies with his head enclosed in a transparent plastic canopy, sealed off by foam plastic straps around the neck. Air is pumped in and out of the canopy at equal rates so that the pressure inside of the canopy is the same as outside except for the patient's breathing. This allows a spirometer, attached to the canopy, to record the volume of each breath. Thus this instrument can be used both for indirect calorimetry and to record breathing patterns. On-line transmission of electrical signals from the spirometer and O_2 and CO_2 analyzers monitoring the expired gases permits computer analysis and display of the data. This system has served as a prototype for some of the commercial instruments currently available (Chapter 6). A recording of VO_2, VCO_2, and R, typical for such patients, obtained from this system is illustrated in Figure 5.14. When the patient is first placed in the canopy, VO_2 and VCO_2 are at maximum values and then subside slowly over 5 to 15 minutes to a fairly stable plateau, which is maintained to the end of the measurement at 40 minutes. Since body O_2 stores are small compared to VO_2 (Table 2.14), this high value of VO_2 represents an increase in tissue O_2 consumption and therefore an increase in REE. The maximal value for VCO_2 is proportionally higher then for VO_2. This is because there was initial hyperventilation as well as increased REE. Since body CO_2 stores are proportionally much larger than O_2 stores, they become depleted during hyperventilation as excess CO_2 is blown off; during this period, R, representing respiratory gas exchange, is higher than RQ, representing tissue gas exchange. Subsequently, after ventilatory rate returns to normal, body CO_2 stores are repleted and R drops below RQ, although this is not always perceptible. During the final 20 to 30 minutes VO_2, VCO_2 and R remain reasonably constant, although they may show minute-to-minute or even longer term variations, changes in VO_2 and VCO_2 tend to go together, R remains more constant, and there are no long-term trends. The constant steady-state value of R indicates that during this time it truly represents RQ, the gas exchange taking place at the cellular level. This last 20 to 30 minutes is averaged to derive steady state-values of VO_2 and VCO_2, and the first 5 to 10 minutes is ignored. Of course, should the patient move about or become excited during this period it will be readily apparent and will invalidate the measurement. It should be kept in mind that the example shown in Figure 5.14 is only an example and that there are almost infinite variations in the recordings made from different patients and at different times. Nevertheless, Chikenji et al. (25), found that 3-5 such measurements, evenly distributed throughout the day, were sufficient to determine 24-hour REE, with an error averaging less than 5%. Thus, it takes far longer, 150 to 240 minutes, to measure 24-hour REE in patients who are breathing naturally than the 30 minutes required for ventilated patients.

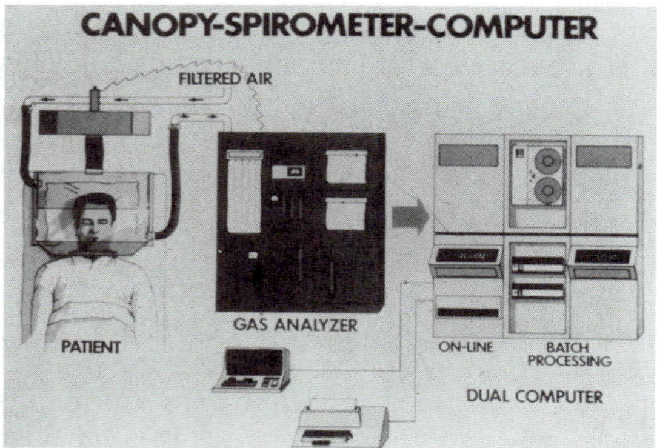

Figure 5.13. Reproduced from Kinney JM, Askanazi J, Gump FE et al.: Use of the ventilatory equivalent to separate hypermetabolism from increased dead space ventilation in the injured or septic patient. *J Trauma*20:111-119, 1980. With permission of the *Journal of Trauma.*Canopy system for simultaneous measurement of gas exchange and spirometry.

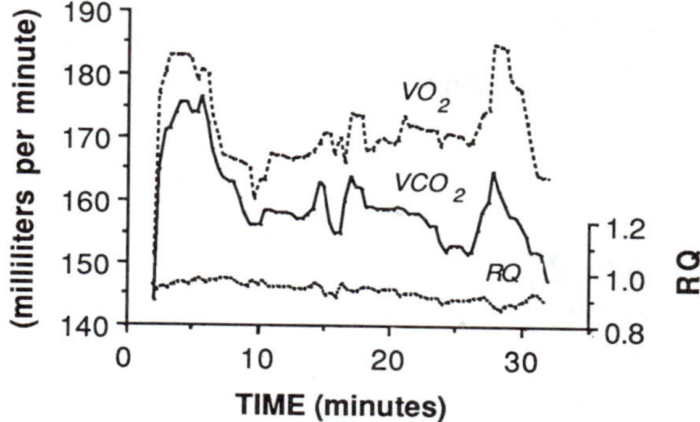

Figure 5.14. Continuous measurement of VO_2, VCO_2, and RQ using the canopy system described in Figure 5.13.

An even more suitable system for indirect calorimetry for naturally breathing patients, is the open canopy system. This consists of a flexible plastic cone or tent surrounding the patient's head and shoulders sufficiently that all expired gases will be captured by the airflow pumped through the tent to the gas analyzers (Figs. 5.15-5.16). This does not restrict the patient in any way and permits continuous monitoring of the subject over periods much longer than can be used with a closed canopy. Furthermore since the patient is not put into it, and need not be aware that measurements are being taken, the initial hyperventilation and increased energy expenditure seen with the closed canopy does not occur. Of course, as an open system, it cannot be used for simultaneous spirometric measurements.

Determination of Methodological Errors

The above discussion shows that in both ventilated and spontaneously breathing patients, it is possible to determine 24-hour REE within about 5% of actual values using equipment now available to the ICU (Chapter 6). This presupposes that the accuracy of each individual measurement is good enough to draw these conclusions. Properly calibrated and properly used, the commercial equipment available to the ICU is capable of this kind of accuracy. Errors in individual determinations are of the order of 2% or less. However, even the best equipment goes out of calibration or suffers malfunction from time to time, and instruments for indirect calorimetry are no exception. The most common malfunctions are leaks, followed by the detector drifting out of calibration, and then by more serious malfunctions of detectors, pumps, etc. Since such malfunctions may occur at any time, all patient data

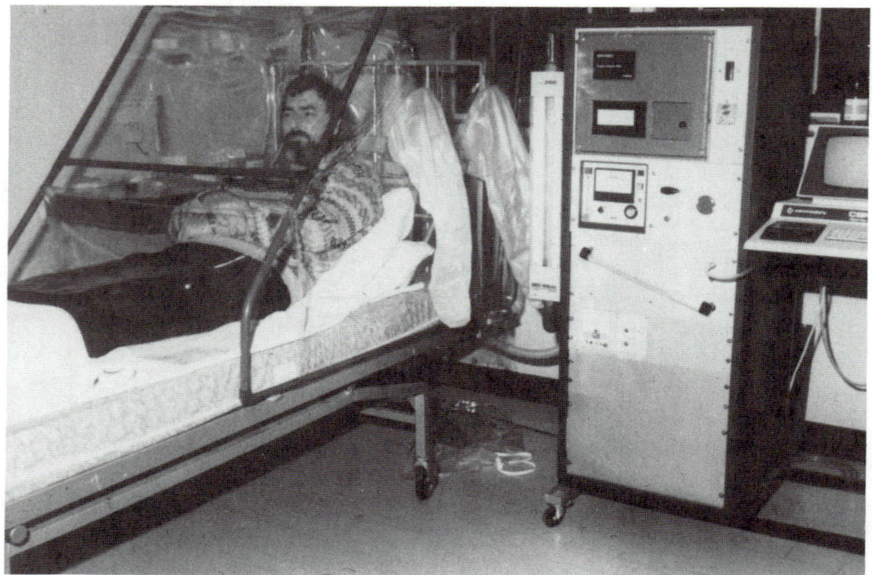

Figure 5.15. Courtesy of Dr. Marinos Elia. Open canopy system used at the Dunn Nutritional Centre, Cambridge, England. The volume of the hood is about 1000 liters and the airflow is 75 liter/min. These conditions are adequate to prevent any loss of expired air, even with a moving subject.

should be examined to see whether there are signs of them. Even if the equipment is functioning properly, it may be improperly used, for instance, in a patient who is either hyper- or hypoventilating.

The first way to look for error is to examine the data, together with other information such as diet, disease, and weight to see if they are internally consistent. Is the value for REE consistent with the size, condition, and diet of the patient? Is it consistent with previous or subsequent measurements in the same patient? Is the RQ consistent with dietary intake, both current and past? Failure to check or think through these questions may lead to inappropriate management of the patient and to misleading information presented in the literature. As an example, consider a patient who has been maintained on a hypocaloric diet for several days for whom an R value of 1.10 is obtained. If R is taken to be equal to RQ, it would mean that the patient was converting substantial amounts of carbohydrate to fat, which is impossible on this diet. The high R value might be because the patient was hyperventilating, because either the O_2 or CO_2 analyzers were out of calibration or possible other reasons. These possibilities should then be systematically investigated, measurements in other patients before and after this one should be examined for inconsistencies,

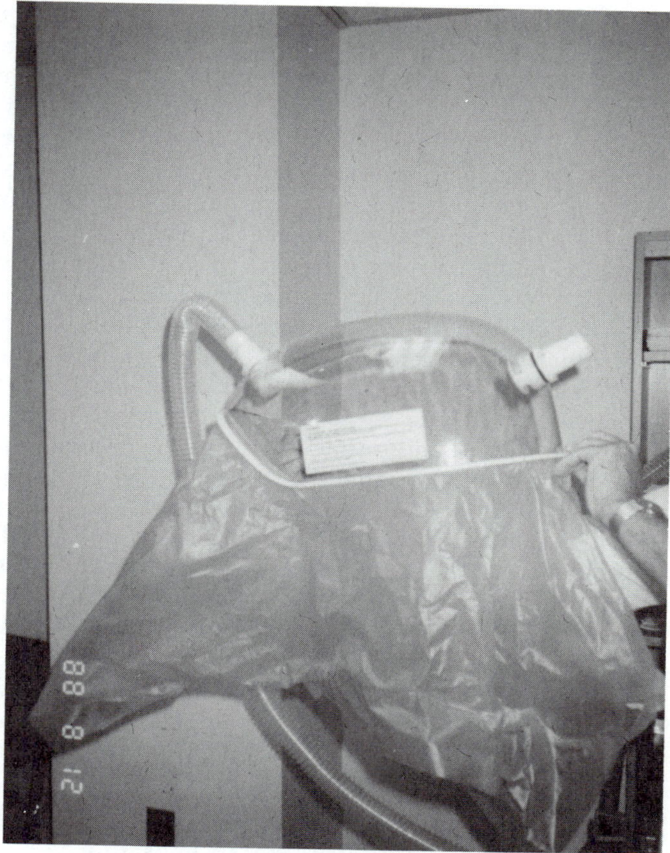

Figure 5.16. Open canopy system used with the Datex Deltatrac gas analyzer (see Chapter 6).

and the calibration of the equipment checked. What should not be done is to report the R of 1.1 as an RQ. That many investigators do not adequately check their data is attested by reports in the literature of RQs below 0.65 or above 1.40, well out of the range of values for which there is any reasonable physiological explanation.

Fuel Utilization

Nitrogen Excretion and Balance

For physiological reasons, N excretion is not as useful for establishing nutrient requirements as is energy expenditure. There is a direct relation between energy expenditure and energy requirements. It is true that energy expenditure is affected by diet, but compared to N excretion, this effect is small. If one measures REE, in a patient receiving 2 liters per day of 5% dextrose, to be 1800 kcal (7531 kJ) per day, then, depending on the type of patient, one can expect an increase of 10% to 20% in REE, to 2000-2200 kcal (8368-9205 kJ), when the patient receives an adequate nutrient intake. If, however, one finds N excretion to be 12 g per day in a patient on 5% dextrose, it provides little information as to what it will be on an adequate diet; depending on the composition of the diet it might be more or less than 12 g. This is because N balance and N excretion relate in a complex way to both N intake and total energy intake (Chapter 3). Another example is the severely stressed, bedridden patient receiving TPN containing 2400 kcal (10,042 kJ) and 10 g N per day, whose REE is 2200 kcal (9205 kJ), and N excretion is 13 g per day. Since he or she is in positive energy balance there is no urgent need to provide additional energy. If the patient is not malnourished, providing an additional 5 g N per day would probably increase excretion by 4.5 g improving N balance from -3 to -2.5 g per day. If the patient is malnourished, N excretion may go up by only 3.5 g, improving N balance to -1.5 g per day. These predictions can be checked by measuring N balance, and on the next day further modification of the diet can be made if it seems appropriate. In either case, however, if and as the stress decreases, the patient will achieve zero or positive N balance on either the 10 g or the 15 g N diet. Thus accurate determination of N excretion is not very useful in establishing appropriate N or energy intake, but can be useful as a check on whether the diet is adequate, and in fine tuning the N requirements.

However, accurate determination of N excretion is very difficult to achieve. For one thing N excretion is very variable; in a single patient on a constant diet it may vary by 2-3 g or more from day to day. Thus to provide a guide to nutrition, one requires 2-3 days of accurate measurements. But accurate measurements are hard to obtain. Collection of 24-hour urine is very difficult and, even if this is achieved, prediction of total N excretion from urinary urea can easily be in error by 2 g N per day (26). Determination of total N in all excreta by traditional Kjeldahl methods is time consuming and rarely available for clinical use, although important for research considerations. Recent introduction of chemiluminescent methods for total N (Chapter 3) may improve this situation. They are easy to use with urine and have a rapid turnaround time of a few minutes to a few hours. Stool and drainage samples can also be analyzed, but with greater difficulty. If the problem of accurate collection of 24-hour urines can be solved, instrumentation for this procedure, available for about $15,000, may greatly facilitate accurate estimation of N excretion in time to be of use for patient care purposes. Nevertheless, even when accurately and rapidly determined, measurement of N excretion is much less useful for predicting nutritional requirements than is measurement of energy expenditure.

Carbohydrate and Fat Oxidation

Accurate values for carbohydrate and fat oxidation require accurate determinations of VO_2, VCO_2, and urinary N excretion (Chapter 2). Since accurate values of VO_2 are necessary for accurate estimation of REE, and since almost all equipment for measuring gas exchange will provide as accurate values for VCO_2 as for VO_2, these will be available whenever accurate values of REE are obtained. However, as discussed above, accurate values of N excretion are more difficult to obtain and are not necessary for REE. It seems unlikely that unless they are measured in order to estimate N balance, N determinations can be justified for estimating rates of carbohydrate and fat oxidation for purposes of patient care. The amount of total energy in the diet should preferably be based on measurements of energy expenditure. The amount of N in the diet will be based on energy expenditure and the type of patient, and may or may not be fine tuned by measurements of N excretion. The proportions of carbohydrate and fat, which provide the nonprotein energy of the diet, should be determined by considerations largely unrelated to their rates of oxidation on any particular day (Chapter 7). Thus, for purposes of nutritional care of the patient, there is no point in measuring rates of oxidation of carbohydrate and fat.

As discussed in Chapter 4, stressed patients tend to burn more fat and less carbohydrate than normal subjects or malnourished patients. Their response to increased glucose loads is to increase energy expenditure more and to decrease fat oxidation less than do other subjects. Response to a glucose challenge could be a useful tool in determining the degree of stress in injured or septic patients.

Summary

We may summarize this section by repeating that measurement of energy expenditure by indirect calorimetry is very useful for predicting nutritional requirements of critically ill or malnourished patients who require parenteral or enteral nutrition. As discussed at more length in Chapter 7, measurement of energy expenditure combined with our present knowledge of the responses of malnourished and stressed patients to nutrients can provide a reasonable guide for deciding on the amount of total energy, and the proportions of protein, carbohydrate, and fat to be provided. Measurement of the amounts of each of these fuels which are utilized in a particular patient on a particular day does not provide significant additional help for this purpose. This is partly because of the difficulties in obtaining N excretion measurements which are sufficiently accurate and rapid to be of practical use; improvements in N measurements may make this a more desirable determination in the future. Nevertheless, the actual amounts of each nutrient oxidized, in a particular patient on a particular day, are inherently of less use than is energy expenditure. This is because, while measured energy expenditure provides a direct guide as to the desirable energy intake, measured values of protein, fat, and carbohydrate oxidation merely reflect what was eaten or administered on that particular day and do not indicate what would be a desirable intake. More important is our general understanding of how sick patients respond to nutrients, of the general requirements for each nutrient, and of the undesirable side effects of each nutrient. Such general information is, of course, derived from research into the energy metabolism and nutrient requirements in such patients, a major part of which concerns evaluation of N balance and fuel utilization. However, since this research has already been performed, it largely obviates the need to repeat the same measurements in each individual patient.

REFERENCES

1. Margaria R, Edwards HT, Dill DS: The possible mechanisms of contracting and paying the oxygen debt and the role of lactic acid in muscular contraction. *Am J Physiol* 106:689-715, 1933.
2. Bock AV, Dill DB, Edwards HT et al.: On the partial pressure of oxygen and carbon dioxide in arterial blood and in alveolar air. *J Physiol* 68:277-291, 1929.
3. Glaser P, Bursztein S: *Etude Synchronique de la Regulation de l'Equilibre Acido-basique dans les Suites de la Chirurgie Abdominale*. Edizioni Fondazione Prof Ganassini, Milano, 1971.
4. Bursztein S, Taitelman U, De Myttenaere S et al.: Reduced oxygen consumption in catabolic states with mechanical ventilation. *Crit Care Med* 6:162-164, 1978.
5. Consolazio CF, Johnson RE, Pecora LJ: *Physiologic Measurements of Metabolic Functions in Man*. New York, McGraw-Hill, 1963, pp 313–339.
6. Bursztein S, Saphar P, Glaser P et al.: Determination of energy metabolism from respiratory function alone. *J Appl Physiol* 42:117-119, 1977.
7. Tissot J: Nouvelle methode de mesure et d'inscription du debit et des mouvements respiratoires de l'homme et des animaux. *J Physiol et Pathol Gen* 6:688-700, 1904.
8. Benedict FG: A portable apparatus for clinical use. *Boston Med Surg J* 178:667-678, 1918.
9. Krogh A: Determination of standard (basal) metabolism of patients by a recording apparatus. *Boston Med Surg J* 189:313-317, 1923.
10. Fowler WS, Blackburn CM, Helmholz HF: Determination of basal rate of oxygen consumption by open and closed circuit methods. *J Clin Endocrinol* 17:786-796, 1957.

11. Van Slyke DD, Neil JM: The determination of gases in blood and in other solutions by vacuum extraction and manometric measurements. *J Biol Chem* 61:523-573, 1926.
12. Natelson S: Routine use of ultramicro methods in the clinical laboratory. *Am J Clin Path* 21:1153-1172, 1951.
13. Liggett SB, St John RE, Lefrak SS: Determination of resting energy expenditure utilizing the thermodilution pulmonary artery catheter. *Chest* 91:562-566, 1987.
14. Osborn JJ, Elliot SE, Segger FJ, Gerbode F: Continuous measurement of lung mechanics and gas exchange in the critically ill. *Med Res Eng* 8:19-23, 1969.
15. Davis NJH, Denison DM: The measurement of metabolic gas exchange and minute volume by mass spectrometry alone. *Resp Physiol* 36:261-267, 1979
16. Scholander PF: Analyzer for accurate estimation of respiratory gases in one-half cubic centimeter samples. *J Biol Chem* 167:235-250, 1947.
17. Parbrook GD, Davis PD, Parbrook EO: *Basic Physics and Measurement in Anesthesia*, London, Heinemann Medical Books, 1982, p 227.
18. Berger J, Riess I, Tanhauser DS: Dynamic measurements of oxygen diffusion in indium-tin oxide. *Solid State Ionics* 15:225-231, 1985.
19. Ellis RF, Nunn JF: The measurement of gaseous oxygen tension utilizing paramagnetism: An evaluation of the Servomex O. A.150 analyser. *Br J Anaest* 40:569-578, 1968.
20. Weissman C, Kemper M, Askanazi J et al.: Resting metabolic rate of the critically ill patient. Measured versus predicted. *Anesthesiology* 64:673-679, 1986.
21. Van Lanschot et al.: Extrapolation accuracy of intermittent metabolic gas exchange recordings and its relation to diurnal variations of critically ill patients. *Crit Care Med* 16:737-742, 1988.
22. Ultman JS, Bursztein S: Analysis of error in the determination of respiratory gas exchange at varying FIO_2. *J Appl Physiol: Resp Envir Exer Physiol* 50:210-16, 1981.
23. Kinney JM, Morgan AP, Dominguez FJ, Gildian KJ: A method for continuous measurement of gas exchange and expired radioactivity in acutely ill patients. *Metabolism* 13:205-211, 1964.
24. Spencer JL, Zikria AB, Kinney JM et al.: A system for the continuous measurement of gas exchange and respiratory function. *J Appl Physiol* 33:523-528, 1972.
25. Chikenji T, Elwyn DH, Gil KM et al.: Effects of increasing glucose intake on nitrogen balance and energy expenditure in malnourished adult patients receiving parenteral nutrition. *Clin Sci* 72:489-501, 1987.
26. Shaw-Delanty SN, Elwyn DH, Jeejeebhoy KN et al.: Components of nitrogen excretion in hospitalized adult patients on intravenous diets. *Clin Nutr* 6:257-266, 1987.

CHAPTER

6

Evaluation of Metabolic Measurement Equipment

The recent revolution in microelectronics has fostered a major change in the instruments used to measure oxygen consumption and carbon dioxide production. These changes have made these measurements a commonly used clinical tool especially in exercise studies. This chapter will review these technological advances as well as examine how to evaluate the capabilities and accuracy of the new generation of instruments.

BACKGROUND

The measurement of oxygen consumption and carbon dioxide production is one that requires much accuracy. In addition, the measurement of gases requires close attention to pressure and temperature (Boyle's, Charles' and Gay-Lussac's laws). The measurement conditions must also be carefully controlled so that accuracy is maintained. Therefore, when making such measurements, it is extremely important to know the capabilities and limitations of the instrumentation. Also, strict adherence to protocol during the measurement period is needed to insure accurate measurements.

MEASUREMENT THEORY

The evaluation of instruments designed to measure oxygen consumption and carbon dioxide production is performed both in vitro and in vivo. Before describing the actual evaluation methods, a review of measurement theory is in order:

The objective of evaluating such an instrument is to access a variety of functions. These include:

1. Accuracy (validity)—How closely does the measurement approach the real value (1) or in practical terms, the "gold standard?"
2. Reproducibility (precision or reliability)—How consistent are the measurements over time, i.e., are they stable?
3. Range—Under what conditions is the instrument accurate and/or precise, e.g., is it accurate in pediatric as well as adult patients?
4. Long-term stability—Does the instrument provide accurate and precise values over minutes, hours, days, or months? When does it require calibration, adjustment, and maintenance?

In general, evaluation of such an instrument allows one to characterize the errors inherent in the method. Error can be defined as the degree to which the measurement differs from the real value (1). Errors can be systematic or random. Systematic errors are those that cause a consistent and measurable difference and thus, if recognized, can either be compensated for or resolved. For example, if one uses a ruler that is improperly marked in that a measurement of 10.5 inches is really 10 inches, one can routinely subtract 0.5 inch from a measurement that reads 10.5 inches.

One way to eliminate systematic errors is to calibrate an instrument. Of course, the elimination of such error is only as good as the accuracy of the calibration standard. For example, when calibrating a gas analyzer, the calibration is no better than the accuracy with which we know the true concentration of calibrating gas. Other systematic errors include range and scale errors (2). The former type of error occurs when the true measurement is outside the instruments useful measurement range. This error can present in a variety of ways. For example, introduction of 9% CO_2 into a CO_2 analyzer with a range of 0%-6% can result in a number of possible scenarios: a reading of 6% (clipping) where the observed measurement remains at a lower level because the instrument cannot report a higher value than the limits of its meter; a reading of 8% if the instrument is inaccurate above a specific range; or no reading, if the instrument's circuits are unable to handle or interpret the large signal. Scale errors are errors that occur during the reading of a scale. This is important in gas exchange measurements where resolving power—the ability to measure finer parts of the measurements—are very important. For example, when calculating oxygen consumption, it is important to use values that are accurate to the fourth significant figure. At a 40 liter min^{-1} canopy airflow, an error of .05% O_2 leads to an error of 20 ml min^{-1} in the VO_2 calculation.

Random errors can be much more difficult to compensate for than systematic ones. Random errors arise from three sources (2); drift, linearity, or noise. Drift refers to time-dependent changes in an instruments' operating characteristics. The cause of drift may be inherent to the instrument (i.e., electronic instability) or be caused by external factors such as temperature, vibration, or moisture accumulation. Often one can eliminate errors of drift with calibration. It is useful to know the degree of drift so that calibrations or other maneuvers can be instituted at the appropriate times to lessen inaccuracies.

Linearity is defined as the characteristics of an instrument to give equal increments of output for equal increments of input. Often instruments are nonlinear in their measurements (e.g., infrared CO_2 analyzers), requiring that the results be linearized to maintain accuracy. Many instruments are linear only within a specific range. It is important to recognize that range prior to making measurements. Calibration at two points within the range to be measured prior to making measurements often can improve accuracy.

Noise is the change in an instrument's output that is not related to the change in input. Noise can come from the environment (e.g., AC interference at 60 Hz) or the instrument itself. Noise is usually random in nature and contributes to measurement error. To reduce noise, signal averaging is used. Random errors are usually dealt with by increasing the number of observations and averaging them to reduce the effects of the deviations.

It is important to know the effects of drift, linearity, and noise prior to making measurements such as those of VO_2 and VCO_2 that require much accuracy and precision.

EVALUATION

When evaluating an instrument designed to measure VO_2 and VCO_2, it is important to examine components individually. The instruments used to measure VO_2 and VCO_2 using the open circuit method generally consist of the following components: an oxygen analyzer, a carbon dioxide analyzer, a volume measurement device, a mixing chamber, and a computer. Descriptions of the first four of these components can be found in Chapter 5.

Most investigators have found that the component that needs the most attention has been the O_2 analyzer. The oxygen analyzers in use are of a variety of technologies, including polarographic electrodes, fuel cells, and zirconium oxide and paramagnetic analyzers. Polarographic electrodes and fuel cells consume oxygen as they make their measurements and, therefore, after a period of time may lose their accuracy or precision and need replacement. Yet, these analyzers have a rapid response (especially important for exercise measurements) and are a proven, easy to use technology. Until the recent introduction of "solid state" versions, paramagnetic analyzers, were sensitive to shock and dirt. The infrared carbon dioxide analyzers tend to be accurate, provided they are properly linearized and that compensation for oxygen (and nitrous oxide concentration) is made.

In Vitro

Prior to first using an instrument for clinical measurements, it is important to characterize its capabilities as well as its limitations. Evaluation of a gas measurement instrument initially requires in vitro examination of its individual components.

One should start by reading the manufacturers specifications. For gas analyzers, they will often indicate the type of technology used, the environmental conditions (temperature, humidity) under which the instrument should be used and operating specifications such as the range over which the instrument can make accurate measurements (e.g., CO_2, 0%-10%; O_2, 21%-100%) and the response time (the time it takes to respond to a change in concentration). Accuracy is often listed but may mean a number of things. It may mean the sum of errors from various sources such as drift, linearity, and noise or it may be the resolution of the analyzer meter. It is, therefore, important to ask the manufacturer what is meant by accuracy. The manufacturer may also specify the amount of drift and the range over which the instrument is linear. In general, it is important to realize that these specifications were developed by the manufacturer under ideal conditions. It is often useful to confirm these specifications prior to using the instrument. A number of procedures may be carried out to confirm them under working conditions. Some of these procedures are simple, requiring no additional equipment, while others require various pieces of equipment.

The initial set of in vitro studies include those that simply examine the reliabilty of the instrumentation.

Drift and noise can be tested for simply by calibrating the instrument as instructed by the manufacturer and then at specific intervals reintroducing the calibration signal. This can be performed for volume as well as gas measurements. To illustrate: If the manufacturer recommends calibrating the CO_2 analyzer with 0% and 4% CO_2, one should calibrate at set intervals,e.g., 5 minutes, reinfuse the calibration gas, and determine the stability of the calibration. This simple test will allow rather easy determination of drift and noise. The length of this test should be equal to the planned interval between calibrations. If drift is noted then the amount of drift over time should be examined and the interval between calibrations reduced accordingly. If there is noise, i.e., unstable readout, then its cause must be determined. Causes can include 60 Hz interference and vibration. The latter is not infrequent in metabolic devices since they have pumps that tend to vibrate. Another test that can be performed is a study of the linearity. After calibration, a known quantity, different than that used for calibration, is introduced and the accuracy examined. For example, if one calibrates a volume measurement device at 2 liters, then introducing 1 and 3 liters will be helpful in assessing linearity. It is important to be very confident in the accuracy of the test signals that are introduced. If one finds alinearity, then its extent must be further evaluated and the point of calibration, in view of the range to be measured, reassessed. For example, a CO_2 analyzer calibrated at 1.2% CO_2 may result in alinear readings between 0.5% and 1% CO_2. Calibrating at 0.75% may markedly improve the linearity (3). The above tests should be repeated at set weekly or monthly intervals to see if, with use and wear, drift, linearity, or noise increase.

In addition to these tests, it is often important to characterize the capabilities of the whole instrument. An instrument designed for use in adults may not have the accuracy needed for pediatric measurements, while an instrument designed for room air exercise studies may need modification for measurements made on mechanically ventilated patients breathing at elevated FIO_2. The traditional method of characterizing such instruments has been in vitro simulation (3,4). Such simulation of oxygen consumption and carbon dioxide production is performed using a nitrogen dilution technique for the former and a carbon dioxide infusion technique for the latter. The simulation for mechanical ventilation is accomplished by infusing a precisely measured amount of nitrogen or CO_2 into a jar or bag that is being simultaneously ventilated. For a canopy, the CO_2 or nitrogen are added to the through flow of air. Carbon dioxide production is equal to the amount of carbon dioxide being infused per minute (equation 1).

$$VCO_2\,(measured) = VCO_2\,(added) \tag{1}$$

It is important to remember that both sides of the equation need to be corrected for water vapor pressure, temperature, and barometric pressure. The instruments frequently report VCO_2 in STPD while flowmeters or mass flow controllers are calibrated at room temperature (ATPD).

Oxygen consumption is simulated by infusing nitrogen to dilute the expired oxygen content thus creating a difference between inspired and expired oxygen concentrations (equation 2).

$$FEO_2 = \frac{VI \times FIO_2}{VI + VN_2} + \frac{VI \times FIO_2}{VE} \tag{2}$$

When performing such in vitro simulations, it is important to insure there are no leaks in the test system, that the mass flow controllers or flowmeters are calibrated properly, and that the equipment supplying ventilation to the test equipment provides a stable minute ventilation. It is also important to wait until there is adequate mixing of the infused gas (N_2 or CO_2) with the ventilator-delivered inspired volume or the canopy airflow. It is possible to infuse CO_2 and N_2 simultaneously and this simulates a respiratory quotient as well as VO_2 and VCO_2. The respiratory quotient can be validated by completely combusting a fuel that consumes a known amount of oxygen and produces a known amount of CO_2 (Figure 6.1b). Methanol or ethanol each of which has an RQ of 0.67 are used frequently. Other organic fuels with different RQ's such as acetone may also be used. The fuel may be burned qualitatively, only examining RQ, or quantitatively so that the amount of O_2 consumed and CO_2 produced may also be assessed. These in vitro simulation methods have been used by many investigators and are considered the major validation technique. When performing such in vitro studies, it is important to simulate the situations that might be encountered in the clinical environment as closely as possible. These include varying inspiratory oxygen concentration, tidal volume, ventilatory frequency, inspiratory and expiratory flow rates, inspiratory pressures, and positive end-expiratory pressure (PEEP). Testing of various inspiratory pressures and levels of PEEP is needed since most oxygen analyzers measure partial pressures and are, thus, very sensitive to changes in pressure. The addition of humidification is also important since handling of humidity can seriously affect accuracy. Ideally, the values obtained from the instruments should be within ± 5% of those calculated from the known gas infusions.

Another important aspect of evaluating metabolic measurement equipment is assessing the instrument's method of sampling and analyzing inspired oxygen concentration. Browning et al. (5) demonstrated that some mechanical ventilators do not provide a stable FIO_2 and this requires either that an external blender be attached to both the air and oxygen intakes or that there be continuous sampling of the FIO_2 and that an average be taken to determine the mean FIO_2. It is useful to assemble the ventilator and metabolic measurement apparatus and determine the stability of the FIO_2 at various tidal volumes, inspiratory pressures, inspiratory wave forms, respiratory frequencies, and PEEP levels with and without humidification. If there are wide swings in concentration, an external blender should be introduced and the evaluation repeated.

In vitro evaluations, although tedious, allow the user to understand the technical aspects of an instrument's operation so that in the clinical environment, measurements can be made with some degree of proficiency and confidence.

In Vivo

In vivo evaluation studies must be designed not only to examine accuracy and precision but also safety, efficiency, and economy.

It important to remember Lord Kelvin's measurement rule: The measurement itself must not alter the event being measured. For instance, a mouthpiece plus noseclip can alter respiratory pattern (6) and make the individual uncomfortable. Therefore, noninvasive canopy systems were developed (7). Changing the mechanical ventilation environment, i.e., changing from one ventilator to another for the period of the measurements or changing the FIO_2, may also affect the results.

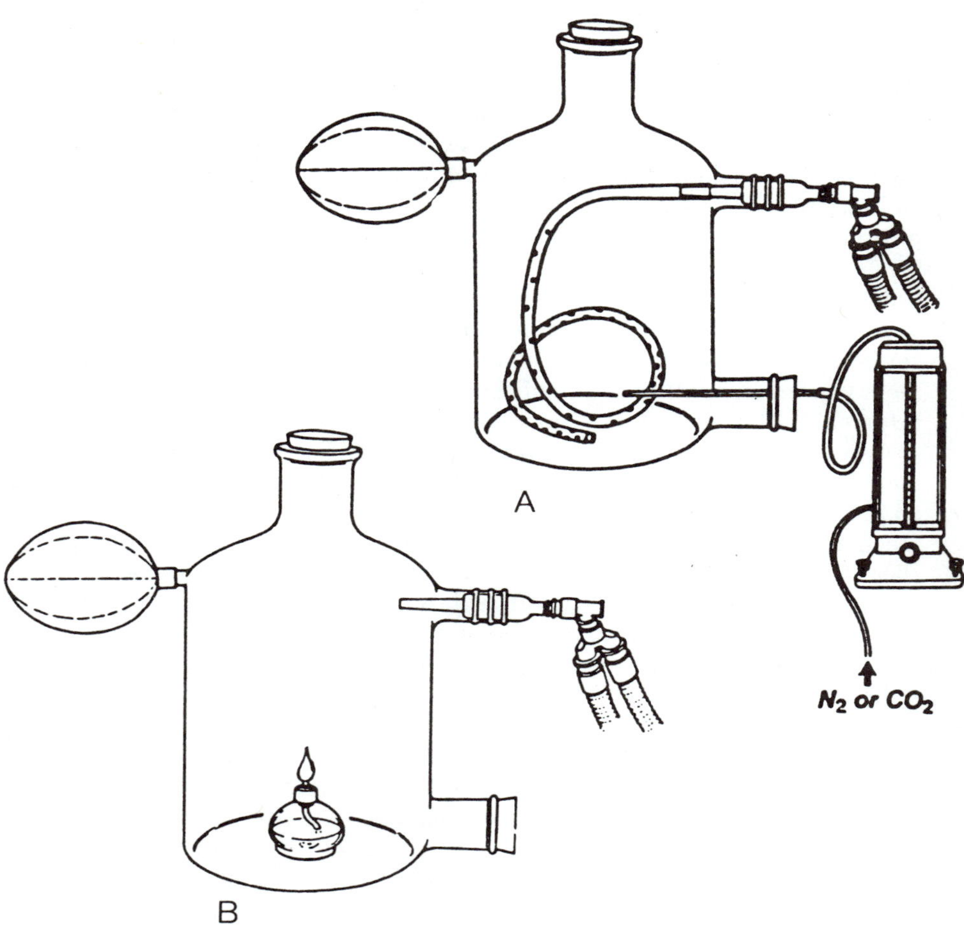

Figure 6.1. Reproduced from Damask MC, Weissman C, Askanazi J et al.: A systematic method for validation of gas exchange measurements. *Anesthesiology* 57: 213-218, 1982. With permission of *Anesthesiology*. (a) Lung model used for simulation of oxygen consumption and carbon dioxide production. The lung model is ventilated by a mechanical ventilator while nitrogen and/or carbon dioxide are infused into the jar. (b) Lung model adapted for combustion of methanol (RQ=0.067) for use in validation of RQ measurements.

In vivo validation is rather difficult to perform since it usually involves comparing the results obtained with one system to those obtained with another one. It is therefore important to be confident in the "reference" system. In vivo validations have been performed against finely tuned research systems (8,9) in the case of exercise. In general, the traditional reference system has been the Douglas bag technique (Figure 6.2). This technique (described in Chapter 5) must be employed with utmost caution since it has many sources of error and therefore validation studies employing it must be looked upon critically. Another validation method has been to compare values obtained with a gas exchange instrument to those obtained using the Fick method (Chapter 5). This requires the presence of a pulmonary artery catheter. Cardiac output is measured using either the thermodilution or dye dilution method. Arterial and mixed venous oxygen contents must also be measured. This can be accomplished either by measuring the contents directly using the Van Slyke method or by calculating from measurements of hemoglobin (Hb), oxygen saturation (SO_2), and partial pressure of oxygen (PO_2):

$$CO_2 = SO_2 \times Hb \times 1.38 + 0.003 \times PO_2 \tag{4}$$

VO_2 is then calculated using the Fick equation:

$$VO_2 = CO\ (CaO_2 - CvO_2) \tag{5}$$

where

CO = cardiac output
CaO_2 = arterial oxygen content
CvO_2 = mixed venous oxygen content

It is important to realize that there are many problems associated with using the Fick method as a reference method. Measurements of cardiac output by the thermodilution method are only accurate to about ± 15%, and are affected by the phase of the respiratory cycle when injections are made. Also, the Fick method gives only a single snapshot measurement of VO_2.

Ideally, when performing in vivo validation studies, the measurements should be performed simultaneously with the two systems. However, this is often impossible to do and it is, therefore, important to insure that the subject is at a similar steady state during measurements made with either system. Since there are limitations to the reference system method, another simple method to examine accuracy superficially is to examine the results obtained in the clinical setting

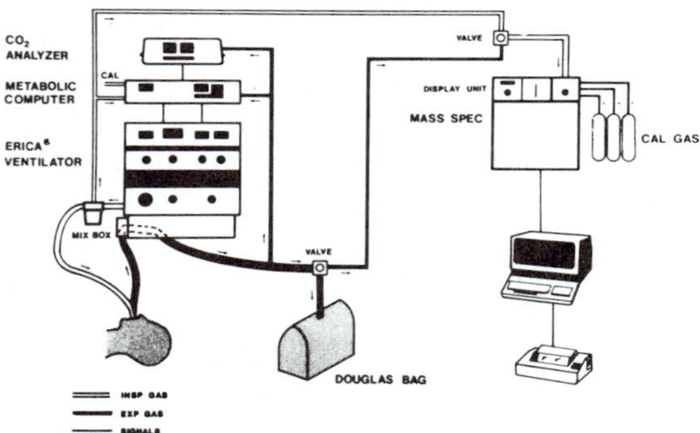

Figure 6.2. Reproduced from Bredbacka S, Kawachi S, Norlander O, Kirk B: Gas exchange during ventilator treatment. A validation of a computerized technique and its comparison with the Douglas bag method. *Acta Anaesthesiol Scand* 28: 462-468, 1984. With permission of *Acta Anaesthesiologica Scandinavica.* An example of a set up for in vivo validation studies. The patient is intubated or tracheostomized. Inspired gas samples are taken from the mixing box at the inspiratory side to an Engstrom Metabolic Computer (EMC) and the mass spectrometer (CMS). Expiratory gas is collected in a Douglas bag and sampled by the EMC and carbon dioxide analyzer (ELIZA). The mixed expiratory gas in the Douglas bag is analyzed by the mass spectrometer and the bag volume is independently determined.

critically. The objective is to study a patient in the resting or sleeping steady state and examine the results obtained. For example, a patient, 2 days postoperative, who has received only 100-150 gram per day of dextrose (i.e., 100-125 ml hr^{-1} of 5% dextrose) since surgery should have an RQ of 0.74-0.84. This range reflects the semistarved state in which lipid is the predominant fuel. Alternately, a patient receiving carbohydrate for at least 2-3 days in amounts close to or above energy expenditure should have an RQ above 0.90. While performing in vivo evaluations a number of other checks should be performed. A gross check of accurate minute volume quantitation can be performed either by using the minute volume value obtained from the ventilator or from an independent spirometer. The latter check can be performed using either a Wright-type spirometer for coarse measurements or a Tissot spirometer for more accurate measurements. Another gross check is to examine the VO_2 and VCO_2 measurements in relation to body weight and/or surface area. At rest, VO_2 should be 2.5-3.4 ml $min^{-1}kg^{-1}$, while VCO_2 should be 1.7-3.0 ml $min^{-1}kg^{-1}$. Results outside this range need to be further examined in light of the patient's clinical condition and for technical problems. Measurement of metabolic rate using the gas exchange method is an exacting task. Close attention must be paid to details while making the measurements. The clinical arena, especially the ICU, can be a distracting environment. Yet, it is mandatory that attention to detail be maintained. It is necessary to prevent leaks by making sure that all the gas connections are tight. Taping them to prevent leakage and disconnection is often done. The cuff of the endotracheal tube must be inflated to minimize both leakage on inspiration and in patients with high minute ventilations, entrapment of air from above the tube. Inspiratory oxygen concentration must be kept stable and analyzers and other parts of the instrument should be in good working order and properly calibrated. Gas drying must be performed carefully. If used, dessication compounds must be replaced regularly. Attention must be directed toward the activity state of the patient (10) so that one can interpret the measurements. Results that are outside the physiological range or are not consistent with the patient's clinical condition must be evaluated with the appropriate suspicion (11). Maintenance should be performed in accordance with the manufacturers' suggestions.

METABOLIC MEASUREMENT EQUIPMENT

Over the last few years, a number of commercially manufactured instruments capable of measuring VO_2 and VCO_2 have become available. The short history of commercial instrumentation has been one of increasing sophistication and reliability. Many of the instruments were initially designed for exercise testing and were then modified for use in conjunction with mechanical ventilators. More recently, instruments designed specifically for use on mechanically ventilated patients have been developed. Another recent development has been the introduction of canopy systems for noninvasive (no mouthpiece or mask) measurements in spontaneously breathing patients. The commercially manufactured instruments currently in clinical use are briefly described below.

Beckman Metabolic Measurement Cart (Beckman Instruments, Fullerton, CA)

This is one of the original instruments designed to measure oxygen consumption and carbon dioxide production. It was originally designed for use in exercise-testing but software is available for measurements during mechanical ventilation. The Beckman Metabolic Measurement Cart (MMC I) is a self-contained mobile cart that includes an LB-2 infrared CO_2 analyzer, an OM-II polarographic O_2 analyzer, a turbine for volume measurements, a mixing chamber, and a

Monroe calculator. Expired gas entering the MMC passes into the mixing chamber and then through the turbine. A constant aliquot of expired gas (usually 500 ml min^{-1}) is sampled from the mixing chamber and flows through a dessication tube containing Dryerite prior to analysis for O_2 and CO_2 concentration. There is a bias flow (12 liters min^{-1}) through the turbine to minimize the effects of inertia. It then returns to the mixing chamber. The instrument requires much user interface as all the calibration procedures are manual, but the simple and accessible plumbing system allows for easy troubleshooting. Specifications of both analyzers have a response time that is rapid, 100 ms, with a resolution of 0.01%. The linearity of the OM-II is ± 0.1% for an oxygen concentration of 0%-99%. The CO_2 analyzer has an accuracy of ± 0.2% over a 0%-10% CO_2 range. The volume transducer has an adequate accuracy of ± 2% over a flow range of 6-600 liters min^{-1}. The turbine specifications are for accuracy above 6 liters min^{-1} so the machine is not generally used on children or infants.

A canopy with an adjustable blower (20-50 liters min^{-1}) is available for use in performing measurements in resting, nonventilated patients. Validation studies have been performed. Wilmore et al. (9) compared the MMC to a reference exercise system and found excellent agreement. Damask et al. performed an in vitro validation study and found less than a ± 5.5% difference at FIO_2 of 0.21-0.80, between measured and predicted (12). Validation of RQ with methanol combustion found little error. Similarly, the canopy system has been validated using in vitro techniques and comparison with a reference system (3). This instrument has been used extensively in scientific investigations, including nutritional and critical care studies (10,13-15).

SensorMedics Horizon Metabolic Measurement Cart (SensorMedics, Anaheim, CA)

This instrument is the successor to the Beckman MMC I and represents the transition to microprocessor-based systems. It can be used in the exercise, canopy, and bedside (ventilator) modes. It is a self-contained mobile unit that consists of a LB-2 infrared CO_2 head with an improved digital linearizing system, a polarographic O_2 analyzer, and a turbine volume measurement device (Figure 6.3). Unlike the original MMC, there is no bias flow; instead there is a computer algorithm that takes into account the effects of inertia at the start of each breath.

All signals are processed by a dedicated INTEL 8085 microprocessor. The system contains two floppy disk drives for program input and data storage. A thermal printer-plotter allows for digital and graphic output while a single-line alphanumeric display assists user interface. Control of

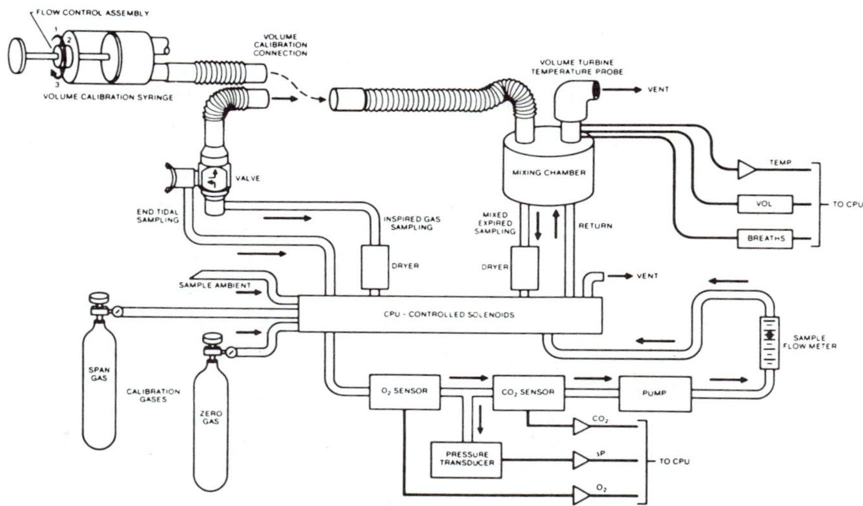

Figure 6.3. Reproduced from Jones NL: Evaluation of a microprocessor-controlled exercise testing system. *J Appl Physiol* 57: 1312-1318, 1984. With permission of the *Journal of Applied Physiology*. Schematic diagram of the Horizon Metabolic Measurement Cart.

the instrument is through a full typewriter keyboard that also has some special function keys. Temperature is measured at the mixing chamber while barometric pressure must be entered manually. A special gas calibration system ("micro-cal") performs frequent checks for oxygen sensor drift and recalibrates the cell if needed. The instrument has automatic gas calibration using tanks mounted on the rear of the instrument. Volume calibration is performed manually with a built-in calibration syringe (850 ml). The drying of the sampled gases is accomplished using a proprietary drying agent that, unlike calcium sulfate, does not selectively and differentially retain O_2 and CO_2. It is built for user servicing, with the gas plumbing system and circuit boards easily accessible. The software provides diagnostic messages. This instrument was one of the first to provide customized reports and to print graphics. It also can be interfaced with an external microcomputer and can accept analogue inputs from peripheral devices such as oximeters and cardiac (ECG) monitors. The accuracy and resolution of the analyzers and the volume measurement equipment are similar to those of the MMC I. In vitro validation studies have revealed an operating ability similar to that of the MMC I in both respirator and canopy modes. Results of in vivo validation of the canopy and respirator modes were similar to those of the

MMC I (C. Weissman, unpublished observations). The Horizon MMC has been used extensively in clinical studies (10,16).

Utah Metabolic Gas Monitor 2 (Utah Medical, Utah)

The MGM-2 is a small portable instrument designed for use in mechanically ventilated patients as well as those spontaneously breathing room air at rest (4). Expired gas is drawn into a 2.8 liter mixing chamber, expired volume is measured with an ultrasonic vortex-shedding transducer, an infrared sensor is used to measure CO_2 concentration, and oxygen concentration is measured with a zirconium oxide sensor (Figure 6.4). A built-in dedicated microprocessor system acquires all the data and performs the necessary calculations. Water vapor partial pressure is compensated for by passing all gas samples through a 5 ° C metal block (Peltier cooler); this removes or adds water as needed so that the water vapor content of inspired, expired and calibration gas are very similar (6 torr). The zirconium oxide sensor has a 120 msec response time and a resolution of 0.02% O_2 with an accuracy of 1% of the reading. The CO_2 sensor's accuracy is 1% of full scale and a response time of 100 msec. Calibration of the sensors is performed automatically by the microprocessor. A printer attached via a serial port allows for a permanent record. A pediatric version is available.

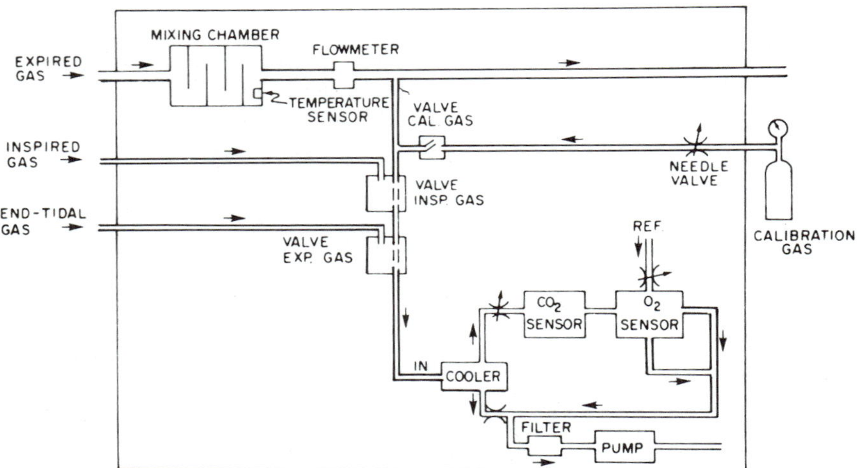

Figure 6.4. Reproduced from Westenkow DR, Cutler CA, Wallace WD: Instrumentation for monitoring gas exchange and metabolic rate in critically ill patients. *Crit Care Med* 12:183-187, 1984. With permission of *Critical Care Medicine.* Diagram of the MGM-2.

Engstrom Metabolic Computer (Gambro-Engstrom, Bromma, Sweden)

This instrument differs from those already described in that it is designed to specifically interface with an Engstrom ERICA ventilator, and thus can be used only with mechanically ventilated patients. The components of the system include an ERICA mechanical ventilator, an ELIZA infrared CO_2 analyzer, and an Engstrom Metabolic Computer (EMC). The EMC contains an oxygen fuel cell and a microprocessor. The latter acquires inspiratory volume data from the ELIZA. Inspiratory gas is sampled from a Venturi meter in the ERICA (absolute accuracy of ± 5%) and CO_2 data from the ELIZA. Inspiratory gas is sampled from a mixing chamber on the inspiratory limb and expired gas is sampled distal to the respirator's 3-liter bag expiratory measurement device. Both the inspiratory and expiratory gases are sampled through special plastic tubing (Aridus), which allows for equilibration of water vapor and gas temperature with ambient air. Specifications call for a relative humidity of within 1% and temperature within 0.5% of ambient air in both inspiratory and expiratory samples. The oxygen cell is calibrated using room air and the CO_2 analyzer using 5% CO_2. A printer attached to a digital output port provides for tabular data output. In vitro and in vivo validation studies have been performed (17,18). One study compared direct Fick measurements to those obtained with the EMC and found a mean difference of about 6.6% with a correlation coefficient of 0.91 (18). Another in vivo validation study using Douglas bags revealed differences of 4.3 ± 8.4% (SD), 2.4 ± 9.1% and -1.98 ±7.1% in VO_2, VCO_2 and RQ, respectively. In vitro validation studies (19) found VO_2 measurements to be within ± 6% of predicted values with excellent reproducibility (coefficient of variation = 2.7%).

Gould 9000 IV Computerized Pulmonary Function Cart (Gould Electronics, Inc., Dayton, Ohio)

The Gould 9000 IV is an automated system designed for performing measurements of oxygen consumption and carbon dioxide production in patients breathing room air. Its components include a paramagnetic O_2 analyzer, an infrared CO_2 analyzer, a dry rolling seal spirometer, and a 32k RAM computer with a CRT display. Expired gas is collected in the spirometer and samples from the spirometer flow through a tube containing Drierite and thence to the analyzers. The spirometer is emptied after collecting about 3 liters. The manufacturer's specifications for the oxygen analyzer are a resolution of 0.01% and accuracy of ± 0.1% over 0%-25% oxygen concentration; from 0%-100% O_2, resolution is 0.04% and accuracy ± 0.2%. The CO_2 analyzer has a resolution of

0.01% with an accuracy of ± 0.1% over a 0%-10% CO_2 range. The spirometer has specifications of tidal volumes of up to 10 liters and determination of expired minute ventilation is accurate to ± 0.025 liters (20). Volume is calibrated using a 3-liter syringe. Gas temperature is measured by the instrument while barometric pressure must be entered. The expired and inspired gas concentrations are measured alternately, each for 30 seconds (20). The instrument has been modified for use with mechanical ventilators and a validation study performed (20). This study revealed that when the analyzers were calibrated with room air and 5% CO_2, 49.56% O_2 and 79.87% O_2, there was an increasing error in VO_2 as FIO_2 increased. Errors in measured VO_2 were 2.6%, 3.5%, 5.9%, and 16.9% at FIO_2 values of 0.22, 0.40, 0.60, and 0.80, respectively. VCO_2 accuracy was ± 2.6%.

Gould 2900 Metabolic Measurement Cart

This instrument is designed for use during exercise and in mechanically ventilated patients. It can also be used in the canopy mode using a built-in blower. The unit is a self-contained cart that includes a paramagnetic oxygen analyzer, an infrared CO_2 analyzer, a mixing chamber and a hot-wire anemometer for volume measurements. A built-in microprocessor system acquires the data and transmits it to a commercially available microcomputer (Epson or IBM-AT) for final processing. The instrument features automated gas calibration and manual volume calibration. Graphic capabilities are available both on the microprocessor and unit printout.

Waters MRM-6000 Metabolic Analyzer (Waters Instruments, Inc. Rochester, MN)

This self-contained, rather large instrument is a closed circuit spirometer system. It can be used with mechanically ventilated patients as well as spontaneously breathing ones. The instrument contains a bellows that is filled with 100% oxygen, a volume measurement device (a dry rolling type respirometer), and an infrared CO_2 analyzer. Specifications of the volume device include a range of 2-40 liters min^{-1}, a resolution of 3.3 ml, and an accuracy of 2% of the reading. The CO_2 analyzer has a resolution of 0.004% CO_2 with an accuracy of 1.5% of the reading. Oxygen consumption is measured by quantitating the rate of disappearance of 100% O_2 from the bellows. CO_2 production is calculated from the measurement of volume and the expired CO_2 concentration. Measurement in mechanically ventilated patients involves attaching the mechanical ventilator tubing directly to the MRM-6000. The ventilator thus drives the bellows of the MRM-6000 and the patient therefore is ventilated with 100% oxygen. There is a built-in PEEP valve in the circuit of the MRM-6000. A microprocessor assists in calibration, data acquisition, and calculations.

Datex Deltatrac (Datex Instrument Corp., Helsinki, Finland)

The Deltatrac is a small, compact instrument designed for use in mechanically ventilated and spontaneously breathing patients. It can also be used in the canopy mode. Measurements are performed with the aid of a fast differential paramagnetic O_2 analyzer, an infrared CO_2 sensor, a mixing chamber, and a built-in microprocessor. The specifications for the oxygen analyzer include a variation of the differential gain as a function of reference gas concentration of less than $\pm$ 1%. The instrument contains a flow generator that provides a stable output of 40-45 liters min^{-1}. In the canopy mode this flow is drawn through the canopy and into the instrument, where it is sampled for O_2 and CO_2 concentration. With mechanical ventilators and spontaneously breathing patients, the flow generator is used as part of a unique gas dilution system to determine expired volume. The latter is determined by measuring expired CO_2 concentration prior to and following dilution with a precisely controlled airflow. The instrument allows for real time graphics of VO_2, VCO_2, and V_E on an integral video screen. Hard copies can be obtained from an attached printer.

Other instruments, designed specifically for exercise studies but that can also be used for resting studies in spontaneously breathing patients, include the Med Graphics, the Morgan Magna Metabolic Cart (PK Morgan Ltd., Kent UK), and the EOS Sprint (E. Jaeger, Rockford IL).

Undoubtedly, further advances in ventilator design, volume measurement equipment, and gas analyzers will facilitate metabolic measurements in the near future.

REFERENCES

1. Norton AC: Accuracy in pulmonary measurement. *Resp Care* 24:131-137, 1979.
2. Rubin SA: *The Principles of Biomedical Instrumentation*. Chicago, Yearbook Medical Publishers, 1987, pp 50–64.
3. Weissman C, Damask MC, Askanazi J et al.: Evaluation of a noninvasive method for the measurement of metabolic rate in humans. *Clin Sci* 69:135-141, 1985.
4. Westenkow DR, Curler CA, Wallace WD: Instrumentation for monitoring gas exchange and metabolic rate in critically ill patients. *Crit Care Med* 12:183-187, 1984.
5. Browning JA, Lindberg SE, Turney SZ, Chodoff P: The effects of a fluctuating FIO_2 on metabolic measurements in mechanically ventilated patients. *Crit Care Med* 10: 82-85, 1982.
6. Weissman C, Askanazi J, Milic-Emili J et al.: Effect of respiratory apparatus on respiration. *J Appl Physiol* 57:475-480, 1984.

7. Spencer JL, Zikria BA, Kinney JM et al.: A system for continuous measurement of gas exchange and respiratory functions. *J Appl Physiol* 33:523-528, 1971.
8. Jones NL: Evaluation of a microprocessor-controlled exercise testing system. *J Appl Physiol* 57:1312-1318, 1984.
9. Wilmore JH, Davis JA, Norton AC: An automated system for assessing metabolic and respiratory function during exercise. *J Appl Physiol* 40:619-624, 1976.
10. Weissman C, Kemper M, Damask MC et al.: The effect of routine intensive care interactions on metabolic rate. *Chest* 86: 815-818, 1984.
11. Weissman C: Measuring oxygen uptake in the clinical setting. In Bryan-Brown CW, Ayres SM (eds), *New Horizons: Oxygen Transport and Utilization.* Fullerton, Society of Critical Care Medicine, 1987, pp 25–64.
12. Damask MC, Weissman C, Askanazi J et al.: A systematic method for validation of gas exchange measurement. *Anesthesiology* 57:213-218, 1982.
13. Rodriguez JL, Weissman C, Damask MC et al.: Physiologic requirements of rewarming: Suppression of the shivering response. *Crit Care Med* 11: 490-497, 1983.
14. Hunker FD, Burton CW, Hunker EM et al.: Metabolic and nutritional evaluation of patients supported with mechanical ventilation. *Crit Care Med* 8: 628-632, 1980.
15. White RH, Frayn KN, Little RA et al.: Hormonal and metabolic responses to glucose infusion in sepsis studied by the hyperglycemia glucose clamp technique. *JPEN* 11:345-353, 1987.
16. Robertson CS, Lifton GL, Grossman RG: Oxygen utilization and cardiovascular function in head injured patients. *Neurosurgery* 15:307-314, 1984.
17. Bredbacka S, Kawachi S, Norlander O, Kirk B: Gas exchange during ventilator treatment: A validation of a computerized technique and its comparison with the Douglas bag method. *Acta Anaesthesiol Scand* 28:462-468, 1987.
18. Behrendt W, Weiland CHR, Kalff J, Giani G: Continuous measurement of oxygen uptake. *Acta Anaesthesiol Scand* 31:10-14, 1987.
19. Quinn T, Weissman C, Kemper MC: Continuous trending of Fick variables in ICU patients: A role for VO_2. Anesthesiology. In press, 1988.
20. Eccles RC, Swinamer DL, Jones RI, King EG: Validation of a compact system for measuring gas exchange. *Crit Care Med* 64:807-811, 1986.

CHAPTER

7

Guidelines for Parenteral and Enteral Nutrition

Why ? Evidence of the Necessity for Nutritional Support
  Nutrition and Morbidity and Mortality
  Interaction of Nutrition and the Respiratory System
How Much ?
  Measurement or Estimation of Energy Expenditure
  Criteria for Nutritional Recommendations for Artificial Nutrition
What ?
  Carbohydrate and Fat
  Parenteral Preparations
  Enteral Preparations
When ?
  Preoperative Artificial Nutrition
  Artificial Nutrition for Postoperative, Injured, Septic, and Burned Patients
How ?
  Enteral Nutrition
  Parenteral Nutrition
How Long?
  Preoperative Patients
  Postoperative, Injured, Burned, and Critically Ill Patients.

In this chapter we would like to answer the following practical questions: Why? How much? What? When? How? and How long?

Why ? Is there real and objective evidence that nutrition is an indispensable part of patient management?

How much ? When energy expenditure is known and protein breakdown is evaluated, what is the optimal relationship between measured or estimated caloric loss and caloric supply, between nitrogen loss and nitrogen supply, and between nitrogen and caloric intake?

What ? When the assumed right decision about quantities to be supplied is made, which type of calories (carbohydrate or fat) and of proteins, and in which proportions, should be given to various types of patients?

When ? Should nutritional support start before, during, or immediately after an elective surgical procedure? In severely injured patients when should it be initiated?

How ? Which is the best route for supplying artificial nutrition? Peripheral veins, central veins? Or is the enteral route, when possible, the best way?

How long ? What are the criteria that will allow a correct decision to discontinue artificial nutritional support?

WHY? EVIDENCE OF THE NECESSITY FOR NUTRITIONAL SUPPORT

To be fed is an absolute human right, that should be extended to hospitalized patients and to all human beings who for one reason or another, have difficulties in consummating this physiological obligation. It seems only a matter of common sense, as recently pointed out by Seltzer, that nutrients have to be supplied to everybody "virtually always" (1). The need for us to pose this question, Why does nutritional support have to be provided to sick people? arises from historical reasons and relatively recent history at that. Thirty years ago a person who could not eat was doomed to die of starvation, since it was only in the 1960's that it became technically possible to provide adequate nutrition by vein. However, by then physicians were used to not feeding patients adequately, and long-standing traditions in medicine as in other fields are very hard to change. Since Seltzer's statement is not generally accepted in medical practice, we shall present some general considerations, hoping to convince the reader that an adequate energy and protein supply is necessary under all circumstances.

Nutrition and Morbidity and Mortality

Even before the era of nutritional support a few publications pointed out the relation between nutritional status and postoperative complications. In 1936, an increased rate of complications was shown after gastric surgery in patients who lost more than 20% of their body weight (2). In 1944, a relation between reduced protein levels and infection rate was demonstrated (3), and more recently a clinical study claimed that patients with preoperative serum albumin levels below 2.5 g per dl before surgery had four times as many complications and a mortality rate six times higher than patients with serum albumin levels above 2.5 g (4,5). This relation between low albumin levels and increased mortality rate has been shown or disputed by others, some claiming for instance, that total serum protein level is a better predictor of postoperative sepsis than serum albumin in cancer patients (6,7). One of the striking effects of the introduction of adequate parenteral nutrition has been the reduction in mortality of patients with multiple abdominal fistulas. Prior to the 1960's, mortality rates were in the range of 80% to 90%. With appropriate use of artificial nutrition this has dropped to approximately 10%-20%. Some of the improvement may be due to other factors, but most of it must come from improved nutrition.

Body Weight and Serum Albumin as Nutritional Markers

Most of the examples cited above used loss of body weight and serum albumin concentration as nutritional markers. Both are very useful for this purpose but must be interpreted carefully. Loss of body weight from the subject's own normal weight is the best single indicator of protein energy malnutrition. Comparison to tables of ideal weight is not very useful since there is an enormous variation of normal weights. In addition, changes in weight reflect not only nutritional effects on body cell mass and fat, but also changes in retention of sodium and extracellular water due to both nutritional and non-nutritional effects. There is an important nutritional component to the level of serum albumin concentration, but the direct effects of nutrition, acting through changes in rates of protein synthesis and degradation, act very slowly, over weeks to months. Short-term changes in serum albumin concentration primarily reflect changes in its distribution between blood and extravascular, extracellular water.

These relationships are illustrated by a study of Starker et al. in two groups of undernourished surgical patients who received TPN during two weeks prior to major abdominal surgery (8).

Group 1 : 16 patients had a mean decrease in body weight from 127.9 to 124.6 lbs with, at the same time, an increase of serum albumin concentration from 3.21 to 3.46 g dl^{-1}. In this group only one patient showed a postoperative complication.

Group 2 : 16 patients had a mean increase of body weight from 119.3 to 121.3 lbs, and a decrease in serum albumin concentration from 3.14 to 3.00 g dl^{-1}. In this group eight patients presented a total of fifteen postoperative complications.

Nitrogen balance was positive and about the same in both groups. This clinical study shows that body weight and albumin level may provide, during preoperative nutritional support, an important indication of postoperative complications. But in this case, loss of body weight was a good sign representing loss of extracellular fluid, and the increase in albumin concentrations also resulted from loss of extracellular fluid, and not from increased rates of protein synthesis. Nitrogen balance was a poor prognostic sign since it was the same in both groups. Our knowledge today allows us to make the following statements: (*a*) Serum albumin and total protein concentration are related to nutritional status. A number of visceral proteins, such as retinol binding protein and transferrin, turn over very rapidly, and give quicker indications of changes in rates of visceral protein synthesis than can be obtained with albumin (9,10). (*b*) In depleted patients a redistribution of body fluids increases the proportion of extracellular fluid, decreasing serum albumin level, without necessarily reducing the total pool of albumin. This is augmented by the presence of acute sepsis, severe trauma, severe burns, and in all situations where high amounts of crystalloids or colloids are administered for volume load or for fluid challenge (11). In these situations the low albumin level is a consequence of an expanded extracellular space that may result in local edema in the wound area, delayed healing, if not provoking wound dehiscence or suture leaks, local infection, and low pressure pulmonary edema (12). This type of edema is not easy to reduce and should not be treated obsessively with diuretics since it will usually last as long as severe infection, trauma, or burns persist. The overuse of diuretics to reduce this type of edema will mainly reduce intravascular space, endangering the patient and often inducing hemodynamic instability, that will require vasoactive drugs, and acute renal failure, which will often necessitate hemodialysis. (*c*) Albumin and other serum proteins are correlated with postoperative complications, morbidity, and mortality.

Preoperative Nutrition and Postoperative Complications

There is evidence that when nutrition is supplied preoperatively in depleted patients there is an impressive improvement in postoperative outcome, which correlates closely with serum levels of albumin and of other indicators. The morbidity described in these patients is mainly related to infectious complications, as delayed wound healing, respiratory failure, or generalized sepsis, and these complications can be avoided, or at least substantially reduced, when nutritional support is supplied for enough time. Administration of TPN for three days preoperatively was shown to be of little benefit (13), whereas when supplied for more than one week there was a marked reduction in complication rate (14).

In order to objectively evaluate the importance of preoperative nutritional status, a Prognostic Nutritional Index was developed by Buzby et al. (14,15), based on serum proteins, anthropomorphic measurements, and immunological parameters, and proven to be a reliable predictor for post-operative complications after major abdominal surgery. In this index,

$$PNI = 158 - 16.6(ALB) - 0.78(TSF) - 0.20(TFN) - 5.8(DH) \qquad (1)$$

where

ALB = albumin (g dl^{-1})
TSF = triceps skin fold (mm)
TFN = serum transferrin (mg dl^{-1})
DH = delayed cutaneous hypersensitivity to mumps, streptokinase, streptodornase, and candida (graded as: 0 = non reactive, 1 = 2 mm induration, and 2 = 5 mm induration)

The important contribution of this PNI was that the authors could demonstrate that, in patients considered according to this index as high risk (PNI 50), preoperative nutrition resulted in a 2.5-fold reduction in complications, a 7-fold reduction in infection rates and a 5-fold reduction in mortality (14). Similar impressive results have been reported by others (16,17).

Postoperative Nutrition and Morbidity

Postoperative nutrition has been shown to be effective after very severe operations (18). Patients after radical cystectomy were given total parenteral nutrition or 5% dextrose for one week. Mean hospital stay was 24 days for those receiving only dextrose, but only 17 days for those on TPN, a saving of one week. With less severe operations, such as colectomy, no such differences have been observed.

Interaction of Nutrition and the Respiratory System

Specific effects of malnutrition on respiratory muscles were described as early as 1916. In a large study of necropsies, a linear relation was found between body weight loss and diaphragm weight loss; for a mean body weight loss of 23% there was a 22% mean loss of diaphragm weight (19). In a more recent study, for a body weight loss of 32%, the corresponding loss of diaphragm was 43% (20). This respiratory muscle weight loss in malnourished patients was associated with loss of respiratory muscle strength to 37%, vital capacity to 63%, and maximum voluntary ventilation to 41% of normal values (21). In the Minnesota starvation study of Keys et al. (22), the subjects lost 24% of their body weight in 24 weeks and showed a simultaneous progressive decline in vital capacity, which fell to an average of 390 ml. The vital capacity returned to its normal values after twelve weeks of refeeding. Similar relations between lost body weight and respiratory function have been observed in patients with anorexia nervosa (23). In patients with chronic obstructive pulmonary disease (COPD) there is often a progressive loss of weight that can be related to an increase in REE (24,25), or to a reduced caloric intake related to increased effort required for eating and swallowing (26). This body weight loss in COPD patients is associated with an increase in mortality rate (27,28). Providing such patients with adequate artificial nutrition, either enteral or parenteral, for several weeks can reverse this weight loss and improve pulmonary function (28). It remains to be shown whether longer term nutrition can improve mortality.

Mechanically ventilated patients, particularly those with weakened respiratory muscles, will benefit from nutritional support through improvement of muscle function, which will facilitate the weaning procedure (29). However, improvement of respiratory muscle mass and strength is a slow process requiring one to several weeks to obtain significant results (28,30). It should be kept in mind, as discussed in Chapter 4, that administration of large amounts of carbohydrate stimulates ventilation by increasing CO_2 production, to a point that may lead to respiratory distress in critically ill patients (31-33). Substitution of a part of the carbohydrate intake by fat decreases ventilatory demand by reducing CO_2 production, as represented in Figure 7.1 (32).

HOW MUCH?

There is no question, as discussed above, that providing adequate nutrition by parenteral or enteral means greatly improves morbidity and in many instances is essential for patient survival. A much more difficult question to answer is what is the optimal amount to give.

Giving adequate amounts of artificial nutrition, whether called total parenteral nutrition or hyperalimentation, whether given enterally or parenterally, is lifesaving compared to its historical alternative, 100-150 g day^{-1} of glucose, as a 5% dextrose solution; although even 5%

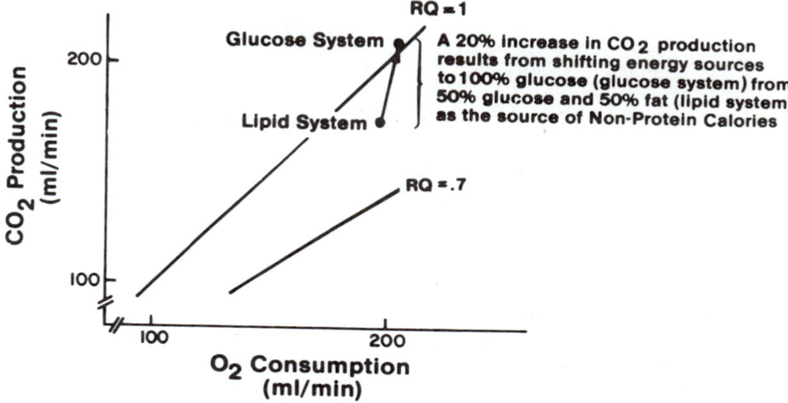

Figure 7.1. Data adapted from Askanazi et al. (32). Reduction of CO_2 production in substituting a part of the carbohydrate intake (glucose system) by fat intake (lipid system).

dextrose, as pointed out by Gamble (34), is a very potent sparer of nitrogen, reducing protein losses by one-half in normal subjects (Fig 7.2), and undoubtedly reducing morbidity as compared to no nutrient intake at all.

In 1969, Dudrick and colleagues published the first impressive results of hyperalimentation supplied to 300 adults receiving between 2400 and 5000 kcal (10,042 and 20,920 kJ) day^{-1} in preoperative, intraoperative and postoperative management of a large variety of diseases (35). In this study, amino acids were infused together with glucose as caloric source. Very good results were obtained, as evaluated by increased body weight, positive nitrogen balance, and clinical results. In 12 newborn infants, growth and normal development were also obtained. Obviously, for Dudrick and his group, evaluating energy expenditure was not a major preoccupation in this study. As with many pioneering advances in the science of nutrition, impressive improvements were obtained in severely ill patients by giving nutrition on largely empirical grounds, nor has it ever been proven harmful to the patients who were treated according to Dudrick's method; on the con-

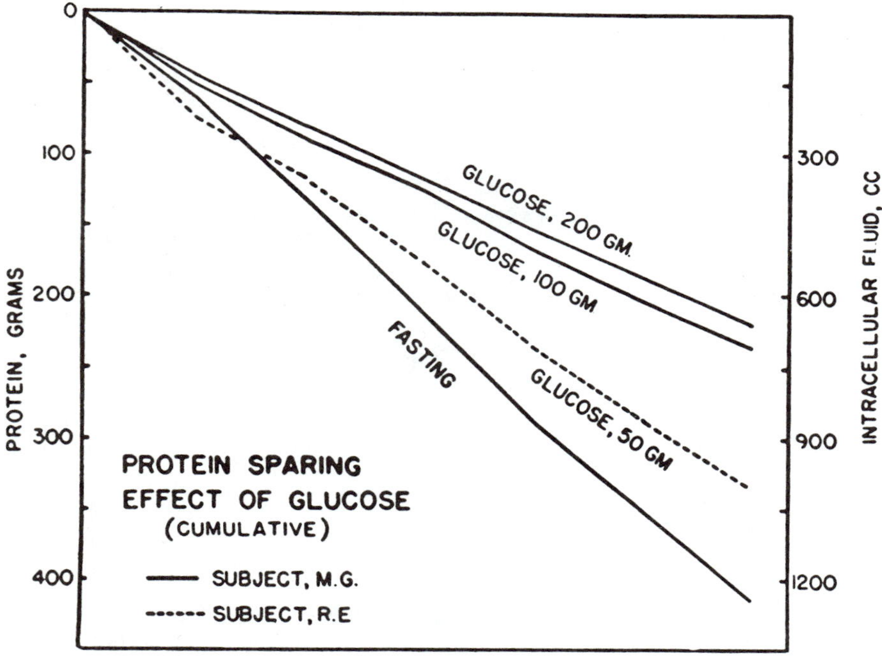

Figure 7.2. From Gamble JL: Physiological information gained from studies on the life raft ration. *Harv Lect* 42:247-273, 1946. With permission of the Harvey Lectures. Influence of glucose intake on nitrogen excretion in healthy young men.

trary, the difference with non-nutritionally supported patients was so huge that this new approach of treating undernourished, or even normally nourished patients unable to be fed orally, represented a genuine revolution in management of severely injured patients and rapidly became part of the management of many pathological states.

Since the pioneering work of Dudrick and the introduction of safe fat emulsions in 1962 by Wretlind (36), all of the macronutrients, fat, carbohydrate, and protein, have been available for parenteral nutrition. With this availability of nutrients and their increasingly widespread use, has come much discussion and many recommendations as to appropriate or optimal amounts of protein and nonprotein energy to give to various kinds of patients.

One such study performed retrospectively by Rutten et al (37) classified the patients according to their degree of catabolism. Urinary urea N was measured in patients receiving no nitrogen intake for 3 days, but at least 100 g carbohydrate day^{-1} (Table 7.1). The recommended amounts of calories to be delivered in order to reach a positive nitrogen balance varied between 1.75 and 2.0 times the resting energy expenditure, calculated by the Harris Benedict formulas, with a calorie-to-nitrogen ratio of 150-200:1. Intake of less than 1.5 x REE was generally not associated with a positive nitrogen balance. Finally, this study attests to the importance of a low calorie-to-nitrogen ratio. With a ratio of 476:1, increasing the caloric intake to 2.7 x REE was still associated with negative nitrogen balance. According to Wilmore, even severely catabolic patients may further improve their nitrogen balance when calories are given in excess of 2.0 x REE with an appropriate calorie-to-nitrogen ratio (38).

Table 7.1.
Recommended intake and presumed increase in energy expenditure based on degree of catabolism as indicated by urea N excretion on a N-free diet.[a]

Degree of Catabolism	Urea Nitrogen Excretion (g day^{-1})	Presumed Increase in REE (%)	Recommended Intake (% REE)
Normal	<5	0	100
Mild	5–10	0–20	120
Moderate	10–15	20–50	165
Severe	>15	>50	180

[a]Adapted from Rutten et al. (37).

These and other publications have proposed a variety of rules or formulas for prescribing nutrition. These include recommended energy intakes of 1.75 times REE, 40 to 60 kcal (167 to 251 kJ) kg^{-1} day^{-1}. Some recommendations are much higher, even up to 8000 kcal (33,500 kJ) day^{-1} for severe burns (39). Others have recommended lower rates, ranging from 1.0 to1.5 times REE (40). Gazzaniga et al. (41) pointed out the importance of measuring REE by indirect calorimetry and basing nutrition on measured values rather than on the various kinds of formulas given above.

Measurement or Estimation of Energy Expenditure

There are two aspects of assessing nutrient requirements. The first is measuring or estimating energy expenditure, which we will consider in the present section. The second is how much to give, once energy expenditure is known. This will be discussed in the following section.

The Harris-Benedict equation or other formulas for estimating energy expenditure (42-45) predict normal values within ± 10 % (Chapter

1). However, injury, sepsis, burns, and malnutrition change the normal values. Kinney and coworkers (46) estimated the magnitude of variations in resting energy expenditure in different pathological situations as represented in Figure 7.3, and these values are widely used as stress correction factors to be added to estimated energy expenditure as calculated from one of the above methods. From Figure 7.3 it can be seen that energy expenditure can be reduced by 30% or even 40% of normal values in starvation, that it is little affected by elective surgery, but that it can increase by up to 30% in severe trauma with multiple fractures, and up to 60% with sepsis. Severe burns can cause more than a doubling of energy expenditure. Anxiety, pain, the patient's temperature, and ambient temperature are other important factors able to increase energy needs. With all these influences, energy expenditure can vary greatly during the course of treatment in acute or chronic diseases, as shown in Figure 7.4 taken from Long et al. (47). Evaluation, based on estimation of resting energy expenditure and corrected according to the type of disease, may, for any single patient, be in error by 20% to 100% each time. This great variability in energy expenditure was demonstrated in ICU patients by Weissman et al. (48). Although the average value of measured energy expenditure was only 5% above that predicted, the individual values ranged from −30% to + 50%.

Some of the problems involved in estimating energy expenditure are illustrated in an analysis of 52 ICU patients taken from data of Singer et al. (49). One measurement of resting energy expenditure was made for each patient, three of whom were brain dead. Of the others, 17 were measured while receiving only 5% dextrose; the other 32 were measured when given adequate nutrition, either enterally or parenterally (Table 7.2). Predicted values were calculated by the Harris-Benedict equation (equations 5 and 6 in Chapter 2). The patients were very ill, with an average simplified APACHE score (50) of 15.5. In the brain-dead patients there was a nearly 50% reduction in REE from predicted values. This was probably partly due to decreased brain metabolism, but mainly due to hypothermia. For patients receiving 5% dextrose, measured REE averaged 14% above predicted, while for those receiving adequate diets it was 23% above. This difference of 2 kcal (8 kJ) kg^{-1} or 155 kcal (649 kJ) per subject is due to diet-induced thermogenesis. Therefore, when measurements made during 5% dextrose administration are used to predict energy requirements when adequate nutrition will be supplied, about 2 kcal (8 kJ) kg^{-1} or 150 kcal (630 kJ) should be added to cover the thermic effects of nutrients.

Although these patients were severely ill as reflected by their APACHE scores, averaging 15.5, the mean value of REE when they were

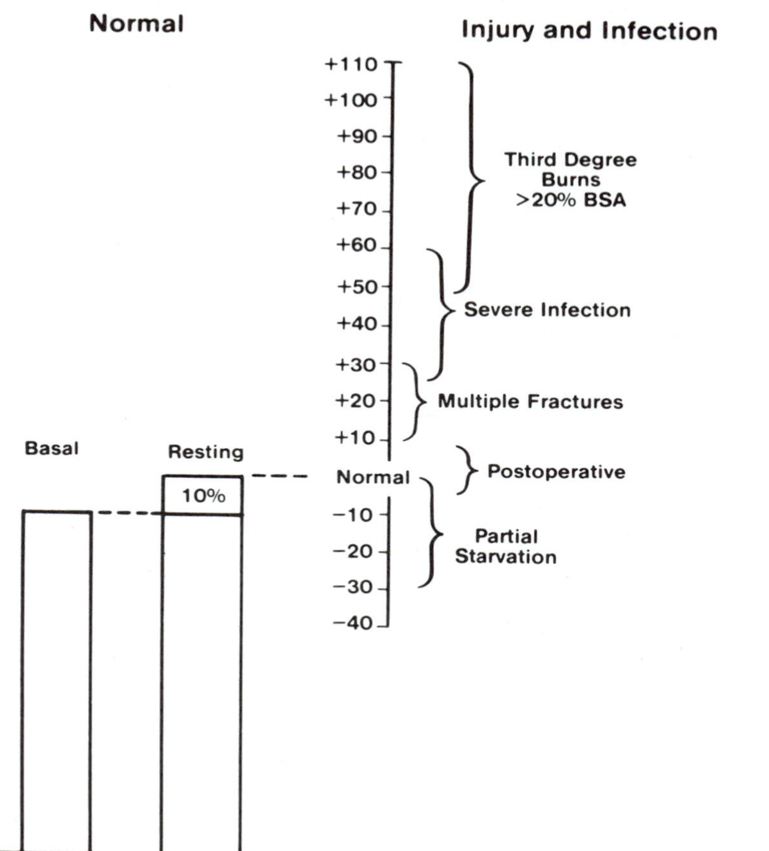

Figure 7.3. Based on data of Kinney et al. (46). Reproduced from Elwyn DH: Nutritional requirements of surgical patients. *Crit Care Med* 8:9-20, 1980. With permission of *Critical Care Medicine*. The effects of injury, sepsis, and nutritional depletion on resting energy expenditure.

adequately nourished was only 340 kcal (1423 kJ) day^{-1} or 4.8 kcal (20 kJ) kg^{-1}day^{-1} above predicted values. There are several ways that we can add to the predicted values in order for the mean predicted value to be equal to the mean measured value. One way is to calculate the predicted value for each individual patient and add the mean difference, from Table 7.2, as either 340 kcal (1423 kJ) or 4.8 (20 kJ) kcal kg^{-1}. A more esthetically satisfying procedure is to calculate the expected change due to in-

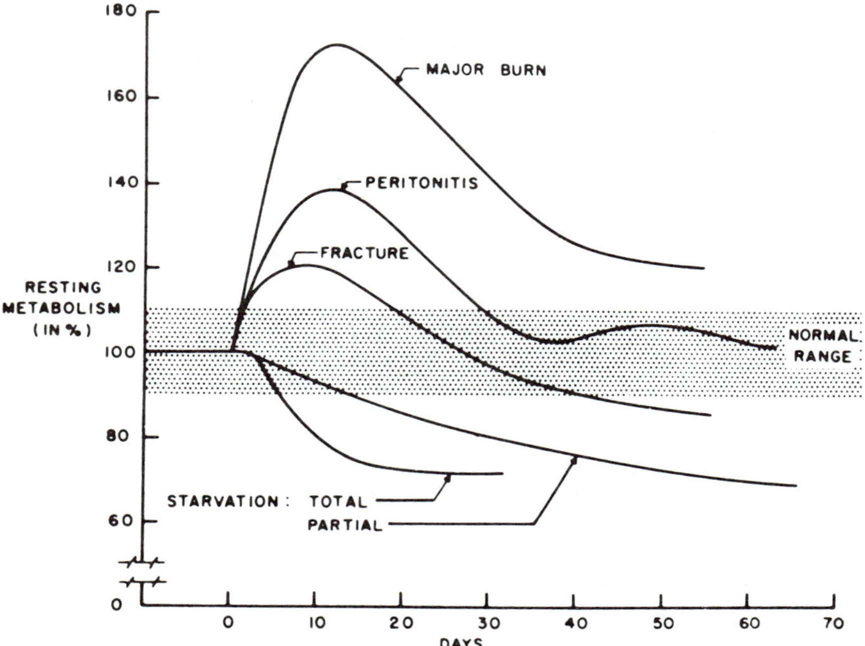

Figure 7.4. Reproduced from Long CL: *Am J Clin Nutr* 30:1301-1310, 1977. With permission of the *American Journal of Clinical Nutrition.* Changes of resting energy expenditure in different pathological states over 60 days.

jury, sepsis, or starvation and add it to each individual Harris-Benedict prediction. This was done in this study by taking the most extreme value for each condition from Kinney's data, shown in Figure 7.3, adding them if there were more than one, and then dividing by 2. Thus if a patient was accidentally injured, septic, and malnourished, the percentage increase was taken to be (30+60-30)/2, or 30%. How good the different methods are can be judged by how accurately they predict each individual patient's REE, since each method gives the same mean REE as the measured value. The average errors in prediction as percentage above or below each measured value are shown in Table 7.3. All the methods used give about the same error, 16% to 19%. There is no advantage in calculating a stress score for each patient, as in procedure 1. There is no advantage in calculating per kg instead of per subject. There is not even any advantage in calculating a predicted value for each patient, since assuming an average value of 1839 kcal (7694 kJ) day^{-1} for all subjects is as good as any other procedure, and much simpler.

What the data in Table 7.3 do show is that measuring energy expen-

Table 7.2.
Comparison of measured values of resting energy expenditure (single measurement) to values predicted by the Harris-Benedict equation in 52 critically ill patients. Mean ± SEM.[a]

	Patients		
	Brain Dead (N=3)	Dextrose 5% (N=17)	Adequate Nutrition (N=32)
$\frac{\text{kcal}}{\text{kJ}}$ subject^{-1} day^{-1}			
Energy intake	750±650 3138±2720	429±131 1795±548	1945±568 8138±2377
REE measured	955±92 3996±3856	1647±421 891±176	839±468 7694±1958
REE predicted	1650±247 6904±1033	1462±247 6117±1033	1504±242 6293±1013
Measured minus predicted	-695±154 -2908±644	185±393 774±1644	340±423 1423±1770
$\frac{\text{kcal}}{\text{kJ}}$ kg^{-1} day^{-1}			
Energy intake	9.3±7.2 38.9±30.1	6.1±2.6 25.5±10.9	27.4±9.3 114.6±38.9
REE measured	12.3±1.0 51.5±4.2	22.8±7.0 95.4±29.3	25.5±6.8 106.7±28.5
REE predicted	21.1±1.0 88.3±4.2	19.9±2.7 83.3±11.3	20.7±3.2 86.6±13.4
Measured minus predicted	-8.8±0.8 -36.8±3.3	2.8±6.6 11.7±27.6	4.8±5.9 20.0±24.7

[a]Data of Singer et al. (49).

diture by indirect calorimetry is much more accurate than estimating it. As discussed in Chapter 5, twenty four-hour energy expenditure can be easily measured to better than 5% in each patient, whereas by any method of estimation (Table 7.3), one-half of the values will differ from the actual value by more than 18%, either above or below. We can avoid giving too little to most patients by raising the average intake to 2300 kcal (9623 kJ) day^{-1} (corresponding to 1.5 times Harris-Benedict or 31.3 kcal [131 kJ] kg^{-1} day^{-1}). At this intake only two patients of this group, with REEs of 3100 and 3250 kcal (12,970 and 13,598 kJ), would be seriously underfed. Meanwhile, 5 patients with REEs of about 1200 kcal (5021 kJ) or less would be grossly overfed.

We may conclude that: (*a*) measuring energy expenditure is much

Table 7.3.
Mean error, regardless of sign, in predicting REE by different methods of adding a stress factor to values calculated by Harris-Benedict equations.[a]

Procedure	Average Error of Measured Value (%)
1. Adding an individual estimate for stress to each individual prediction	18
2. Adding 340 kcal day^{-1} to each individual prediction	19
3. Adding 4.8 kcal kg^{-1} day^{-1} to each individual prediction	16
4. Assuming a value of 1,839 kcal day^{-1} for all patients	18
5. Assuming a value of 25.5 kcal kg^{-1} day^{-1} for all patients	19

[a]Data for 32 severely ill patients given adequate nutrition.

more satisfactory than estimating it, and is probably worth the expense of maintaining an indirect calorimeter in any ICU; (*b*) that energy expenditure in the very hypermetabolic patient, who may be at severe risk, will always be underestimated if it is not measured; and (*c*) that if REE is not measured, using an average value for energy intake for all patients is just as good as, and very much simpler than, predicting each individual REE by the Harris-Benedict or other formulas.

Criteria for Nutritional Recommendations for Artificial Nutrition

It would be nice to base recommendations for enteral and parenteral nutrition on prospective studies of well-defined groups of injured, septic, or malnourished patients, in whom morbidity and mortality are correlated with the amounts of protein and energy supplied. However except for a few studies of gross differences, such as the difference between 5% dextrose and TPN, or very fine differences, such as variations in the amounts of the branched chain amino acids, such studies are completely lacking. We must look elsewhere for criteria to help us make recommendations, even though such criteria are less satisfactory than morbidity and mortality data, were they available.

The major sources of criteria are: general nutritional principles, for instance, the widely held opinion that adequate nutrition should be supplied on a daily basis; and studies of the physiological and pathological effects of nutrients, particularly as they apply to injured, septic, or malnourished patients. These topics have been discussed in detail in previous chapters. In this section we will review these concepts only briefly, and only to the extent that they are necessary to the arguments at hand. For further detail, the reader is referred back to Chapters 2,3, and 4.

Given time and facilities it is possible to tailor the amounts of each nutrient to the individual needs of each patient. For instance, the scheme in Figure 3.9 can be used to provide appropriate amounts of energy and nitrogen to restore BCM and fat in malnourished patients in any desired ratio, from zero to infinity. However, it would only be effective if careful monitoring of N and energy balances were also performed. Obviously, this approach is not feasible in the clinical ward or ICU. Therefore, in the following paragraphs we will attempt to derive a few relatively simple rules for the amounts of nutrients to be given enterally or parenterally. Because it makes a difference whether or not energy expenditure has been measured, these rules will be given in two ways: (*a*) when REE has been measured, the amounts of nutrients will be directly related to REE; and (*b* when REE has not been measured, the amounts will be presented as a daily amount per subject or per kg, since, as presented above, calculating predicted values or deriving a stress factor for each individual patient adds little or nothing to the accuracy of the estimated requirement.

As discussed in Chapters 3 and 4, malnourished patients and injured or septic patients respond differently to nutrients, both from each other and from normal subjects. For this reason we will consider the two types of patients separately.

Recommended Amounts of Energy and Protein for Injured and Septic Patients

Injured or septic patients are resistant to nutrients, particularly protein and carbohydrate. Studies of Larssen et al. (Chapter 3) indicate that at least 200 mg N kg^{-1} are required for maximum protein sparing, but that above this N intake has little further effect (Figure 3.10). Since this is only one experiment, we will err on the side of overfeeding and pick 270 mg N kg^{-1} day^{-1} as an appropriate amount for severely injured patients.

In contrast to N intake, increasing energy intake at any level will improve N balance, and even the most severely traumatized patients can probably reach zero N balance if given 2 to 3 times their energy expenditure. However, N balance is not the only criteria for determining energy intake. Fat deposition, with energy intakes of 2 to 3 times expenditure, becomes enormous. The thermic effects of both protein and carbohydrate are of the order of 30% or more when given in excess, so that these enormous amounts of nutrients can raise energy expenditure by 50% or more. Carbohydrate given in excess increases sympathetic activity; causes lipogenesis, fatty liver, and liver dysfunction; and increases ventilation and the work of breathing. Lipid given enterally in large amounts, can increase the metabolic response to burns and reduce host defense (Chapter

4). For these reasons it seems desirable not to give too much energy. The problem is, how to pick an appropriate amount.

In the study of Larssen et al., cited above, daily energy intake was 45-50 kcal (188-209 kJ) kg^{-1}, about 50% above the presumed energy expenditures, and N balance, at N intakes above 200 mg kg^{-1}, was -3.5 g day^{-1}. Losses of this magnitude are tolerable for a few days to weeks in previously well-nourished, stressed patients who will shift to an anabolic phase in time. In a different study, of severely injured multiple trauma patients, Francois et al. (51) provided 200 mg N and 25.5 kcal (106.7 kJ) kg^{-1} day^{-1}, either enterally or parenterally. This level of energy intake was probably 10% to 20% below energy expenditure. These patients were in daily negative N balance of -10 g in the first week, -11 g in the second, -7 g in the third, and -5 g in the fourth week. The total N loss was 231 g in four weeks, corresponding to 7 kg or nearly 20 % of body cell mass. Such losses represent severe morbidity, and it seems worthwhile to increase energy intake above this level. If we arbitrarily choose an energy intake of 1.33 times REE, we will be much closer to the acceptable N balances of Larssen et al. than to the unacceptable ones of Francois et al.

Since energy expenditure averages approximately 30 kcal (126 kJ) kg^{-1} day^{-1} in injured or septic patients (52), slightly higher than the mean shown in Table 7.2 which includes both traumatized and malnourished patients, 1.33 times REE equals 40 kcal(167 kJ) kg^{-1} day^{-1} or 2800 kcal (11,715 kJ) day^{-1} in a 70 kg man. Since our proposed N intake is 270 mg kg^{-1} day^{-1}, or 18.7 g day^{-1}, the calorie-to-N ratio is 150:1.

The recommendations for septic or injured patients are:

1. If energy expenditure is measured, provide energy (carbohydrate, fat, and protein) at 1.33 times REE. The calorie-to-N ratio should be 150 kcal per g N, giving an N intake of 6.67 mg per kcal (1.59 mg per kJ).
2. If energy expenditure is not measured, provide 2800 kcal (11,715 kJ) day^{-1} or 40 kcal (167 kJ) kg^{-1} day^{-1}, with a calorie-to-N ratio of 150 kcal per g N, to give an N intake of 18.7 g day^{-1} or 270 mg kg^{-1} day^{-1}.

Recommended Amounts of Energy and Protein for Malnourished Patients

Malnourished patients tolerate nutrients better than stressed patients or normal subjects. Most important they can achieve positive N balance at zero energy balance (Figure 3.9). Most acutely malnourished patients have lost body cell mass in the ratio of 2 parts BCM to 1 of fat.

To restore tissue in this proportion requires that N intake be in the range of 300 to 350 mg kg^{-1} day^{-1}. Average REE for malnourished patients is about 26 kcal (109 kJ) kg^{-1} day^{-1} (52-54), or, since the weight of such patients averages close to 60 kg, about 1600 kcal (6694 kJ) day^{-1} per subject. In order to restore some fat, we should give energy at 25% above resting expenditure to bedridden patients, and at 50% above resting expenditure to ambulatory patients to allow for activity energy expenditure (54).

These considerations lead to the following recommendations for malnourished patients:

1. If energy expenditure is measured, provide energy at 1.25 times REE for bedridden patients, and at 1.5 times REE for ambulatory patients. The calorie-to-N ratio should be 100 kcal per g N, giving an N intake of 10 mg per kcal (2.4 mg per kJ).
2. If energy expenditure is not measured, provide 2000 kcal (8368 kJ) day^{-1} or 32.5 kcal (136 kJ) kg^{-1} day^{-1} to bedridden patients, and 2400 kcal (10,042 kJ) day^{-1} or 39 kcal (163 kJ) kg^{-1} day^{-1} to ambulatory patients. The calorie-to-N ratio should be 100 kcal per g N, providing 20 g N day^{-1} or 325 mg N kg^{-1} day^{-1} to bedridden patients, and 24 g N day^{-1} or 390 mg N kg^{-1} day^{-1} to ambulatory patients.

Patients who are both malnourished and septic or injured are more catabolic than the malnourished patients and respond better to nutrients than do the well-nourished stressed patients. They should be given energy at the rates recommended for the injured and septic patients but with a calorie-to-N ratio of 100, as used with the malnourished patients.

These recommendations should be used only as guidelines. Obviously, if there are contraindications, such as high blood urea levels or labored breathing, one should reduce the rates of administration of either energy or nitrogen, or both. Furthermore, as can be seen from the arguments by which we derived the recommendations, they are only crude estimates. While they seem reasonable to us on general physiological and nutritional grounds, they are arbitrary, and other arbitrary recommendations may seem equally reasonable to others. Much larger amounts of nutrients have been given by many therapists with great success. Until we have prospective trials of the effects of various amounts of nutrients on morbidity and mortality, uncertainty as to optimal amounts will persist. What is less uncertain is that adequate nutrition should always be supplied on a daily basis except when return to oral feeding is expected within 2 to 3 days.

WHAT?

In the previous section we discussed how much protein and energy should be given, but did not consider what proportions of fat and carbohydrate should be provided, or the forms in which protein, fat, and carbohydrate are to be supplied.

Carbohydrate and Fat

The requirements for fat and carbohydrate were discussed in Chapter 4. Since carbohydrate shows marked N sparing and has other beneficial effects not shared by fat, it was concluded that at least 50% of REE should be given as carbohydrate, except when its effect to increase ventilation becomes critical, either in free-breathing patients with lack of pulmonary reserve, or in weaning patients off ventilators. Excess carbohydrate causes lipogenesis, fatty liver, hepatic dysfunction, increased energy expenditure, and increased sympathetic activity. Therefore carbohydrate should probably not be given in excess of 80% of REE.

At least 5 to 10 g of polyunsaturated fat should be given daily, as either omega-6 fatty acids, mainly linoleic acid, or as omega-3 fatty acids, which include linolenic acid found in vegetable oils, and eicosapentaenoic acid and docosahexaenoic acids found in fish oils. There is much current investigation of the physiological and pharmacological effects of the omega-3 fatty acids (55), but this has not advanced to the point that firm recommendations can be made as to either the amounts, or which ones, to be included in the diet. There is evidence that when lipids, containing either mainly omega-6 or omega-3 fatty acids, are given enterally as 30% or more of calories, they have harmful effects in burned guinea pigs or humans (Chapter 4).

These requirements generally can be met by providing between 50% and 75% of non protein energy as carbohydrate and 25% to 50% as fat.

Parenteral Preparations

Amino Acid Solutions

There are a large number of commercial amino acid solutions available for intravenous feeding, but there are few studies of differences in their effects on N balance or morbidity. One exception has been the study of branched chain-enriched solutions. But, as discussed in Chapter 3, apart from their effects on normalizing plasma amino acid patterns and awakening comatose patients in hepatic encephalopathy, what beneficial effects that have been reported so far do not warrant their general use with injured, septic, or malnourished patients. There is some evidence that solutions of crystalline amino acids are preferable to protein hydrolysates (Chapter 3), but at present there is little basis on which to prefer one or another crystalline amino acid preparation.

Lipid Emulsions

There are a growing number of lipid emulsions on the market. These include preparations containing either 10% or 20% triglycerides, varying triglyceride-to-phospholipid ratios, mixtures of medium-chain triglycerides with long-chain triglycerides, and will shortly include fish oil preparations. There is extensive investigation of the physiological, nutritional and pharmacological properties of these preparations going on at present, and it is probable that there may be important nutritional differences among them. However, as yet these investigations have not reached the point where firm recommendations can be made.

Carbohydrate Solutions

A variety of sugars and polyols, such as xylose, fructose, xylitol, and sorbitol, have been investigated as substitutes for glucose in parenteral nutrition. As far as we know, there is no evidence to make it worthwhile to use these preparations for clinical nutritional therapy.

Enteral Preparations

There are two main types of enteral preparations: *elemental* or *monomeric*, which contain glucose and amino acids and which have very high osmolality; and *polymeric*, containing protein and starches or dextrins, which require digestion before absorption, but do not pose a hyperosmotic problem. In the past, the monomeric preparations have been fashionable. There is presently a growing recognition that in almost all instances in which the gut's absorptive capability is functional, its digestive capability is also functional. Therefore, it is only rarely that polymeric preparations cannot be used. These have a low osmotic load and reduce diarrhea as compared to monomeric diets. Best results are obtained by infusing these preparations continuously over each twenty four hours, rather than giving them in bolus quantities at intervals throughout the day.

WHEN ?

Should nutritional support start before, during, or immediately after an elective surgical procedure? In severely injured patients, when should it be initiated?

Preoperative Artificial Nutrition

At the beginning of this chapter, in analyzing the reasons why artificial nutrition is important in management of all kinds of patients, we presented to the reader a series of studies pointing out the impressive improvement in postoperative morbidity and mortality when nutritional support is provided preoperatively in undernourished patients(1-8,14-17). In one of these studies, the authors demonstrated that preoperative nutrition resulted in a 2.5-fold reduction in complications, a 7-fold reduction in infection rate and a 5-fold reduction in mortality (14). Mullen showed that when TPN was provided preoperatively in malnourished patients for 2-3 days, almost no benefit was obtained, whereas a reduction of morbidity from 50% to 25% was obtained in malnourished patients after administration of TPN during one week or more prior to surgery (56). Malnourished patients, responding to two weeks of TPN with weight loss, increased albumin level, and sodium diuresis indicating a loss of extracellular fluid, had a negligible complication rate, whereas patients who did not lose weight, retaining an expanded extracellular fluid after two weeks of TPN, still had a 50% complication rate, but this could be reduced when TPN was continued until weight loss, increased albumin level, and reduced extracellular fluid was achieved; these studies also demonstrated that positive nitrogen balance was a poor indicator for morbidity as compared to sodium diuresis accompanied by weight loss and increased serum albumin concentration (8, 57).

Enough evidence has been presented in recent years in the medical literature to convince clinicians and mainly surgeons that malnutrition is a disease per se and that in acute illness it may lead to severe complications and increased surgical risk. Nevertheless this aspect of patient management is ignored in many institutions, and nutritional evaluation of hospitalized patients or in preoperative routine examinations is far from becoming a general rule. Routine preoperative tests consist of standard blood and urine analysis, electrocardiogram, and chest X-ray; in the interview the patient will be asked if he noticed a weight loss in the last few months. Additional investigations will be performed only when something obvious is observed by the clinician. In a study entitled *Hospital Malnutrition*, 48% of the patients were found to have a high likelihood of malnutrition on admission and this percentage increased with the length of hospitalization time (58). Earlier, in the seventies, studies of the same kind showed a high incidence of varying degrees of malnutrition in both medical and surgical patients (59,60). For reasons that are not entirely clear these important facts remain as theoretical abstractions and have failed to convince many surgeons that, in most instances, delaying a surgical procedure for 10 or 15 days would be of great benefit for the postoperative course of malnourished patients. The number of postoperative complications related to preoperative malnutrition are probably more frequent than suspected, and when hypoalbuminemia, increased extracellular fluid, and infection are discovered several days after a surgical procedure, only rarely will it be related, by the treating team, to a poor preoperative nutritional status. At this stage active hyperalimentation and antibiotherapy are often ineffective, whereas delaying the surgery until an improvement of nutritional status would have avoided this deterioration of the patient's condition leading in many instances to irreversible states.

Artificial Nutrition for Postoperative, Injured, Septic, and Burned Patients

When dealing with severely ill patients, nutrition is neither an emergency nor a priority. Nevertheless, it must become an integral part of the patient's daily management. In the same manner that water and electrolyte needs are roughly evaluated, in patients who are unable to feed themselves normally, and are supplied according to certain rules, calorie and nitrogen intake deserve the same consideration. Except in regions where starvation is common, people rarely fast for other than religious or philosophical reasons; those who have experimented with one or two days of real fast know that the feeling is usually unpleasant. The sicker the patient, the more harmful are the effects of nutritional deprivation, and the less able is he to feed himself. A critically ill patient with a gastric tube, an endotracheal cannula, ventilated, and unconscious has no possibility either to request food or even to feel that he would like some nutritional support. In treating severely ill patients, most of the life-threatening situations are detected early in the ICU by monitoring devices or by blood analysis. Acute respiratory failure is usually accompanied by dramatic symptoms that will yield to a series of therapeutic measures, that must be performed in emergency. The same considerations hold for cardiac arrhythmias or for all kinds of shock states due to severe bleeding or to sepsis. When urinary output decreases, a series of measures will be taken in order to try to prevent acute renal failure, but if a patient goes into anuric acute renal failure, the situation is less urgent. Although acute renal failure is a life-threatening condition if not taken care of, it is not a high emergency and the team may quietly decide that hemodialysis should be performed the same day or the next day. When dealing with acute hemodynamic or respiratory disturbances the time is usually counted in minutes, whereas when dealing with acute renal failure the time may be counted in hours or up to one or two days. When dealing with the multiple consequences of malnutrition in severely ill patients, whether reduction in host defense mechanisms leading to infection, delayed or non-wound healing, or reduced serum albumin level with water maldistribution, the time is much longer and counted in many days and sometimes in weeks. This is probably the main reason why this aspect of a patient's management is often neglected or totally ignored until the situation becomes catastrophic, although it becomes life threatening long before the alarming signs appear.

After this long introduction, we recommend that in postoperative, injured, septic, or burned patients, nutrition should be provided in all cases where normal oral feeding is absent or seriously reduced for more than two or three days. Usually oral intake is difficult in the first days after surgery or injury and TPN may be initiated for several days until the enteral route becomes available, by normal oral intake or by gastric or jejunal tube. When the patient has a minor problem and it is evident that he will be able to feed himself within two or three days, then 150-200 g dextrose will be sufficient and there is no need to introduce central venous lines or gastric tubes for the purpose of artificial nutrition.

HOW ?

The enteral route is much more physiological than the parenteral route for supplying nutrients and there seems to be a general agreement that enteral nutrition should be used rather than parenteral when it is possible. Naturally, there is not total agreement on what is called possible. For instance, many surgeons and gastroenterologists believe that digestive fistulae or gastroduodenal bleeding are an absolute contraindication for enteral nutrition whereas, on the contrary, others consider enteral nutrition as a therapeutic procedure to control gastrointestinal bleeding and to reduce fluid loss through enterocutaneous fistulae by 25% to 50% (61).

Since the era of artificial nutrition began in the sixties with parenteral nutrition, and the first favorable results published by Dudrick and Wilmore and colleagues dealt exclusively with parenteral nutrition (35), the medical field is much more conscious of the role played by parenteral than by enteral nutrition. This extends even to the use of terms such as TPN, for total parenteral nutrition, or hyperalimentation, when patients are on partial parenteral nutrition. The more general term of artificial nutrition seems more suitable to designate all forms of nutrition other than normal oral intake.

An important initial statement is that recent studies have clearly demonstrated that there are no significant differences between enteral and parenteral nutrition when comparing efficacy of nutrient utilization as estimated by VO_2, VCO_2, RQ, nitrogen balance and energy supply (61-64). However, there is a huge difference in cost since for the same amount of nutrients the price is 5 to 10 times higher when supplied by parenteral than by enteral nutrition (65).

Enteral Nutrition

Patients after abdominal or thoracic surgery, or critically ill patients on ventilatory support, usually have a decompression gastric tube for avoiding stasis, vomiting, and aspiration of gastric juice. For minor problems this tube will remain in place for several days. When the gastric tube is used for nutritional support, or has to remain for prolonged periods of time for other reasons, soft, small-caliber, silastic tubes are preferred to large-caliber polyvinyl tubes. The most frequent mechanical complication with nasogastric tube (NG) insertion is mucosal injury along the introduction tract that can occur at any level and ranges in severity from bleeding to perforation. Another complication during introduction is misplacement of the tube so that it reaches the larynx and the tracheobronchial tree; these complications mainly occur in comatose patients and are most unpleasant when the feeding material arrives in the lungs instead of reaching the stomach. Some authors consider the jejunum as a better location for enteral feeding and techniques for introducing feeding tubes in the jejunum under fluoroscopy have been described (66). Well tolerated for 3-4 weeks, the NG tubes when kept for longer periods of time may cause many complications, the most severe being aspiration, esophagitis followed by stenosis, and suppurative sinusitis (67-70). For these reasons, each time that a patient, who is expected to be fed by the enteral route for more than 2-3 weeks, undergoes a laparotomy, a feeding gastrostomy, duodenostomy, or jejunostomy should be performed, since this avoids all the complications related to the nasopharyngeal and esophageal parts of the NG tube. This is also true for all the patients that undergo surgery of the upper GI tract with a high risk of fistula formation. There is still a lot of argument concerning the justification of a special surgical procedure for performing an enterostomy for nutritional purposes. Feeding pharyngostomies and esophagostomies are used after head and neck surgery and in patients with subtotal gastrectomy or esophagogastrectomy. These have some specific problems such as local irritation, stenosis, esophagitis, and regurgitations. A few cases of carotid artery erosion have also been described (71). The most common enteral feeding methods, after the nasogastric tube, are gastrostomy and jejunostomy performed by various surgical techniques known since the end of the last century, or use of special material such as a double lumen tube allowing simultaneous gastric decompression and jejunal feeding (72). In patients considered as a high risk for laparotomy or anesthesia, a technique of endoscopic percutaneous gastrostomy was developed for enteral nutrition with relatively satisfying results (73). An alternative technique for enteral nutrition that still has many proponents is the fine needle catheter feeding jejunostomy, which has been shown to be efficaceous for supplying elemental diets (74).

The complication rates of these surgical procedures varies between 5% and 10%. Complications include wound infection, stomy disruption and leak of enteral material with peritonitis. The advantages noted in favor of the jejunal approach over the gastric approach are: (*a*) less leakage and fewer skin erosions; (*b*) less gastric and pancreatic secretion because the stomach and the duodenum are bypassed; and (*c*) less nausea and vomiting, and reduced risk of pulmonary aspiration. A problem that may occur with jejunal feeding is that there may be inadequate mixing with bile and pancreatic enzymes resulting in incomplete digestion and reduced nutrient absorption. This inconvenience seems to be avoided when elemental diets are used.

The enteral route, besides being more physiological then the parenteral route, has a protective effect on the gut mucosa. Nevertheless, whatever technique of administration is used, the most frequent problem encountered in enteral nutrition is diarrhea. This will often lead to replacement of the enteral route by the intravenous one. Some antidiarrhetic products, such as carrot or carob powder, or tapioca, increase the viscosity of the administered enteral feeding. This can, in most instances, overcome the problem of diarrhea when given as 2% to 6% of the enteral mixture (61). Also reducing the osmolarity of the administered products by increasing the proportion of water can help.

Enteral preparations vary, according to the beliefs of the treating team, from blended normal food to highly sophisticated elemental diets. There is also controversy whether to provide continuous administration over 24 hours with simple infusion pumps, to use specialized refrigerated pumps instilling cold fluids into the GI tract, or to give the enteral regimen by bolus of several hundred milliliters at fixed hours, since this method is closer to the normal way of absorbing meals at fixed times of the day. The literature of nutrition has a multitude of papers violently defending each of the methods, but clinical experience tends to be in favor of continuous drip administration of well-balanced diets as stated in a previous section of this chapter.

Parenteral Nutrition

Mostly for historical rather than for rational reasons, parenteral nutrition is more frequently used than enteral nutrition in the United States, whereas in Western Europe the enteral route seems to be more often preferred.

Critically ill, surgical, and trauma patients usually have peripheral and central venous lines used for hemodynamic and respiratory monitoring. Once these functions have been stabilized, these lines become available to supply nutritional mixtures. Intensivists, surgeons, and nutritional teams in general are thus often more familiar with parenteral than with enteral nutrition (64). Central venous catheterization by the subclavian or the internal jugular veins has become a common practice for supplying parenteral nutrition, since the high blood flow allows the use of hypertonic solutions and reduces local infection rate. Various complications are related to these techniques, such as pneumothorax, hemothorax, air embolism, thrombosis, and sepsis; as well as more severe complications, like arterial laceration, cardiac perforation, and migration of portions of the venous catheters. Major complications can be avoided when the procedure is performed by experienced physicians; nevertheless catheter sepsis occurs in about 5% of the cases; this can be usually corrected by removing the catheter. The use of silicon catheters, of Broviac or Hickman type, seem to be better tolerated than polyvinyl (PVC) catheters, and some reports state that these catheters can be tolerated for more than one year without becoming infected (75). In trying to reduce infection rate, subclavian catheters were introduced with long subcutaneous tunnels, but a careful study did not demonstrate a reduction in catheter-related sepsis (76).

In order to prevent the above-mentioned complications, peripheral vein cannulation is used in many instances when the energy to be supplied is relatively low, although iso-osmotic lipid emulsion solutions can greatly increase the amount of calories that can be safely infused through peripheral veins. For hypercatabolic patients Massar et al. (77) showed that the calories that can be supplied by peripheral veins are insufficient to meet energetic requirements, even in previously well-nourished patients. The incidence of phlebitis seems to increase when the osmolarity of the infused solution is higher than 600 milliosmolar and is not prevented by the addition of heparin (78).

The literature on enteral and parenteral nutrition is full of reports emphasizing the advantages of one method over another, based on reduction of infection rate or thrombosis, improved nitrogen balance, etc., but as in many fields the more one reads on this topic, the more difficult is it to decide between the many options. We will attempt to summarize our own attitude, based on our clinical experience by the following:

Enteral feeding when possible is the most physiological (after oral feeding), the safest, and the most economic way to supply artificial nutrition.

TPN should be administered by central lines introduced carefully by well-trained physicians. When central venous puncture is unsuccessful, one must never try the contralateral access without having verified the absence of pneumothorax by a chest X-ray in the sitting position. Fever of unexplained origin requires removal of central venous lines and their introduction in other sites.

Since many severely ill patients behave like insulin-resistant diabetic patients, major complications of TPN, even in patients treated with high amounts of insulin, are hyperosmolar states that may lead to irreversible brain damage. Thus blood sugar levels and electrolytes have to be monitored daily, and sometimes two or three times per day in severely unstable patients, in order to detect disorders as quickly as possible. When measured or calculated serum osmolarity reaches values above 330 , artificial nutrition should be reduced or discontinued until glucose and sodium levels return close to normal values.

HOW LONG ?

Preoperative Patients

In malnourished patients, preoperative nutritional support has substantially reduced postoperative morbidity and mortality as discussed in earlier sections of this chapter. The length of time required to achieve nutritional improvement varies markedly from patient to patient and is dependent in part on the criteria chosen for estimating nutritional improvement. Reduction in extracellular fluid or in extracellular-to-intracellular ratio correlates better with improved postoperative morbidity than does nitrogen balance, and this can be evaluated by reduction in body weight and by increased serum albumin levels (57). This kind of improvement may be achieved in one to two weeks, but sometimes may take longer or even be impossible to obtain. This improvement is probably not strictly an improvement in nutrition, but rather an improvement in underlying infection or inflammation, which is otherwise not readily apparent. Adequate nutrition is permissive, allowing the inflammation or sepsis to resolve, whereas with inadequate nutrition it may never resolve. Other criteria evaluating host defense mechanisms during artificial nutrition may show an improvement only after three or four weeks and are also correlated with a reduction in postoperative morbidity and mortality, as shown many years ago (79,80).

Postoperative, Injured, Burned, and Critically Ill Patients

The best criteria for deciding to discontinue artificial nutrition is when the patient is obviously able to feed himself orally in sufficient quantity with balanced proportions of protein, carbohydrate, and fat. For patients on TPN, recent studies demonstrate a delay in gastric-emptying, inducing a reduction in appetite and so retarding the onset of normal oral feeding. This reduction of appetite may last from a few days up to one week. The nature of this mechanism is still not understood, but this retarded gastric-emptying seems to be reduced by the use of high concentrations of branched chain amino acids (81).

Using body weight as an indicator of nutritional improvement in postoperative or stressed patients is relatively useless since improvement in body cell mass may be masked by loss of extracellular water.

Keeping in mind that it is a human right to be fed every day, and that this rule should be extended to all humankind, including sick people, common sense and appropriate concern will probably do as well as strict indications.

REFERENCES

1. Seltzer MH. Specialized Nutrition Support: A Human Right. *Nutr Intern* 3:35-36, 1987.
2. Studley HO: Percentage of weight loss: A basic indicator. *JAMA* 106:458-460, 1936.
3. Cannon PR, Wissler RW, Woolridge RL et al.: The relationship of protein deficiency to surgical infection. *Ann Surg* 120:514-525, 1944.
4. Seltzer MH, Bastidas JA, Cooper DM et al.: Instant nutritional assessment. *JPEN* 3:157-159, 1979.
5. Seltzer MH, Slocum BA, Cataldi-Betcher EL et al: Instant nutritional assessment: Absolute weight loss and surgical mortality. *JPEN* 6:218-221, 1982.
6. Reinhardt GF, Myskofski JW, Wilkens DB et al.: Incidence and mortality of hypoalbuminemic patients in hospitalized veterans. *JPEN* 4:357-359, 1980.
7. Bozetti F, Migliavacca S, Gallus G et al.: "Nutritional" markers as prognostic indicators of postoperative sepsis in cancer patients. *JPEN* 9: 464-470, 1985.
8. Starker PM, Lasala PA, Askanazi J et al.: The response to TPN, A form of nutrional assessment. *Ann Surg* 198:720-724, 1983.
9. Shetty PS, Jung RT, Watrasiewicz, James WPT: Rapid-turnover transport proteins: An index of subclinical protein-energy malnutrition. *Lancet* 2:230-232, 1979.
10. Young GA, Collins JP, Hill GI: Plasma proteins in patients receiving intravenous amino acids or intravenous hyperalimentation after major surgery. *Am J Clin Nutr* 32:1192-1199, 1979.
11. Insel J, Elwyn DH: Body composition. In Askanazi J, Starker PM, Weissman C (eds): *Fluid and Electrolyte Management in Critical Care.* Boston, Butterworths, 1986, pp 3–37.
12. Daly JN, Vars HM, Dudrick SJ: Effects of protein depletion on strength of colon anastomosis. *Surg Gyn Obst* 134:15-21, 1972.
13. Holter AR, Fischer JE: The effect of perioperative hyperalimentation on complications in patients with carcinoma and weight loss. *J Surg Res* 23: 31-34, 1977.
14. Mullen JL , Buzby GP, Matthews DC et al.: Reduction of operative morbidity and mortality by combined preoperative and postoperative nutritional support. *Ann Surg* 192:604-613, 1980.
15. Buzby GP, Mullen JL, Matthews DC et al.: Prognostic nutritional index in gastrointestinal surgery. *Am J Surg* 139:160-167, 1980.

16. Heatley RV, Williams RHP, Lewis MH. Preoperative intravenous feeding- A controlled trial. *Postgrad Med J* 55: 541-545, 1979.
17. Muller JM, Brenner U, Dienst C, Pichlmaier H: Preoperative parenteral feeding in patients with gastrointestinal carcinoma. *Lancet* i:68-71, 1982.
18. Askanazi J, Hensle TW, Starker PA et al.: Effect of immediate postoperative nutritional support on lengths of hospitalization. *Ann Surg* 203:236-239, 1986.
19. Fromme H: Systematische untersuchungen uber die Gewichtsverhaltnisse des Zwerchfells. *Virchows Arch* 221: 117-155, 1916.
20. Arora NS, Rochester DF: Effect of body weight and muscularity on human diaphragm muscle mass, thickness and area. *J Appl Physiol* 52:63-70, 1982.
21. Arora NS, Rochester DF: Respiratory muscle strength and maximal voluntary ventilation in undernourished patients. *Am Rev Respir Dis* 126:5-8, 1982.
22. Keys A, Brozek J, Henschel A et al.: *Biology of Human Starvation.* Minneapolis, University of Minnesota Press, 1950, pp 601–606.
23. Cravetto C, Carelli E, Cardellino G, Garbagni R: Osservazioni sulla funzione respiratoria nella anoressia mentale. *Minerva Med* 57:3498-3501, 1966.
24. Heymsfield SB, Head A, Grossman G et al.: Mechanism of cachexia in chronic obstructive pulmonary disease (Abstract). *JPEN* 5:562, 1981.
25. Openbrier DR, Irwin MM, Dauber JH et al.: Factors affecting nutritional status and the impact of nutritional support in patients with emphysema. *Chest* 85: 67S-69S, 1984.
26. Thurlbeck WM: Diaphragm and body weight in emphysema. *Thorax* 33:483-487, 1978.
27. Vandenbergh E, Van de Woestijne KP, Gyselen A: Weight changes in the terminal stages of chronic obstructive pulmonary disease: Relation to respiratory function and prognosis. *Am Rev Respir Dis* 95: 556-566, 1967.
28. Goldstein S, Thomashow B, Kvetan V et al.: Nitrogen and energy relationships in malnourished patients with emphysema. *Am Rev Respir Dis*. In press, 1988.
29. Larca L, Greenbaum DM: Effectiveness of intensive nutritional regimes in patients who fail to wean from mechanical ventilation. *Crit Care Med* 10:297-300, 1982.
30. Goldstein SA, Thomashow B, Askanazi J: Functional changes during nutritional repletion in patients with lung disease. *Clin Chest Med* 7:141-151, 1986.
31. Covelli HD, Black JW, Olsen MV et al.: Respiratory failure precipitated by high carbohydrate loads. *Ann Int Med* 95: 579-581, 1981.
32. Askanazi J, Nordenström J, Rosenbaum SH et al.: Nutrition for the patient with respiratory failure: Glucose versus fat. *Anesthesiology* 54:373-377, 1981.
33. Askanazi J, Weissman C, Lasala P et al.: Effects of protein intake on ventilatory drive. *Anesthesiology* 60:106-110, 1984.
34. Gamble JL: Physiological information gained from studies on the life raft ration. *Harvey Lect* 42: 247-273, 1946.
35. Dudrick SJ, Wilmore DW, Vars HM, Rhoades JE: Can intravenous feeding as the sole means of nutrition support growth in the child and restore weight loss in an adult? An affirmative answer. *Ann Surg* 169: 974-984, 1969.
36. Wretlind A: Parenteral nutrition. *Surg Clin North Am* 58:1055-1070, 1978.
37. Rutten P, Blackburn GL, Flatt JP et al.: Determination of optimal hyperalimentation infusion rate. *J Surg Res* 18: 477-483, 1975.
38. Wilmore DW, Long JM, Mason AD et al: Catecholamines: Mediator of the hypermetabolic response to thermal injury. *Ann Surg* 180:653-669, 1974.
39. Barzilai E, Weksler N, Lesmes C et al.: Continuous hemofiltration: Our experience in septic (hypercatabolic and oliguric) acute organ system failure patients. In *Re-*

cent Advances in Anesthesia, Pain, Intensive Care and Emergency, A. P. I. C. Instituto Policatedra di Anesthesia, Rianimazione e Terapia Antalgica, Ospedale di Cattinara, Trieste, Italy, 1987, pp 311–314.

40. Elwyn DH: Nutritional requirements of adult surgical patients. *Crit Care Med* 8: 9-20, 1980.
41. Gazzaniga AB, Polachek JR, Wilson AF, Day AT: Indirect calorimetry as a guide to caloric replacement during total parenteral nutrition. *Am J Surg* 136:128-134, 1978.
42. Harris JA, Benedict FG: *A Biometric Study of Basal Metabolism in Man*. Washington D.C., Carnegie Inst Wash, Publ No 279, 1919.
43. Boothby WM, Berkson J, Dunn HL: Studies of the energy metabolism of normal individuals. *Am J Physiol* 116:468-484, 1936.
44. Aub JC, Du Bois EF: Clinical calorimetry. The basal metabolism of old men. *Arch Int Med* 19:823-831, 1917.
45. Fleisch A: Le metabolisme basal standard et sa determination au moyen du "Metabocalculator" *Helv Med Acta* 18:23-44, 1951.
46. Kinney JM, Duke JH Jr, Long CL, Gump F: Tissue fuel and weight loss after injury. *J Clin Path* 23 (Suppl 14):65-72, 1970.
47. Long CL : Energy balance and carbohydrate metabolism in infection and sepsis. *Am J Clin Nutr* 30:1301-1310, 1977.
48. Weissman C, Kemper M, Askanazi J et al.: Resting metabolic rate of the critically ill patient: Measured versus predicted. *Anesthesiology* 64:673-679, 1986.
49. Singer P, Irving CS, Elwyn DH et al.: The reliability of estimated energy expenditure in critically ill patients. In preparation.
50. LeGall JR, Loirat P, Alperowitch A et al.: A simplified acute physiology score for intensive care patients. *Crit Care Med* 13:173-177, 1985.
51. Francois G, Bouffier C, Dumont JC, Penalver F: Protein catabolism in trauma patients. *Ann Fr Anesth Rean* 2:387-391, 1983.
52. Nordenström J, Askanazi J, Elwyn DH et al.: Nitrogen balance during total parenteral nutrition. *Ann Surg* 197:27-33, 1983.
53. Chikenji T, Elwyn DH, Gil KM et al.: Effect of increasing glucose intake on nitrogen balance and energy expenditure in malnourished adult patients receiving parenteral nutrition. *Clin Sci* 72:489-501, 1987.
54. Elwyn DH, Gump FE, Munro HN et al.: Changes in nitrogen balance of depleted patients with increasing infusions of glucose. *Am J Clin Nutr* 32:1597-1611, 1979.
55. Leaf A, Weber PC: Cardiovascular effects of n-3 fatty acids. *N Engl J Med* 318:549-557, 1988.
56. Mullen JL: Consequences of malnutrition in the surgical patient. *Surg Clin North Am* 61: 465-487, 1981.
57. Starker PM, LaSala PA, Askanazi J et al.: The influence of preoperative TPN on morbidity and mortality. *Surg Gyn Obst* 162:569-574, 1986.
58. Weinsier RL, Hunker EM, Krumdieck CL et al.: Hospital malnutrition. A prospective evaluation of general medical patients during the course of hospitalization. *Am J Clin Nutr* 32:418-426, 1979.
59. Bistrian BR, Blackburn GL, Vitale J et al.: Prevalence of malnutrition in general medical patients. *JAMA* 235:1567-1570, 1976
60. Hill GL, Pickford I, Young GA et al.: Malnutrition in surgical patients. An unrecognized problem. *Lancet* i: 689-692, 1977.
61. Levy E, Malafosse M: La reanimation enterale continue appliquee au traitement des grandes denutritions. In Levy E (ed): *Reanimation Enterale a Faible Debit Continu.* Paris, INSERM, 1977, pp 159–205.

62. Ganger D, Taitelman U, Bursztein S: Comparison of enteral and parenteral nutrition in hypercatabolic states (Abstract). *Crit Care Med* 9:280, 1981.
63. Fletcher JP, Little JM: A comparison of parenteral nutrition and early postoperative enteral feeding on nitrogen balance after major injury. *Surgery* 100:21-24, 1986.
64. Grote AE, Elwyn DH, Takala J et al.: Nutritional and metabolic effects of enteral and parenteral feeding in severely injured patients. *Clin Nutr* 6:161-167, 1987.
65. Heymsfield SB, Bethel RA, Ansley JD et al.: Enteral hyperalimentation: An alternative to central venous hyperalimentation. *Ann Intern Med* 90:63-71, 1979.
66. Grant JP, Curtas MS, Kelvin FM: Fluoroscopic placement of nasojejunal feeding tubes with immediate feeding using a nonelemental diet. *JPEN* 7:299-303, 1983.
67. Eldar S, Meguid MM: Pneumothorax following attempted nasogastric intubation for nutritional support. *JPEN* 8:450-452, 1984.
68. Jeffers SL, Dorr LA, Meguid MM: Mechanical complications of enteral nutrition: Prospective study of 109 consecutive patients (Abstract) *Clin Res* 32:233A, 1984.
69. Olivares L, Segovia A, Revuelta R: Tube feeding and lethal aspiration in neurological patients: A review of 720 autopsy cases. *Stroke* 5:654-657, 1974.
70. Cataldi-Belcher EL, Seltzer MH, Slocum BA, Jones KW: Complications occurring during enteral nutritional support: A prospective study. *JPEN* 7:546-552, 1983.
71. Balkany TJ, Jafek BW, Wong ML: Complications of feeding esophagotomy. *Arch Otolaryngol* 106:122-123, 1980.
72. Meguid MM, Eldar S,Wahba A: The delivery of nutritional support. *Cancer* 55:279-289, 1985.
73. Ponsky TL, Gauderer WL, Stellato TA: Percutaneous endoscopic gastrostomy: A review of 150 cases. *Arch Surg* 118:913-914, 1983.
74. Dunn EL, Moore EE, Bohus RW: Immediate postoperative feeding following massive abdominal trauma: The catheter jejunostomy. *JPEN* 4:393-395, 1980.
75. Thomas JH, MacArthur RI, Pierce GE, Hermreck AS: Hickman-Broviac catheters: Indications and results. *Am J Surg* 140:791-796, 1980.
76. Von Meyenfeldt MM, Stalpert J, Jong PCMD et al.: TPN catheter sepsis: Lack of effect of subcutaneous tunneling of PVC catheters on sepsis rate. *JPEN* 5:514-517, 1980.
77. Massar EL, Daley JM, Copeland EM et al.: Peripheral vein complications in patients recieving amino acid/dextrose solutions. *JPEN*: 7:159-162, 1983.
78. Gazitua R, Wilson K, Bistrian BR, Blackburn GL: Factors determining peripheral vein tolerance to amino acid infusions. *Arch Surg* 114:897-901, 1979.
79. Law DK, Dudrick SJ, Abdou NI: Immunocompetence of patients with protein-calorie malnutrition. The effect of nutritional repletion. *Ann Intern Med* 79:545-550, 1973.
80. Dionigi R, Zonta A, Dominioni L et al.: The effects of TPN on immunodepression due to malnutrition. *Ann Surg* 185:467-474, 1977.
81. Bursztein-De Myttenaere S, Gil KM, Heymsfield S et al.: Post absorptive control of food intake in healthy humans (Abstract). *Faseb J* 2:A1795, 1988

Index

Page numbers in *italics* denote figures; those followed by "t" denote tables.